人卫3D
人体解剖图谱

PMPH 3D ATLAS OF HUMAN ANATOMY

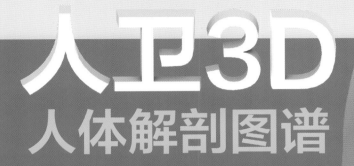
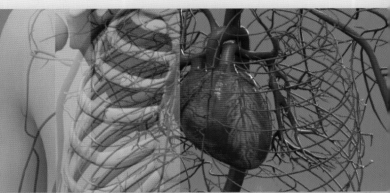

主　编　王　凡

副主编　董立华　李　华

 人民卫生出版社

图书在版编目（CIP）数据

人卫 3D 人体解剖图谱 / 王凡主编. —北京：人民
卫生出版社，2019

ISBN 978-7-117-27924-6

Ⅰ. ①人… Ⅱ. ①王… Ⅲ. ①人体解剖学—图谱
Ⅳ. ①R322-64

中国版本图书馆 CIP 数据核字（2019）第 139693 号

| 人卫智网 | www.ipmph.com | 医学教育、学术、考试、健康，购书智慧智能综合服务平台 |
| 人卫官网 | www.pmph.com | 人卫官方资讯发布平台 |

人卫 3D 人体解剖图谱

主　　编：王　凡
出版发行：人民卫生出版社（中继线 010-59780011）
地　　址：北京市朝阳区潘家园南里 19 号
邮　　编：100021
E - mail：pmph @ pmph.com
购书热线：010-59787592　010-59787584　010-65264830
印　　刷：人卫印务（北京）有限公司
经　　销：新华书店
开　　本：889×1194　1/16　　印张：19
字　　数：423 千字
版　　次：2019 年 12 月第 1 版　2024 年 9 月第 1 版第 5 次印刷
标准书号：ISBN 978-7-117-27924-6
定　　价：98.00 元
打击盗版举报电话：010-59787491　E-mail：WQ @ pmph.com
质量问题联系电话：010-59787234　E-mail：zhiliang @ pmph.com

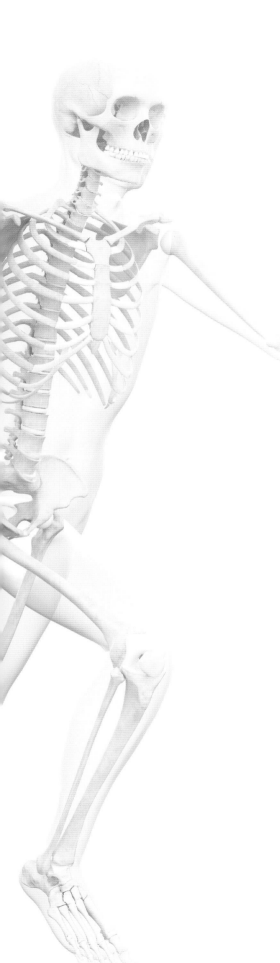

内容提要

　　全书共分为 14 章，目录的编排与人民卫生出版社出版的最新版国家级规划教材《系统解剖学》相辅相成，提纲挈领、层次清晰、详略有方。书中共有 500 余幅图，内容丰富、全面和系统。

　　书中插图均为计算机绘制的人体结构 3D 图。不同于经典的图谱用前、后位和侧位展示结构，本书充分利用 3D 模型的特点，采用左、右前侧位、镜像位和透明或隐藏方式来显示结构，更好地展示人体结构的三维立体形态和相互之间的空间关系，便于读者理解并建立位置关系。

　　该图谱与数字化素材融合，用移动终端扫描标有 AR 图标的图片，即可体现增强现实的三维图像，并能对其进行旋转、放大、缩小、隐藏和透明等操作，有助于读者对人体结构的进一步认知。

　　本书图注和引线扼要、精练和准确，每幅图的解剖学名词按中英文标注，书后附有中英文名词对照索引，便于学习和使用，是医学生、临床医师和解剖学教学人员难得的工具书。

序言

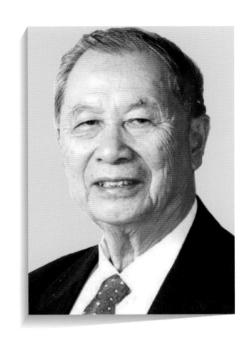

"近水楼台先得月"，三年前，我有幸为创新驱动成果，王凡教授团队主编的《人卫 3D 解剖学系统》教学软件写过序。"独留巧思传千古"，今天这个团队又编著和出版了《人卫 3D 人体解剖图谱》，这是国内第一本整合数字技术的 3D 人体解剖学图谱。

"没有金刚钻，不揽磁器活"，《人卫 3D 人体解剖图谱》用计算机技术绘制 3D 标本并整合 AR 三维展示进行图谱的编著，无愧于"中国医药学术原创精品图书出版工程"这一称呼。这部图谱，遵循科学性、原创性、准确性、艺术性和实用性完美融合，传承了传统图谱的精华，又大胆进行创新，并在创新中超越。

"故为常语谈何易，百炼功纯始自然"，数字医学的发展，使得三维重建、虚拟仿真、3D 打印等前沿性、先进性技术，广泛应用于实际。王凡教授带领的创作团队，历经坎坷、苦心孤诣、标新立异，将该技术应用于解剖学图谱编著，纸数融合。"纸上得来终觉浅，绝知此事要躬行"，给读者们展现耳目一新的内容，让读者们能够身历其境。

"不到园林，怎知春色如许"，作为一位毕生在人体解剖学园地上工作的老园丁，我曾在解剖技术学这一片花圃上播过种、育过苗。现在看见了王凡教授带领的新园丁们精心培育的新品种，已经繁花似锦，五彩缤纷，争奇斗艳，特别欣慰。是为之贺！

原中国解剖学会名誉理事长

中国工程院资深院士

南方医科大学教授

钟世镇

2019 年夏于广州

前言

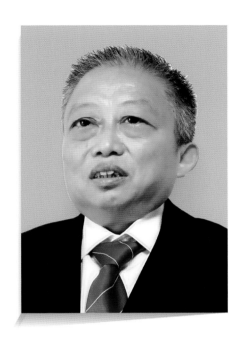

历经坎坷，中国医药学术原创精品图书出版工程《人卫 3D 人体解剖图谱》面市了，它是国内第一本用计算机绘画技术绘制的 3D 人体解剖图谱。

紧密结合人民卫生出版社出版的最新版国家级规划教材《系统解剖学》是编著本图谱的创作理念，创作中将原创性、科学性、准确性、实用性和艺术性完美融合，在读者面前展示出耳目一新和别开生面的画册。

不同于手绘和实物的解剖学图谱，《人卫 3D 人体解剖图谱》借助于 3D 软件绘制人体结构三维模型，更清晰和准确地显示了人体解剖结构的 3D 形态和位置关系。

该图谱也是国内第一本纸数融合的图谱，通过融入计算机数字技术，通过移动终端可对图谱展示的重要解剖结构进行更直观、立体观更强的三维观察，突破了传统图谱的载体局限性，拓展了图谱的功能，带来了更广阔的学习和应用空间。

图谱的出版汇聚了创作团队的智慧和心血。医学团队、美术团队和计算机技术团队卓有成效的配合保障了图谱高质量编写。在此，我向全体参与图谱编著的人员表示衷心的感谢，没有大家齐心协力，图谱只是一个梦，大家的努力使梦想成真。

受制于时间和本人能力，本图谱尚存有不足甚至错误，真诚地恳请广大读者提出批评与建议，这将有助于我们不断地修正，更好地服务于医学教育事业。

王凡

2019 年夏于成都

目录 Contents

第1章 运动系统 骨学 Locomotor System Osteology

第 2 章　运动系统　关节学　Locomotor System　Arthrology

第 3 章　运动系统　肌学　Locomotor System　Myology

第 4 章   内脏学   消化系统   Splanchnology   Alimentary System

第 5 章 内脏学 呼吸系统 Splanchnology Respiratory System

第 6 章 内脏学 泌尿生殖系统 Splanchnology Urogenital System

第 7 章 心血管系统 Cardiovascular System

第 8 章　淋巴系统　Lymphatic System

第 9 章　感觉器　Sensory Organs

第 10 章　周围神经系统　Peripheral Nervous System

第 11 章 中枢神经系统 Central Nervous System

第 12 章　神经系统传导通路　Nervous System Pathways

第 13 章　脑、脊髓的被膜及血管　Meninges and Blood Vessels of the Brain and Spinal Cord

第 14 章　内分泌系统　Endocrine System

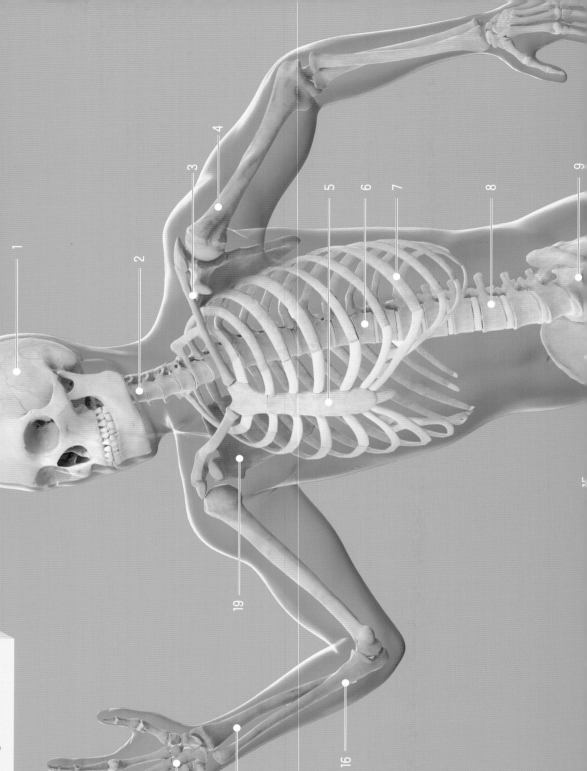

第1章 运动系统 Locomotor System

骨学 Osteology

1

2

3

4

5

6

7

8

9

16

17

18

19

15

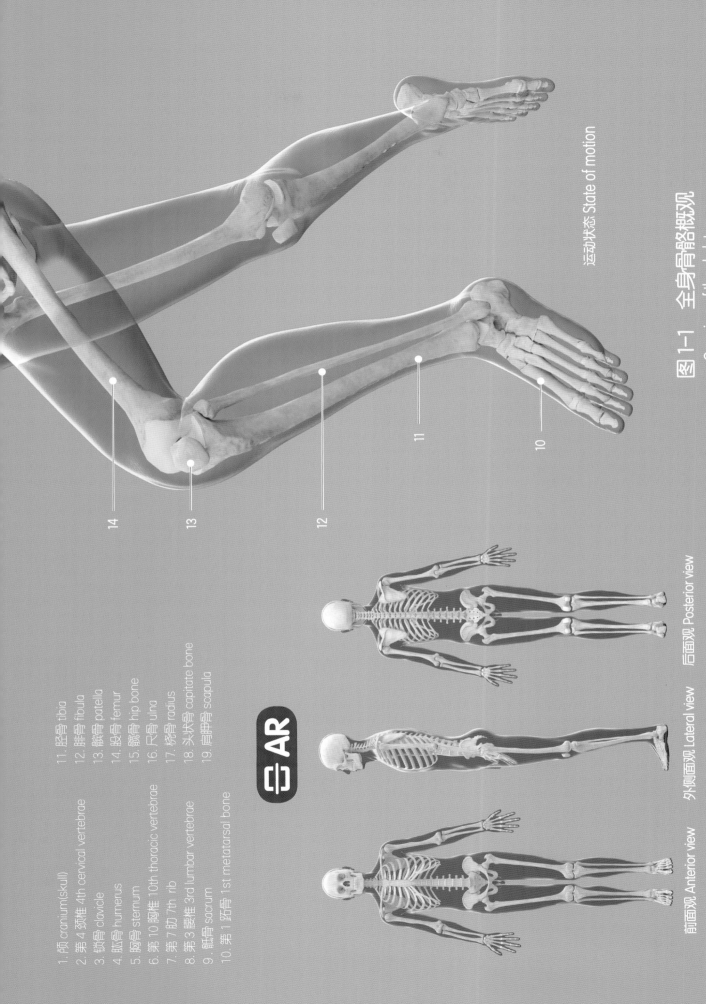

运动状态 State of motion

图1-1 全身骨骼概观
Overview of the skeleton

1. 颅骨 cranium(skull)
2. 第 4 颈椎 4th cervical vertebrae
3. 锁骨 clavicle
4. 肱骨 humerus
5. 胸骨 sternum
6. 第 10 胸椎 10th thoracic vertebrae
7. 第 7 肋 7th rib
8. 第 3 腰椎 3rd lumbar vertebrae
9. 骶骨 sacrum
10. 第 1 跖骨 1st metatarsal bone

11. 胫骨 tibia
12. 腓骨 fibula
13. 髌骨 patella
14. 股骨 femur
15. 髋骨 hip bone
16. 尺骨 ulna
17. 桡骨 radius
18. 头状骨 capitate bone
19. 肩胛骨 scapula

AR

前面观 Anterior view　　外侧面观 Lateral view　　后面观 Posterior view

1. 寰椎 atlas
2. 枢椎 axis
3. 第 7 颈椎 7th cervical vertebrae
4. 第 3 肋 3rd rib
5. 肋软骨 costal cartilage
6. 第 12 肋 12th rib

7. 第 5 腰椎 5th lumbar vertebrae
8. 骶骨 sacrum
9. 尾骨 coccyx
10. 剑突 xiphoid process
11. 胸骨体 body of sternum
12. 胸骨柄 manubrium sterni

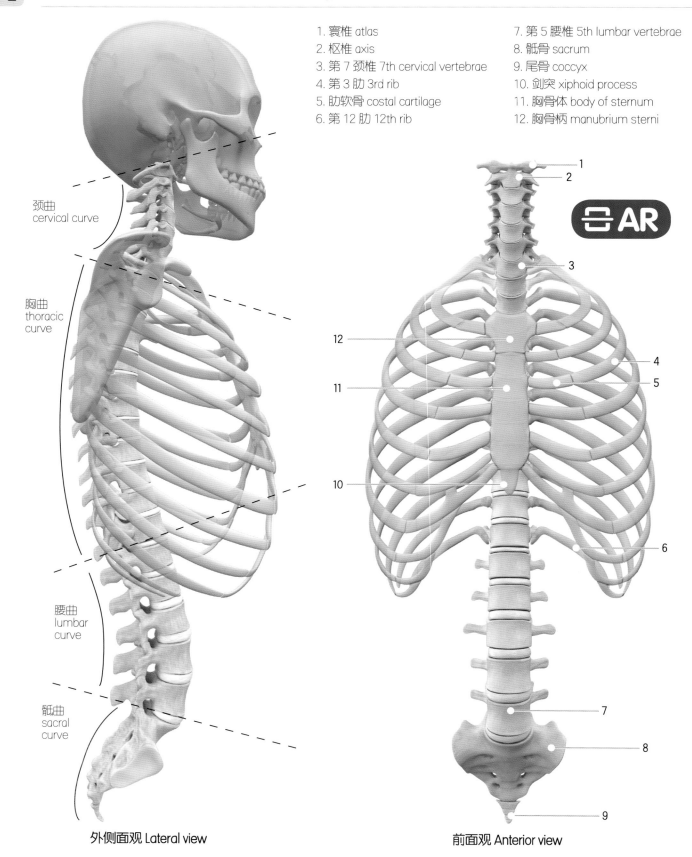

颈曲
cervical curve

胸曲
thoracic
curve

腰曲
lumbar
curve

骶曲
sacral
curve

外侧面观 Lateral view

前面观 Anterior view

图 1-2   中轴骨
Axial skeleton

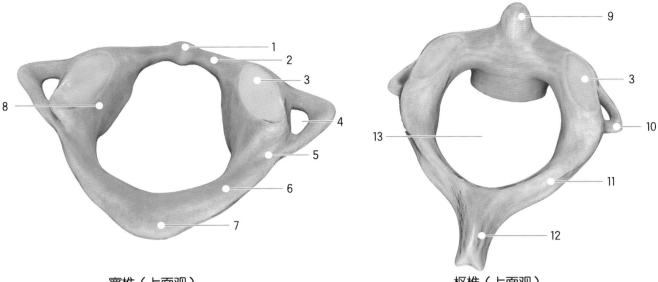

寰椎（上面观）
Atlas (superior view)

枢椎（上面观）
Axis (superior view)

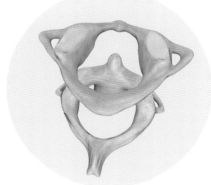

寰椎和枢椎
Atlas and axis

1. 前结节 anterior tubercle
2. 前弓 anterior arch
3. 上关节面 superior articular surface
4. 横突孔 transverse foramen
5. 椎动脉沟 groove for vertebral artery
6. 后弓 posterior arch
7. 后结节 posterior tubercle
8. 侧块 lateral mass
9. 齿突 dens
10. 横突 transverse process
11. 椎弓 vertebral arch
12. 棘突 spinous process
13. 椎孔 vertebral foramen
14. 椎体 vertebral body

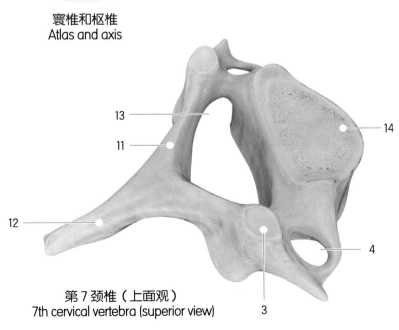

第 7 颈椎（上面观）
7th cervical vertebra (superior view)

图 1-3 颈椎
Cervical vertebrae

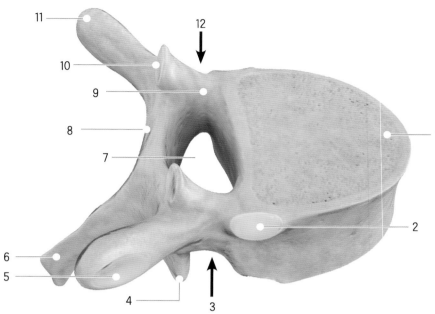

胸椎 （上外侧面观）Thoracic vertebra(superolateral view)

1. 椎体 vertebral body
2. 上肋凹 superior costal fovea
3. 椎下切迹 inferior vertebral notch
4. 下关节突 inferior articular process
5. 横突肋凹 transverse costal fovea
6. 棘突 spinous process
7. 椎孔 vertebral foramen
8. 椎弓板 lamina of vertebral arch
9. 椎弓根 pedicle of vertebral arch
10. 上关节突 superior articular process
11. 横突 transverse process
12. 椎上切迹 superior vertebral notch

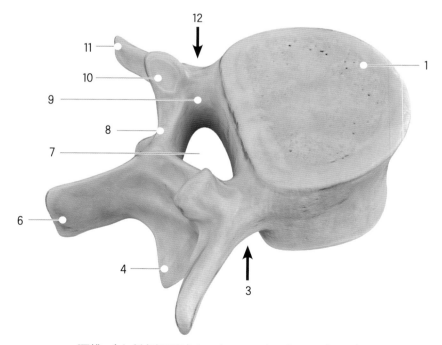

腰椎 （上外侧面观）Lumbar vertebra (superolateral view)

图 1-4 胸椎和腰椎
Thoracic and lumbar vertebrae

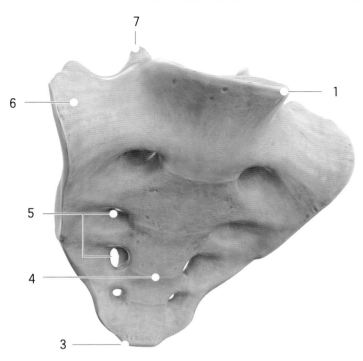

1. 岬 promontory
2. 尾骨 coccyx
3. 骶骨尖 apex of sacrum
4. 横线 transverse line
5. 骶前孔 anterior sacral foramina
6. 骶翼 ala of sacrum
7. 上关节突 superior articular process

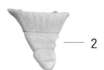

前外侧面观 Anterolateral view

8. 上关节面 superior articular surface
9. 耳状面 auricular surface
10. 骶后孔 posterior sacral foramina
11. 骶外侧嵴 lateral sacral crest
12. 骶中间嵴 intermediate sacral crest
13. 骶正中嵴 median sacral crest
14. 骶管裂孔 sacral hiatus
15. 骶角 sacral cornu
16. 尾骨角 coccygeal cornu
17. 骶粗隆 sacral tuberosity
18. 骶管 sacral canal

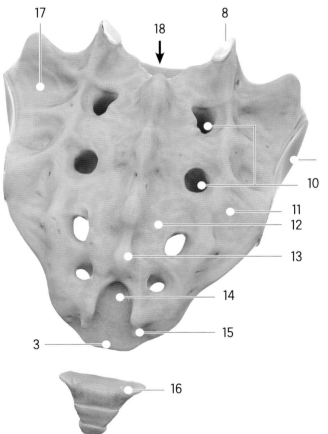

后外侧面观 Posterolateral view

图 1-5　骶骨和尾骨
Sacrum and coccyx

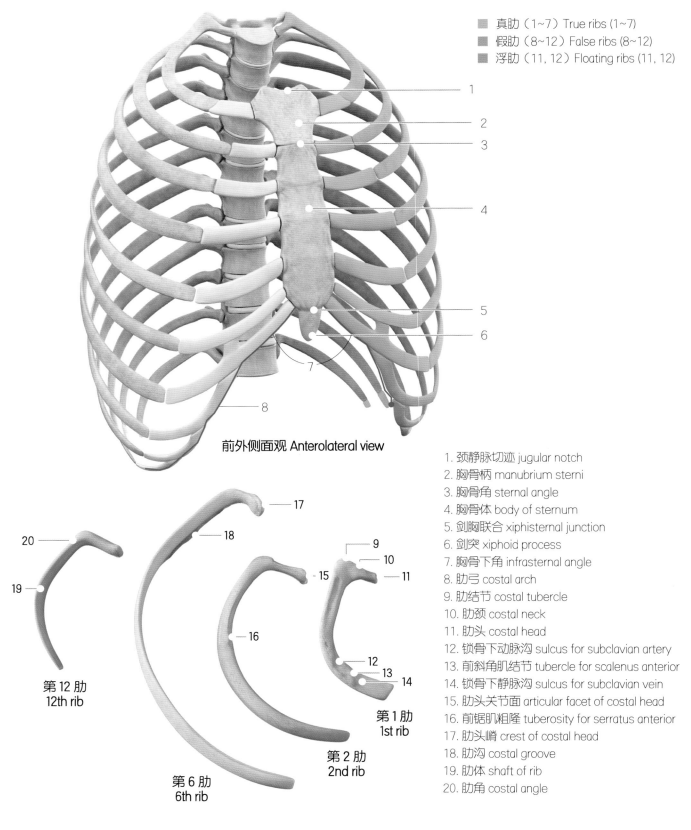

真肋（1~7）True ribs (1~7)
假肋（8~12）False ribs (8~12)
浮肋（11, 12）Floating ribs (11, 12)

前外侧面观 Anterolateral view

1. 颈静脉切迹 jugular notch
2. 胸骨柄 manubrium sterni
3. 胸骨角 sternal angle
4. 胸骨体 body of sternum
5. 剑胸联合 xiphisternal junction
6. 剑突 xiphoid process
7. 胸骨下角 infrasternal angle
8. 肋弓 costal arch
9. 肋结节 costal tubercle
10. 肋颈 costal neck
11. 肋头 costal head
12. 锁骨下动脉沟 sulcus for subclavian artery
13. 前斜角肌结节 tubercle for scalenus anterior
14. 锁骨下静脉沟 sulcus for subclavian vein
15. 肋头关节面 articular facet of costal head
16. 前锯肌粗隆 tuberosity for serratus anterior
17. 肋头嵴 crest of costal head
18. 肋沟 costal groove
19. 肋体 shaft of rib
20. 肋角 costal angle

第 12 肋
12th rib

第 6 肋
6th rib

第 2 肋
2nd rib

第 1 肋
1st rib

图 1-6　胸椎、胸骨与肋骨 1
Thoracic vertebrae,sternum and ribs 1

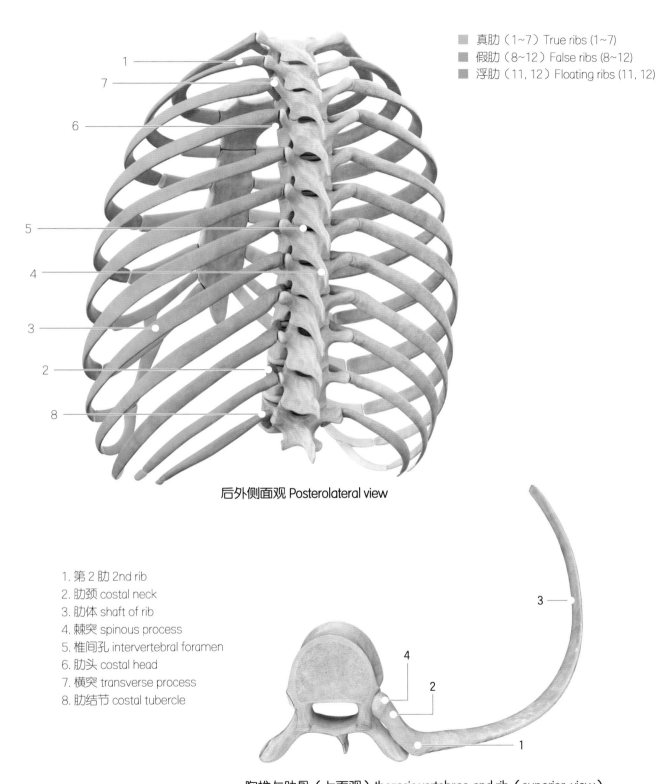

真肋（1~7）True ribs (1~7)
假肋（8~12）False ribs (8~12)
浮肋（11, 12）Floating ribs (11, 12)

后外侧面观 Posterolateral view

1. 第 2 肋 2nd rib
2. 肋颈 costal neck
3. 肋体 shaft of rib
4. 棘突 spinous process
5. 椎间孔 intervertebral foramen
6. 肋头 costal head
7. 横突 transverse process
8. 肋结节 costal tubercle

胸椎与肋骨（上面观）thoracic vertebrae and rib（superior view）

图 1-7　胸椎、胸骨与肋骨 2
Thoracic vertebrae,sternum and ribs 2

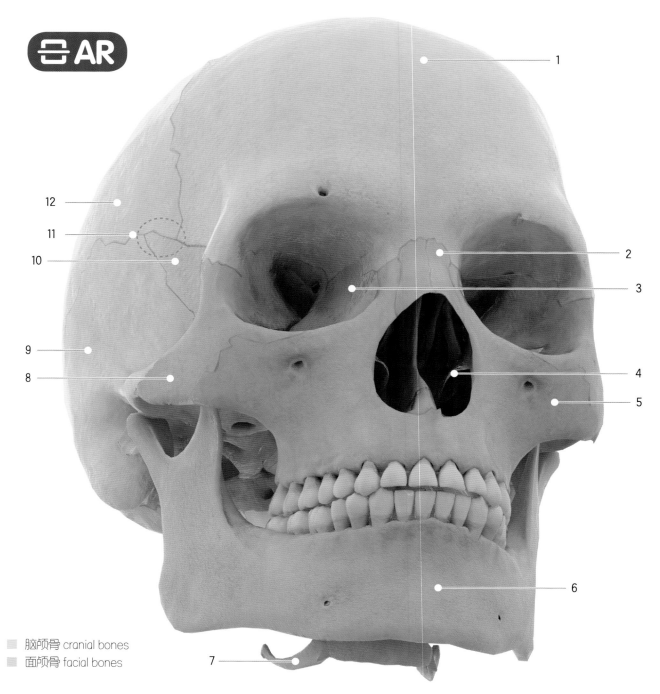

前外侧面观 Anterolateral view

1. 额骨 frontal bone
2. 鼻骨（成对）nasal bone (paired)
3. 筛骨 ethmoid bone
4. 下鼻甲（成对）inferior nasal concha (paired)
5. 上颌骨（成对）maxilla (paired)
6. 下颌骨 mandible
7. 舌骨 hyoid bone
8. 颧骨（成对）zygomatic bone (paired)
9. 颞骨（成对）temporal bone (paired)
10. 蝶骨 sphenoid bone
11. 翼点 pterion
12. 顶骨（成对）parietal bone (paired)

■ 脑颅骨 cranial bones
■ 面颅骨 facial bones

图 1-8　颅
Skull

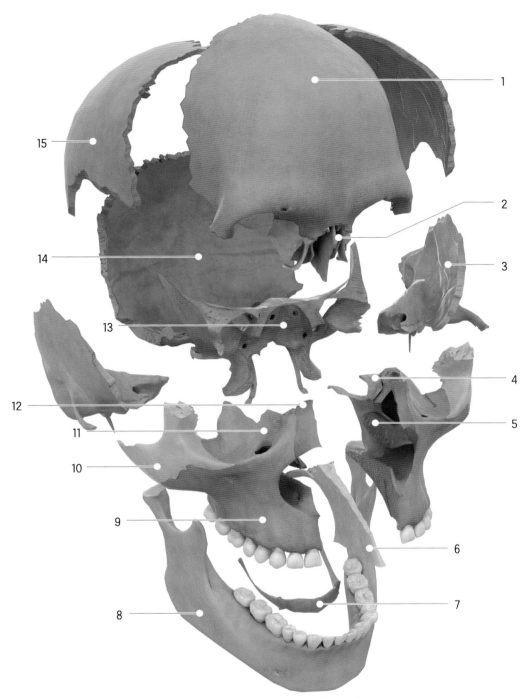

前外侧面观 Anterolateral view

1. 额骨 frontal bone
2. 筛骨 ethmoid bone
3. 颞骨（成对）temporal bone (paired)
4. 腭骨（成对）palatine bone (paired)
5. 下鼻甲（成对）inferior nasal concha (paired)

6. 犁骨 vomer
7. 舌骨 hyoid bone
8. 下颌骨 mandible
9. 上颌骨（成对）maxilla (paired)
10. 颧骨（成对）zygomatic bone (paired)

11. 泪骨（成对）lacrimal bone (paired)
12. 鼻骨（成对）nasal bone (paired)
13. 蝶骨 sphenoid bone
14. 枕骨 occipital bone
15. 顶骨（成对）parietal bone (paired)

图 1-9　分离颅骨
Separation of the skull

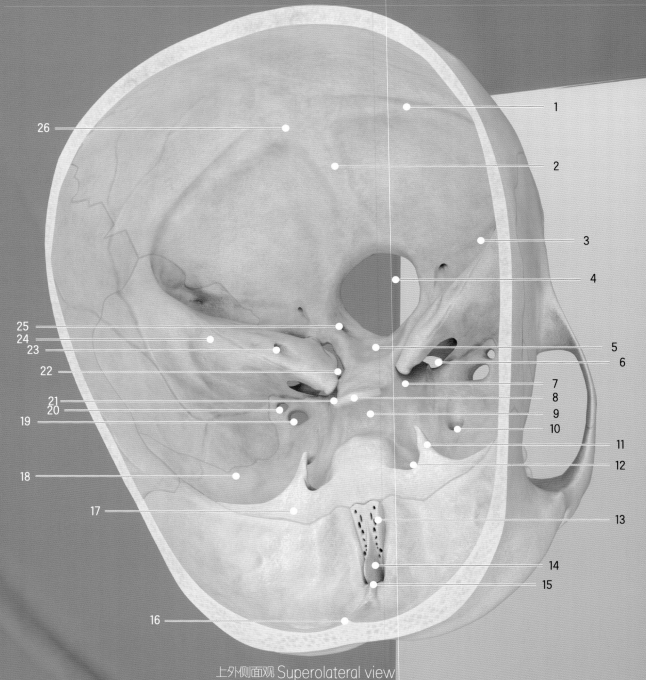

上外侧面观 Superolateral view

1. 横窦沟 sulcus for transverse sinus
2. 枕内嵴 internal occipital crest
3. 乙状窦沟 sulcus for sigmoid sinus
4. 枕骨大孔 foramen magnum
5. 斜坡 clivus
6. 破裂孔 foramen lacerum
7. 颈动脉沟 carotid sulcus
8. 鞍背 dorsum sellae
9. 垂体窝 hypophysial fossa
10. 圆孔 foramen rotundum
11. 前床突 anterior clinoid process
12. 视神经管 optic canal
13. 筛板 cribriform plate
14. 鸡冠 crista galli
15. 盲孔 foramen cecum
16. 额嵴 frontal crest
17. 蝶骨小翼 lesser wing of sphenoid bone
18. 蝶骨大翼 greater wing of sphenoid bone
19. 卵圆孔 foramen ovale
20. 棘孔 foramen spinosum
21. 后床突 posterior clinoid process
22. 颈静脉孔 jugular foramen
23. 内耳门 internal acoustic pore
24. 弓状隆起 arcuate eminence
25. 舌下神经管 hypoglossal canal
26. 枕内隆凸 internal occipital protuberance

图 1-10 颅底内面观
Internal surface of the base of skull

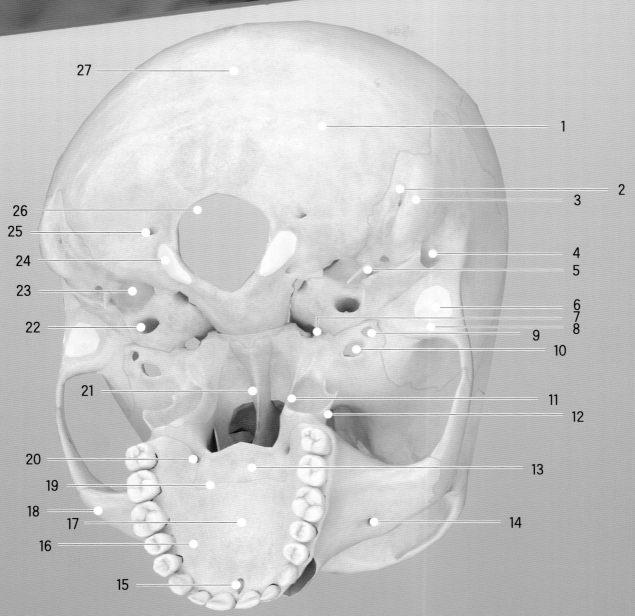

下外侧面观 Inferolateral view

1. 下项线 inferior nuchal line
2. 枕动脉沟 occipital groove
3. 乳突 mastoid process
4. 外耳道 external acoustic meatus
5. 茎突 styloid process
6. 下颌窝 mandibular fossa
7. 破裂孔 foramen lacerum
8. 关节结节 articular tubercle
9. 棘孔 foramen spinosum

10. 卵圆孔 foramen ovale
11. 翼突内侧板 medial pterygoid plate
12. 翼突外侧板 lateral pterygoid plate
13. 腭骨水平板 horizontal plate of palatine bone
14. 眶下孔 infraorbital foramen
15. 切牙孔 incisive foramen
16. 上颌骨腭突 palatine process of maxilla
17. 腭正中缝 median palatine suture
18. 颧骨颞突 zygomatic process

19. 腭横缝 transverse palatine suture
20. 腭大孔 greater palatine foramen
21. 犁骨 vomer
22. 颈动脉管 carotid canal
23. 颈静脉孔 jugular foramen
24. 枕髁 occipital condyle
25. 髁管 condylar canal
26. 枕骨大孔 foramen magnum
27. 枕外嵴 external occipital crest

图 1-11　颅底外面观
External surface of the base of skull

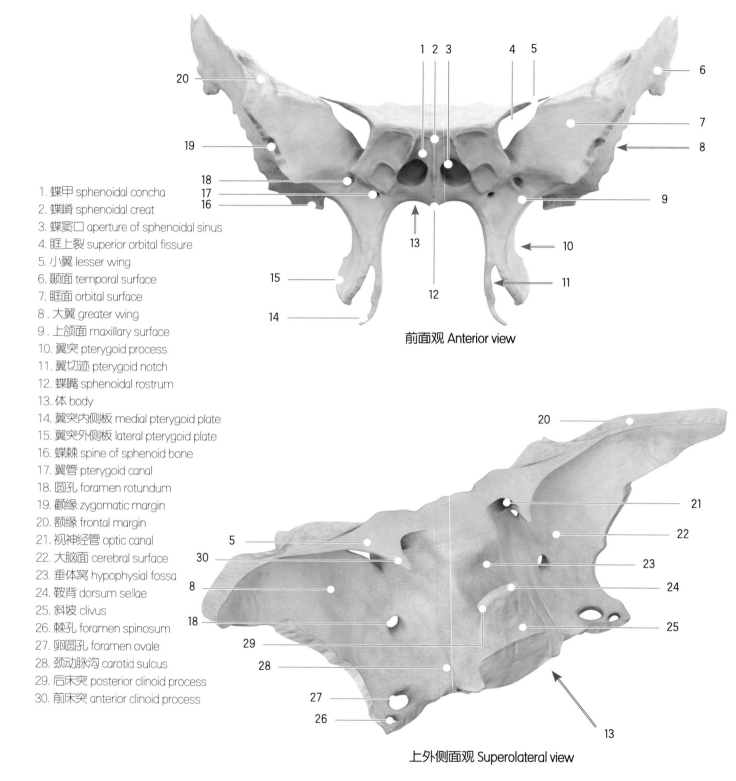

1. 蝶甲 sphenoidal concha
2. 蝶嵴 sphenoidal creat
3. 蝶窦口 aperture of sphenoidal sinus
4. 眶上裂 superior orbital fissure
5. 小翼 lesser wing
6. 颞面 temporal surface
7. 眶面 orbital surface
8. 大翼 greater wing
9. 上颌面 maxillary surface
10. 翼突 pterygoid process
11. 翼切迹 pterygoid notch
12. 蝶嘴 sphenoidal rostrum
13. 体 body
14. 翼突内侧板 medial pterygoid plate
15. 翼突外侧板 lateral pterygoid plate
16. 蝶棘 spine of sphenoid bone
17. 翼管 pterygoid canal
18. 圆孔 foramen rotundum
19. 颧缘 zygomatic margin
20. 额缘 frontal margin
21. 视神经管 optic canal
22. 大脑面 cerebral surface
23. 垂体窝 hypophysial fossa
24. 鞍背 dorsum sellae
25. 斜坡 clivus
26. 棘孔 foramen spinosum
27. 卵圆孔 foramen ovale
28. 颈动脉沟 carotid sulcus
29. 后床突 posterior clinoid process
30. 前床突 anterior clinoid process

前面观 Anterior view

上外侧面观 Superolateral view

图 1-12　蝶骨
Sphenoid bone

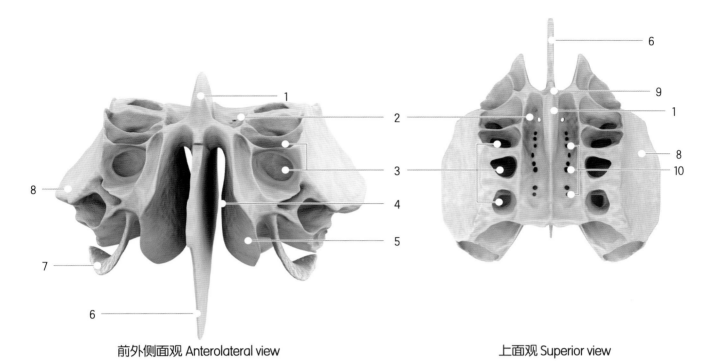

前外侧面观 Anterolateral view　　　　　　　上面观 Superior view

图 1-13　筛骨
Ethmoid bone

1. 鸡冠 crista galli
2. 筛板 cribriform plate
3. 筛窦及筛骨迷路 ethmoidal sinus and labyrinth
4. 鼻道 nasal meatus
5. 中鼻甲 middle nasal concha
6. 垂直板 perpendicular plate
7. 钩突 uncinate process
8. 眶板 orbital plate
9. 鸡冠翼 ala of crista galli
10. 筛孔 cribriform foramina

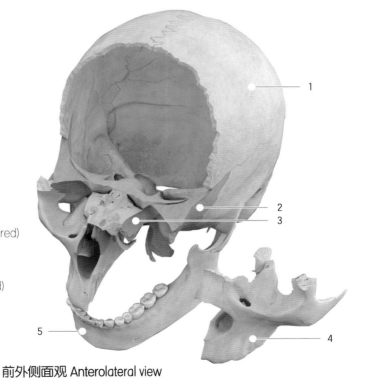

1. 顶骨（成对）parietal bone (paired)
2. 蝶骨 sphenoid bone
3. 筛骨 ethmoid bone
4. 上颌骨（成对）maxilla (paired)
5. 下颌骨 mandible

前外侧面观 Anterolateral view

图 1-14　筛骨与蝶骨的位置
Location of the ethmoid and sphenoid bones

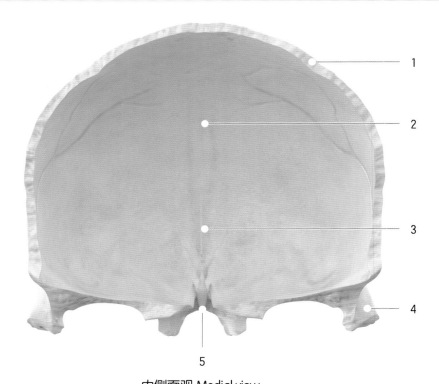

内侧面观 Medial view

1. 顶缘 parietal margin
2. 上矢状窦沟 sulcus for superior sagittal sinus
3. 额嵴 frontal crest
4. 颧突 zygomatic process
5. 鼻棘 nasal spine
6. 颞线 temporal line
7. 眶上缘 supraorbital margin
8. 眉间 glabella
9. 眶上孔 supraorbital foramen
10. 眉弓 superciliary arch
11. 额结节 frontal tuber

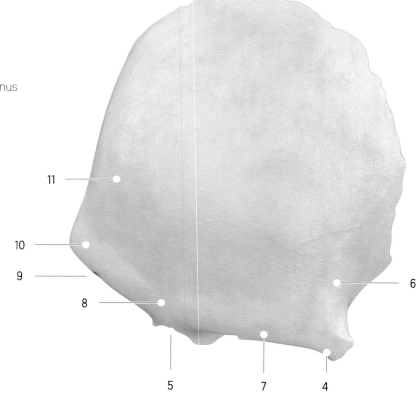

前外侧面观 Anterolateral view

图 1-15　额骨
Frontal bone

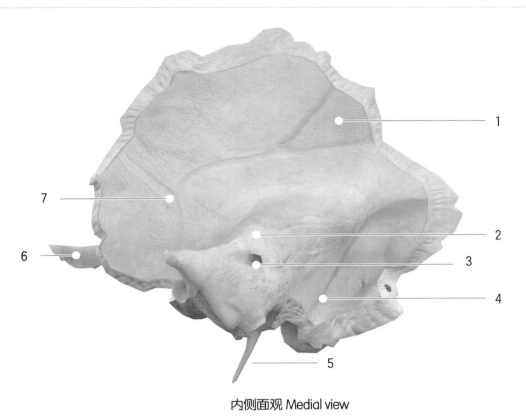

内侧面观 Medial view

1. 鳞部 squamous part
2. 弓状隆起 arcuate eminence
3. 内耳门 internal acoustic pore
4. 乙状窦沟 sulcus for sigmoid sinus
5. 茎突 styloid process
6. 颧突 zygomatic process
7. 脑膜中动脉沟 sulcus for middle meningeal artery
8. 关节结节 articular tubercle
9. 下颌窝 mandibular fossa
10. 鼓部 tympanic part
11. 乳突 mastoid process
12. 外耳门 external acoustic pore

外侧面观 Lateral view

图 1-16　颞骨
Temporal bone

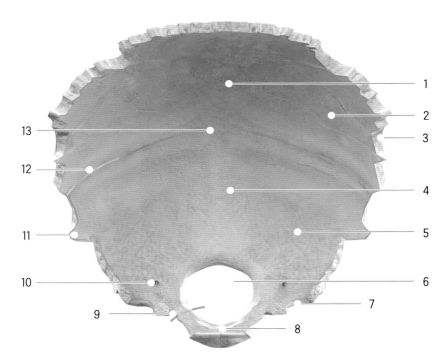

内侧面观 Medial view

1. 上矢状窦沟 sulcus for superior sagittal sinus
2. 大脑窝 cerebral fossa
3. 人字缘 lambdoid border
4. 枕内嵴 internal occipital crest
5. 小脑窝 cerebellar fossa
6. 枕骨大孔 foramen magnum
7. 颈静脉切迹 jugular notch
8. 斜坡 clivus
9. 舌下神经管 hypoglossal canal
10. 髁管 condylar canal
11. 乳突缘 mastoid border
12. 横窦沟 sulcus for transverse sinus
13. 枕内隆凸 internal occipital protuberance

14. 枕外隆凸 external occipital protuberance
15. 上项线 superior nuchal line
16. 下项线 inferior nuchal line
17. 颈静脉突 jugular process
18. 枕髁 occipital condyle
19. 髁窝 condylar fossa
20. 枕外嵴 external occipital crest

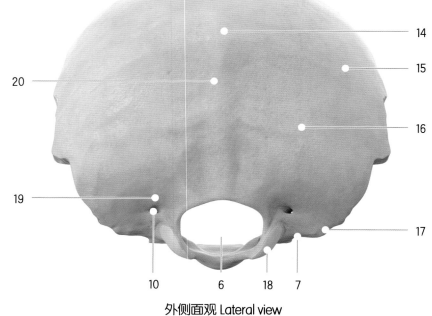

外侧面观 Lateral view

图 1-17 枕骨
Occipital bone

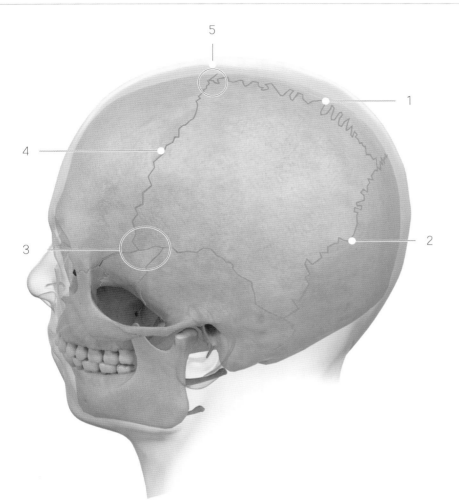

后外侧面观 Posterolateral view

图 1-18　颅顶
Calvaria

1. 矢状缝 sagittal suture
2. 人字缝 lambdoid suture
3. 翼点 pterion
4. 冠状缝 coronal suture
5. 前囟点 bregma

1. 矢状缝 sagittal suture
2. 后囟 posterior fontanelle
3. 人字缝 lambdoid suture
4. 后外侧囟 posterolateral fontanelle
5. 前外侧囟 anterolateral fontanelle
6. 冠状缝 coronal suture
7. 额缝 frontal suture
8. 前囟 anterior fontanelle

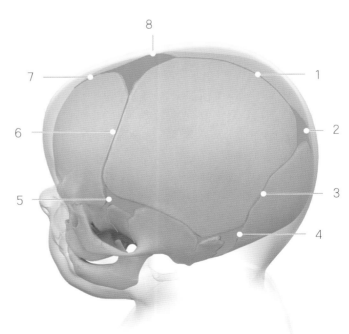

图 1-19　新生儿颅
Infant skull

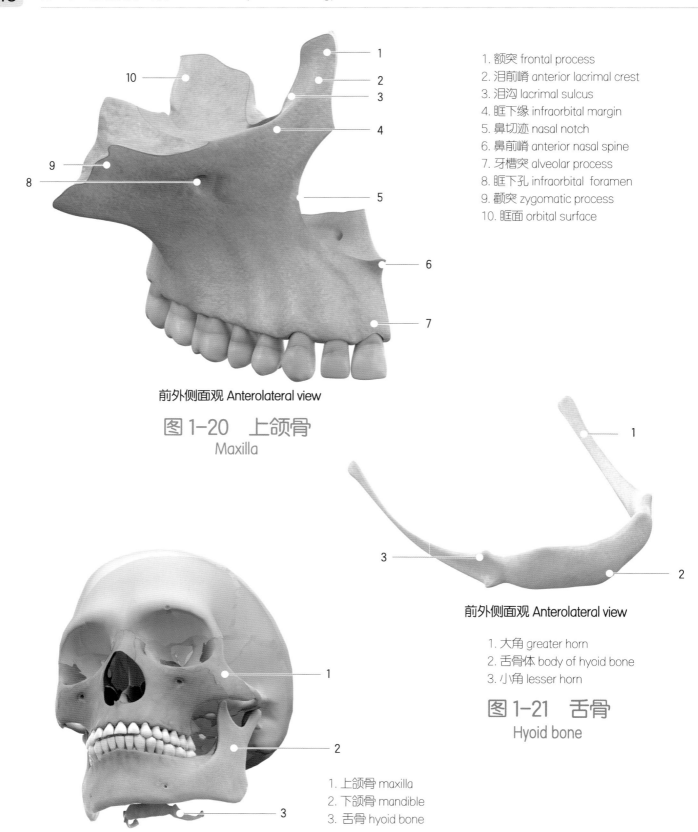

前外侧面观 Anterolateral view

图 1-20 上颌骨
Maxilla

1. 额突 frontal process
2. 泪前嵴 anterior lacrimal crest
3. 泪沟 lacrimal sulcus
4. 眶下缘 infraorbital margin
5. 鼻切迹 nasal notch
6. 鼻前嵴 anterior nasal spine
7. 牙槽突 alveolar process
8. 眶下孔 infraorbital foramen
9. 颧突 zygomatic process
10. 眶面 orbital surface

前外侧面观 Anterolateral view

1. 大角 greater horn
2. 舌骨体 body of hyoid bone
3. 小角 lesser horn

图 1-21 舌骨
Hyoid bone

1. 上颌骨 maxilla
2. 下颌骨 mandible
3. 舌骨 hyoid bone

图 1-22 上颌骨、下颌骨和舌骨的位置
Location of the maxilla, mandible and hyoid bone

1. 髁突 condylar process
2. 下颌头 head of mandible
3. 下颌颈 neck of mandible
4. 下颌支 ramus of mandible
5. 咬肌粗隆 masseteric tuberosity
6. 下颌角 angle of mandible
7. 斜线 oblique line
8. 下颌体 body of mandible
9. 颏孔 mental foramen
10. 下颌底 base of mandible
11. 颏隆凸 mental protuberace
12. 牙槽部 alveolar part
13. 下颌孔 mandibular foramen
14. 下颌切迹 mandibular notch
15. 冠突 coronoid process

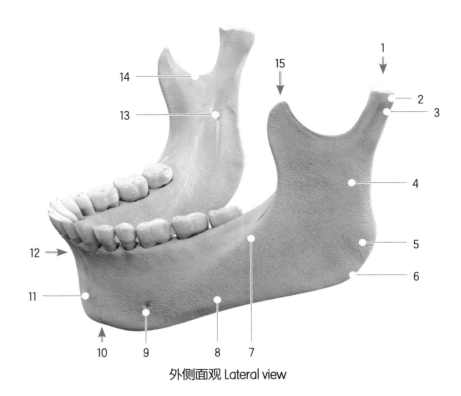

外侧面观 Lateral view

16. 翼肌粗隆 pterygoid tuberosity
17. 下颌管 mandibular canal
18. 下颌下腺凹 submandibular fovea
19. 舌下腺凹 sublingual fovea
20. 颏棘 mental spine
21. 二腹肌窝 digastric fossa
22. 下颌舌骨肌线 mylohyoid line
23. 下颌小舌 mandibular lingula

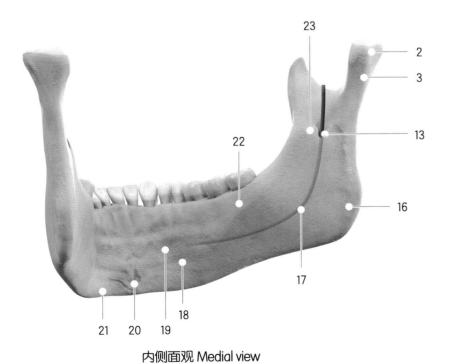

内侧面观 Medial view

图 1-23　下颌骨
Mandible

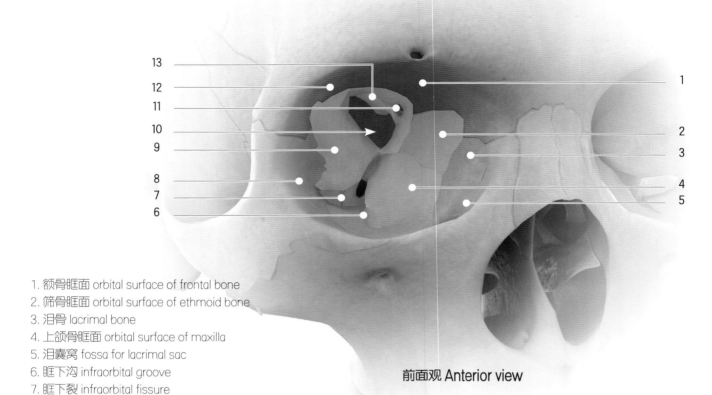

1. 额骨眶面 orbital surface of frontal bone
2. 筛骨眶面 orbital surface of ethmoid bone
3. 泪骨 lacrimal bone
4. 上颌骨眶面 orbital surface of maxilla
5. 泪囊窝 fossa for lacrimal sac
6. 眶下沟 infraorbital groove
7. 眶下裂 infraorbital fissure
8. 颧骨眶面 orbital surface of zygomatic bone
9. 蝶骨大翼眶面 orbital surface of greater wing of sphenoid bone
10. 眶上裂 superior orbital fissure

前面观 Anterior view

11. 视神经管 optic canal
12. 泪腺窝 fossa for lacrimal gland
13. 蝶骨小翼眶面 orbital surface of lesser wing of sphenoid bone

图 1-24 眶
Orbit

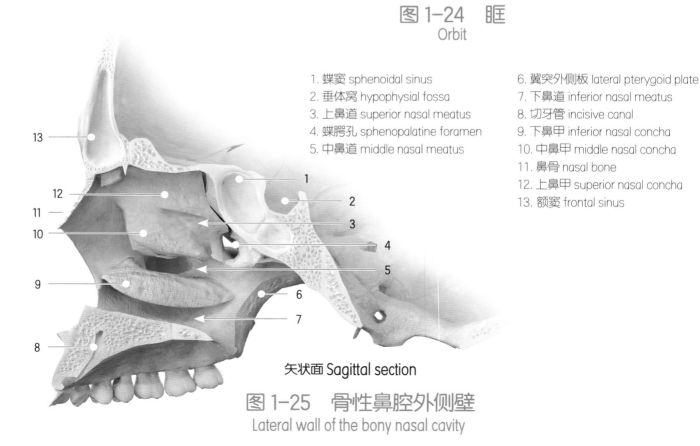

1. 蝶窦 sphenoidal sinus
2. 垂体窝 hypophysial fossa
3. 上鼻道 superior nasal meatus
4. 蝶腭孔 sphenopalatine foramen
5. 中鼻道 middle nasal meatus

6. 翼突外侧板 lateral pterygoid plate
7. 下鼻道 inferior nasal meatus
8. 切牙管 incisive canal
9. 下鼻甲 inferior nasal concha
10. 中鼻甲 middle nasal concha
11. 鼻骨 nasal bone
12. 上鼻甲 superior nasal concha
13. 额窦 frontal sinus

矢状面 Sagittal section

图 1-25 骨性鼻腔外侧壁
Lateral wall of the bony nasal cavity

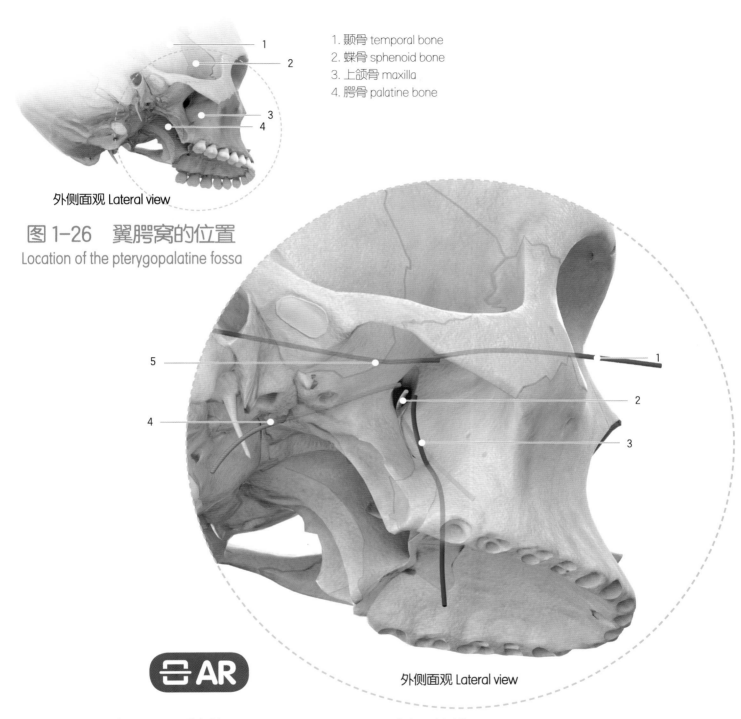

1. 颞骨 temporal bone
2. 蝶骨 sphenoid bone
3. 上颌骨 maxilla
4. 腭骨 palatine bone

外侧面观 Lateral view

图 1-26   翼腭窝的位置
Location of the pterygopalatine fossa

外侧面观 Lateral view

1. 向前经眶下裂通出的探针 a probe that passes through the inferior orbital fissure
2. 向内经蝶腭孔通入鼻腔的探针 a probe that passes through the sphenopalatine foramen into the nasal cavity
3. 向下经腭大管通入翼腭窝的探针 a probe that passes through the greater palatine canal into the pterygopalatine fossa
4. 向后经翼管通入的探针 a probe that passes through the pterygoid canal
5. 向后经圆孔通入颅腔的探针 a probe that passes through the foramen rotundum into the skull

图 1-27   翼腭窝
Pterygopalatine fossa

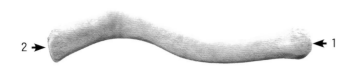

上面观 Superior view

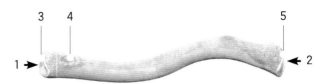

下面观 Inferior view

1. 胸骨端 sternal end
2. 肩峰端 acromial end
3. 胸骨关节面 sternal articular facet

4. 肋锁韧带压迹 impression for costoclavicular ligament
5. 肩峰关节面 acromial articular facet

图 1-28　锁骨
Clavicle

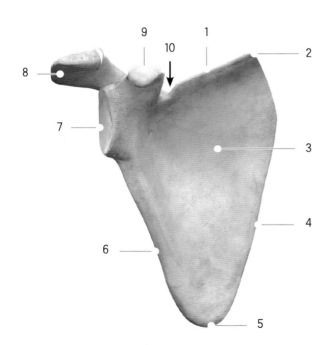

前面观 Anterior view

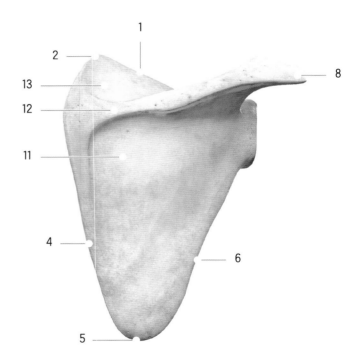

后面观 Posterior view

1. 上缘 superior border
2. 上角 superior angle
3. 肩胛下窝 subscapular fossa
4. 内侧缘 medial border
5. 下角 inferior angle
6. 外侧缘 lateral border
7. 关节盂 glenoid cavity

8. 肩峰 acromion
9. 喙突 coracoid process
10. 肩胛上切迹 suprascapular notch
11. 冈下窝 infraspinous fossa
12. 肩胛冈 spine of scapula
13. 冈上窝 supraspinous fossa

图 1-29　肩胛骨
Scapula

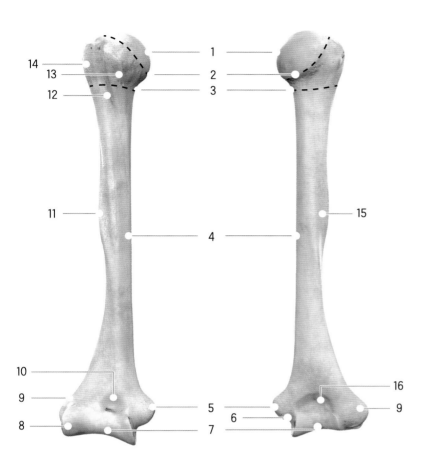

前面观 Anterior view　　　　后面观 Posterior view

1. 肱骨头 head of humerus
2. 解剖颈 anatomical neck
3. 外科颈 surgical neck
4. 肱骨体 shaft of humerus
5. 内上髁 medial epicondyle
6. 尺神经沟 sulcus for ulnar n.
7. 肱骨滑车 trochlea of humerus
8. 肱骨小头 capitulum of humerus

9. 外上髁 lateral epicondyle
10. 冠突窝 coronoid fossa
11. 三角肌粗隆 deltoid tuberosity
12. 结节间沟 intertubercular sulcus
13. 小结节 lesser tubercle
14. 大结节 greater tubercle
15. 桡神经沟 sulcus for radial n.
16. 鹰嘴窝 olecranon fossa

图 1-30　肱骨
Humerus

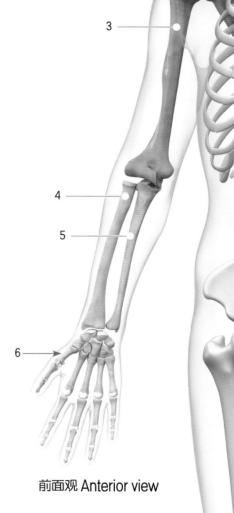

前面观 Anterior view

1. 锁骨 clavicle
2. 肩胛骨 scapula
3. 肱骨 humerus

4. 桡骨 radius
5. 尺骨 ulna
6. 手骨 bones of the hand

图 1-31　上肢骨的位置 1
Location of the upper limb bones 1

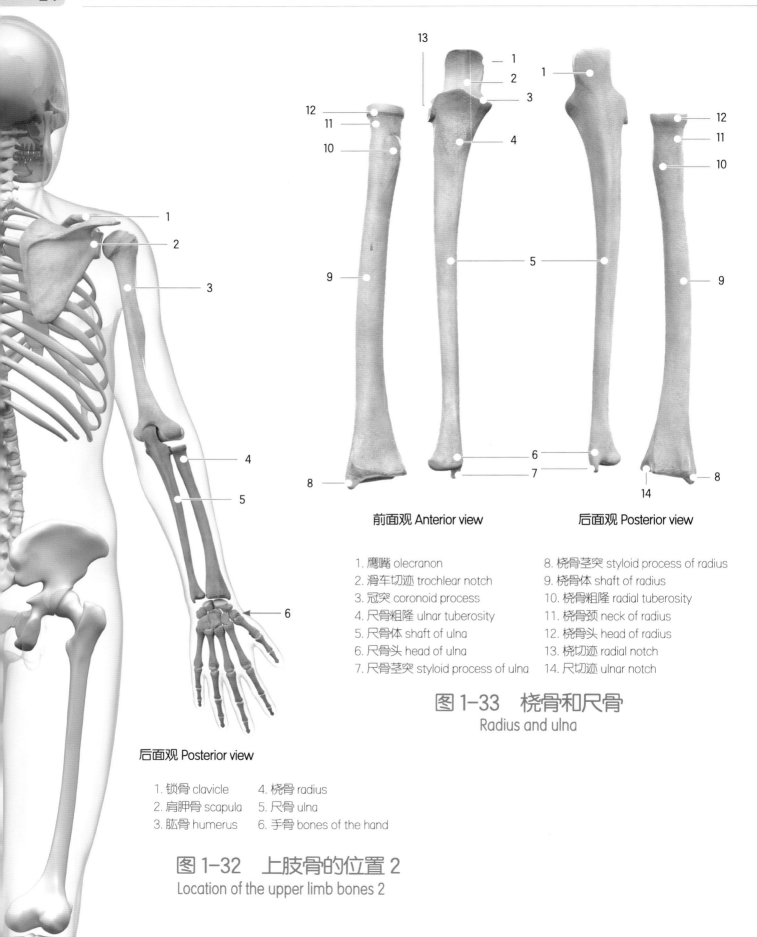

前面观 Anterior view   后面观 Posterior view

1. 鹰嘴 olecranon   8. 桡骨茎突 styloid process of radius
2. 滑车切迹 trochlear notch   9. 桡骨体 shaft of radius
3. 冠突 coronoid process   10. 桡骨粗隆 radial tuberosity
4. 尺骨粗隆 ulnar tuberosity   11. 桡骨颈 neck of radius
5. 尺骨体 shaft of ulna   12. 桡骨头 head of radius
6. 尺骨头 head of ulna   13. 桡切迹 radial notch
7. 尺骨茎突 styloid process of ulna 14. 尺切迹 ulnar notch

图 1-33   桡骨和尺骨
Radius and ulna

后面观 Posterior view

1. 锁骨 clavicle   4. 桡骨 radius
2. 肩胛骨 scapula   5. 尺骨 ulna
3. 肱骨 humerus   6. 手骨 bones of the hand

图 1-32   上肢骨的位置 2
Location of the upper limb bones 2

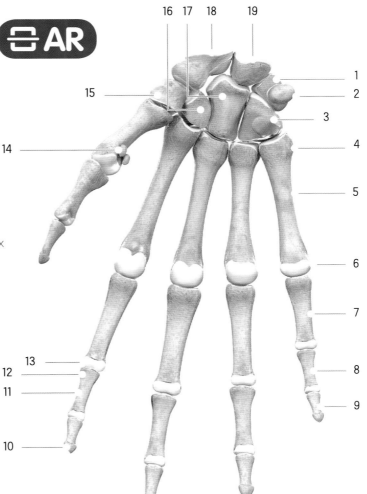

1. 三角骨 triquetral bone
2. 豌豆骨 pisiform bone
3. 钩骨 hamate bone
4. 掌骨底 base of metacarpal bone
5. 掌骨体 shaft of metacarpal bone
6. 掌骨头 head of metacarpal bone
7. 近节指骨 proximal phalanx
8. 中节指骨 middle phalanx
9. 远节指骨 distal phalanx
10. 远节指骨粗隆 tuberosity of distal phalanx
11. 指骨体 shaft of phalanx
12. 指骨底 base of phalanx
13. 指骨滑车 trochlea of phalanx
14. 籽骨 sesamoid bone
15. 大多角骨 trapezium bone
16. 小多角骨 trapezoid bone
17. 头状骨 capitate bone
18. 手舟骨 scaphoid bone
19. 月骨 lunate bone

掌面观 Palmar view

图 1-34　手骨
Bones of the hand

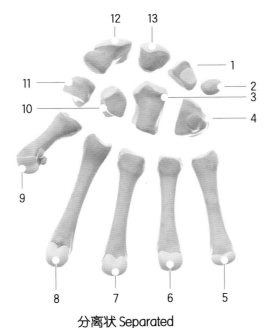

分离状 Separated

图 1-35　腕骨和掌骨
Carpal and metacarpal bones

1. 三角骨 triquetral bone
2. 豌豆骨 pisiform bone
3. 头状骨 capitate bone
4. 钩骨 hamate bone
5. 第 5 掌骨 5th metacarpal bone
6. 第 4 掌骨 4th metacarpal bone
7. 第 3 掌骨 3rd metacarpal bone
8. 第 2 掌骨 2nd metacarpal bone
9. 第 1 掌骨 1st metacarpal bone
10. 小多角骨 trapezoid bone
11. 大多角骨 trapezium bone
12. 手舟骨 scaphoid bone
13. 月骨 lunate bone

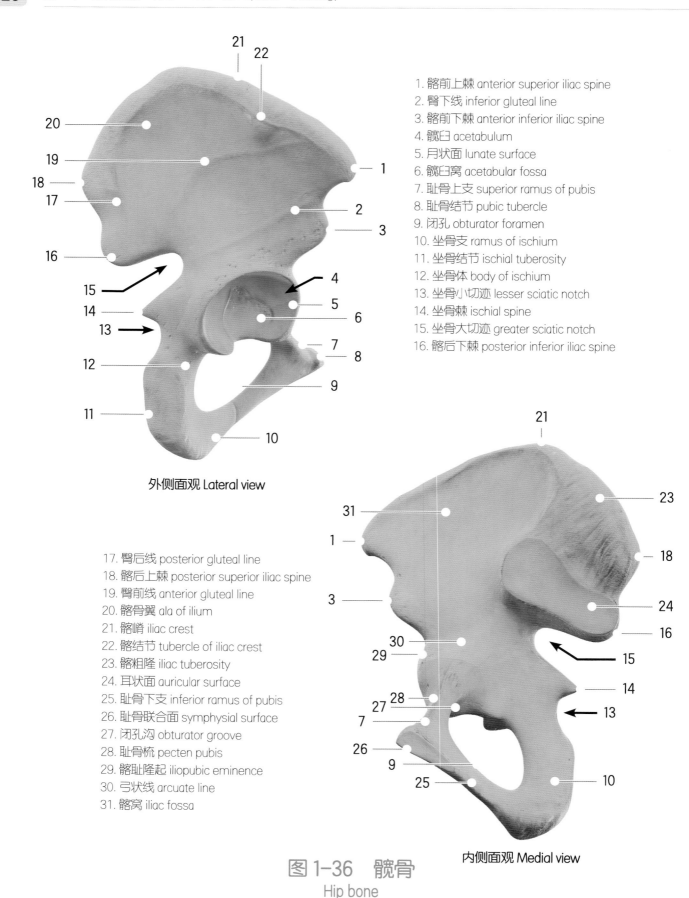

1. 髂前上棘 anterior superior iliac spine
2. 臀下线 inferior gluteal line
3. 髂前下棘 anterior inferior iliac spine
4. 髋臼 acetabulum
5. 月状面 lunate surface
6. 髋臼窝 acetabular fossa
7. 耻骨上支 superior ramus of pubis
8. 耻骨结节 pubic tubercle
9. 闭孔 obturator foramen
10. 坐骨支 ramus of ischium
11. 坐骨结节 ischial tuberosity
12. 坐骨体 body of ischium
13. 坐骨小切迹 lesser sciatic notch
14. 坐骨棘 ischial spine
15. 坐骨大切迹 greater sciatic notch
16. 髂后下棘 posterior inferior iliac spine

外侧面观 Lateral view

17. 臀后线 posterior gluteal line
18. 髂后上棘 posterior superior iliac spine
19. 臀前线 anterior gluteal line
20. 髂骨翼 ala of ilium
21. 髂嵴 iliac crest
22. 髂结节 tubercle of iliac crest
23. 髂粗隆 iliac tuberosity
24. 耳状面 auricular surface
25. 耻骨下支 inferior ramus of pubis
26. 耻骨联合面 symphysial surface
27. 闭孔沟 obturator groove
28. 耻骨梳 pecten pubis
29. 髂耻隆起 iliopubic eminence
30. 弓状线 arcuate line
31. 髂窝 iliac fossa

内侧面观 Medial view

图 1-36　髋骨
Hip bone

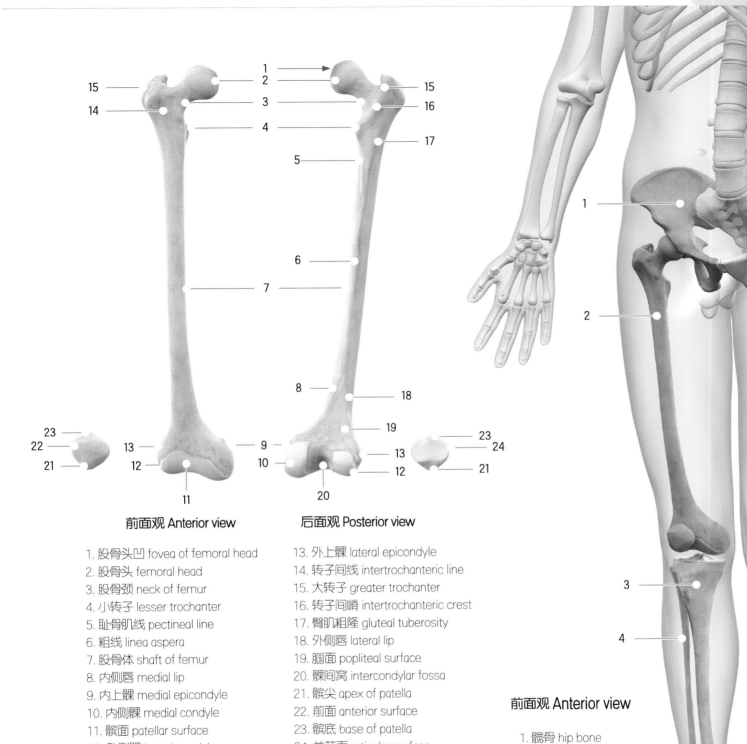

前面观 Anterior view

后面观 Posterior view

1. 股骨头凹 fovea of femoral head
2. 股骨头 femoral head
3. 股骨颈 neck of femur
4. 小转子 lesser trochanter
5. 耻骨肌线 pectineal line
6. 粗线 linea aspera
7. 股骨体 shaft of femur
8. 内侧唇 medial lip
9. 内上髁 medial epicondyle
10. 内侧髁 medial condyle
11. 髌面 patellar surface
12. 外侧髁 lateral condyle

13. 外上髁 lateral epicondyle
14. 转子间线 intertrochanteric line
15. 大转子 greater trochanter
16. 转子间嵴 intertrochanteric crest
17. 臀肌粗隆 gluteal tuberosity
18. 外侧唇 lateral lip
19. 腘面 popliteal surface
20. 髁间窝 intercondylar fossa
21. 髌尖 apex of patella
22. 前面 anterior surface
23. 髌底 base of patella
24. 关节面 articular surface

图 1-37　股骨和髌骨
Femur and patella

前面观 Anterior view

1. 髋骨 hip bone
2. 股骨 femur
3. 胫骨 tibia
4. 腓骨 fibula
5. 足骨 bones of foot

图 1-38　下肢骨的位置 1
Location of the lower limb bones 1

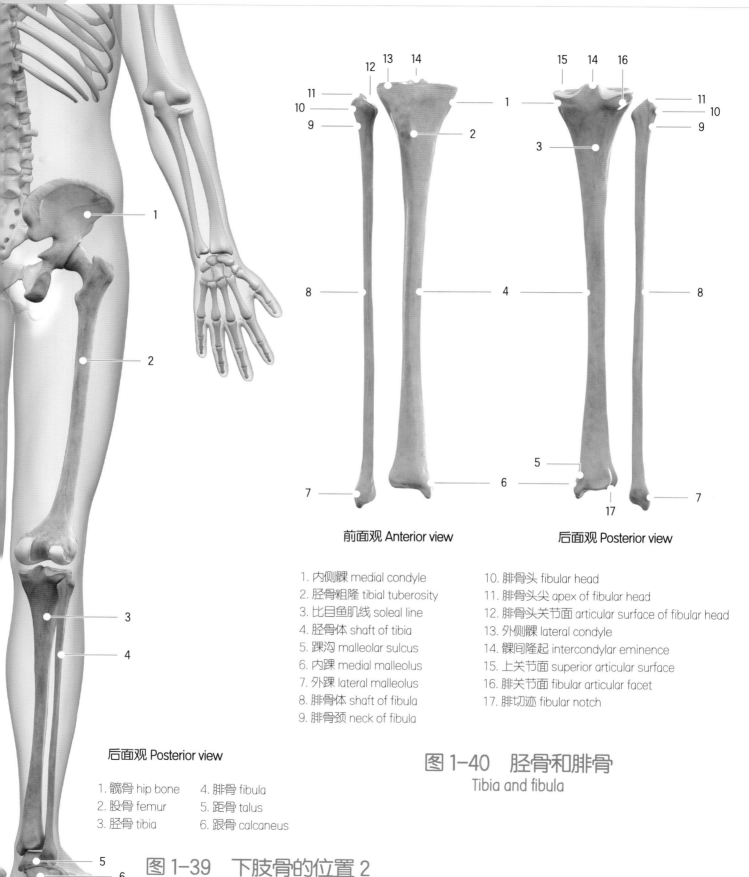

前面观 Anterior view

后面观 Posterior view

1. 内侧髁 medial condyle
2. 胫骨粗隆 tibial tuberosity
3. 比目鱼肌线 soleal line
4. 胫骨体 shaft of tibia
5. 踝沟 malleolar sulcus
6. 内踝 medial malleolus
7. 外踝 lateral malleolus
8. 腓骨体 shaft of fibula
9. 腓骨颈 neck of fibula

10. 腓骨头 fibular head
11. 腓骨头尖 apex of fibular head
12. 腓骨头关节面 articular surface of fibular head
13. 外侧髁 lateral condyle
14. 髁间隆起 intercondylar eminence
15. 上关节面 superior articular surface
16. 腓关节面 fibular articular facet
17. 腓切迹 fibular notch

图 1-40　胫骨和腓骨
Tibia and fibula

后面观 Posterior view

1. 髋骨 hip bone
2. 股骨 femur
3. 胫骨 tibia
4. 腓骨 fibula
5. 距骨 talus
6. 跟骨 calcaneus

图 1-39　下肢骨的位置 2
Location of the lower limb bones 2

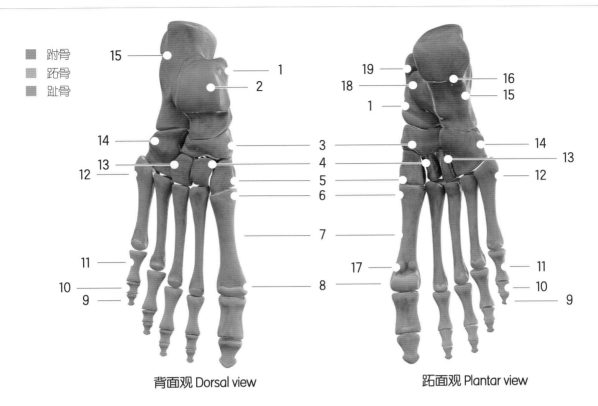

■ 跗骨
■ 距骨
■ 趾骨

背面观 Dorsal view

跖面观 Plantar view

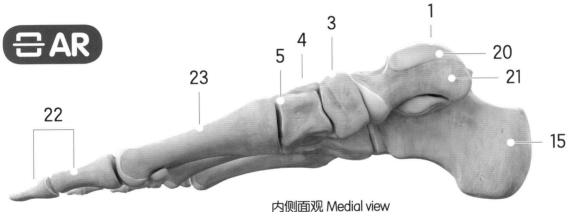

内侧面观 Medial view

1. 距骨 talus
2. 距骨滑车 trochlea of talus
3. 足舟骨 navicular bone
4. 中间楔骨 intermediate cuneiform bone
5. 内侧楔骨 medial cuneiform bone
6. 跖骨底 base of metatarsal bone
7. 跖骨体 shaft of metatarsal bone
8. 跖骨头 head of metatarsal bone
9. 远节趾骨 distal phalanx
10. 中节趾骨 middle phalanx
11. 近节趾骨 proximal phalanx
12. 第 5 跖骨粗隆 tuberosity of 5th metatarsal bone

13. 外侧楔骨 lateral cuneiform bone
14. 骰骨 cuboid bone
15. 跟骨 calcaneus
16. 跟骨结节 calcaneal tuberosity
17. 籽骨 sesamoid bone
18. 载距突 sustentaculum tali
19. 踇长屈肌腱沟 sulcus for tendon of flexor hallucis longus
20. 内踝面 medial malleolar facet
21. 距骨后突 posterior process of talus
22. 趾骨 phalange of toes
23. 第 1 跖骨 1st metatarsal bone

图 1-41　足骨
Bones of the foot

第2章 运动系统 Locomotor System

关节学 Arthrology

1. 颞下颌关节 temporomandibular joint
2. 肩关节 shoulder joint
3. 桡尺近侧关节 proximal radioulnar joint
4. 趾骨间关节 interphalangeal joint
5. 跖骨间关节 intermetatarsal joint
6. 踝关节 ankle joint
7. 膝关节 knee joint
8. 椎间关节 intervertebral joint
9. 胸肋关节 sternocostal joint
10. 胸锁关节 sternoclavicular joint
11. 桡腕关节 radiocarpal joint
12. 拇指腕掌关节 carpometacarpal joint of thumb

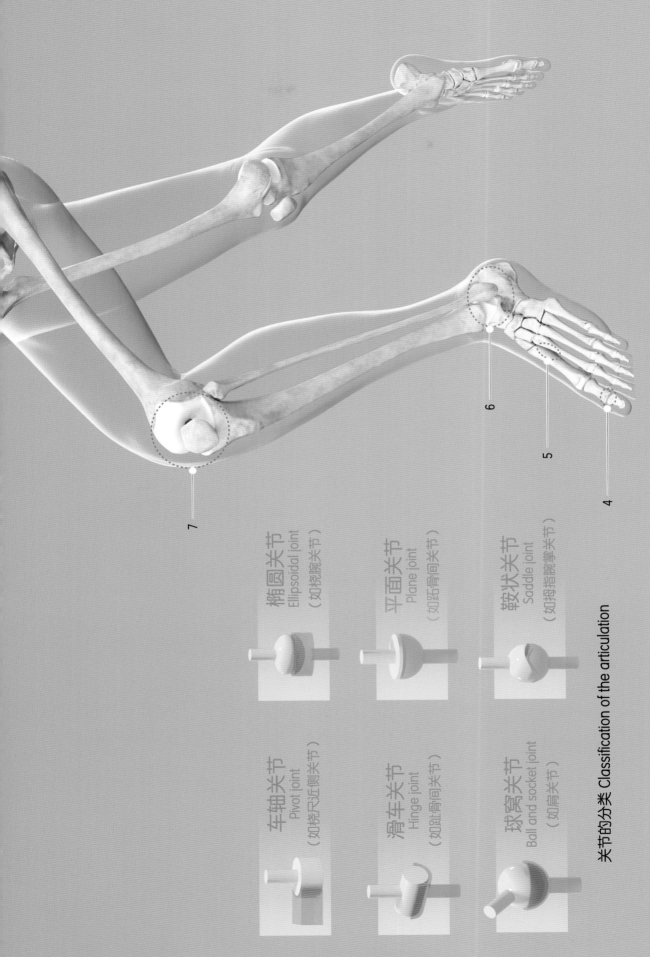

关节的分类 Classification of the articulation

车轴关节
Pivot joint
（如桡尺近侧关节）

滑车关节
Hinge joint
（如趾骨间关节）

球窝关节
Ball and socket joint
（如肩关节）

椭圆关节
Ellipsoidal joint
（如桡腕关节）

平面关节
Plane joint
（如跗骨间关节）

鞍状关节
Saddle joint
（如拇指腕掌关节）

图 2-1　全身关节概观
Overview of the articulation

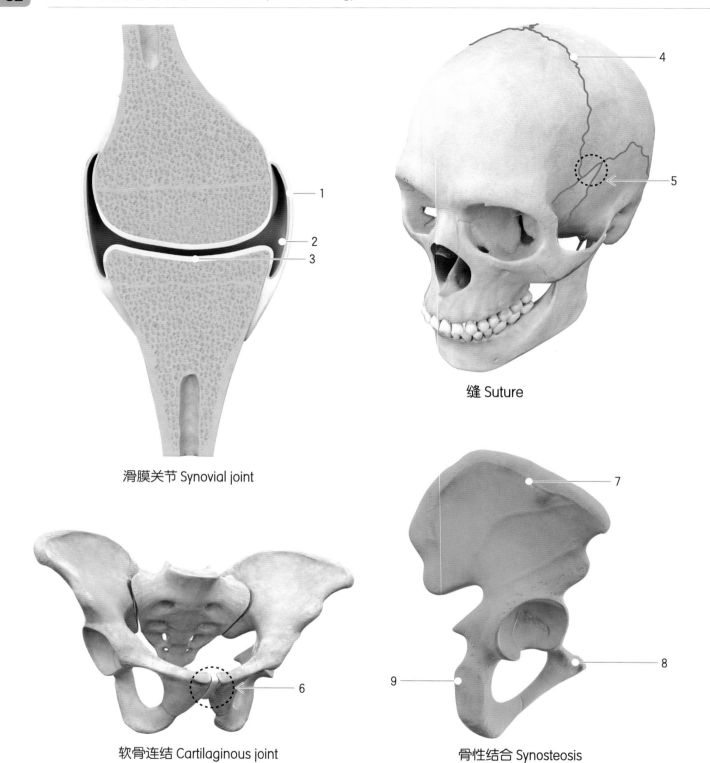

滑膜关节 Synovial joint

缝 Suture

软骨连结 Cartilaginous joint

骨性结合 Synosteosis

1. 关节囊 articular capsule
2. 关节腔 articular cavity
3. 关节面 articular surface
4. 冠状缝 coronal suture
5. 翼点 pterion
6. 耻骨联合 pubic symphysis
7. 髂骨 ilium
8. 耻骨 pubis
9. 坐骨 ischium

图 2-2　骨连结的分类
Classification of the articulation

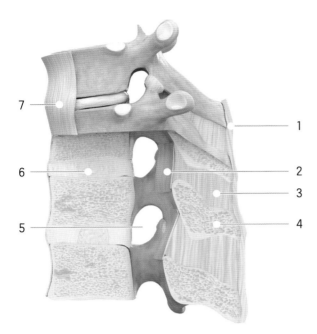

正中矢状面观 Median sagittal view

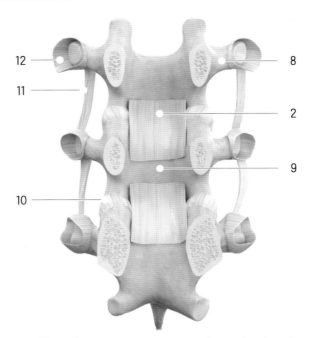

椎弓前面观 Anterior view of vertebral arch

1. 棘上韧带 supraspinal lig.
2. 黄韧带 ligamenta flava
3. 棘间韧带 interspinal lig.
4. 棘突 spinous process
5. 椎间孔 intervertebral foramen
6. 椎间盘 intervertebral disc
7. 前纵韧带 anterior longitudinal lig.
8. 横突 transverse process
9. 椎弓板 lamina of vertebral arch

10. 关节突关节关节囊 zygapophysial articular capsule
11. 横突间韧带 intertransverse lig.
12. 肋横突关节关节囊 costotransverse articular capsule
13. 后纵韧带 posterior longitudinal lig.
14. 椎弓根 pedicle of vertebral arch
15. 髓核 nucleus pulposus
16. 纤维环 anulus fibrosus
17. 肋头辐射状韧带 radiate lig. of costal head
18. 下肋凹 inferior costal fovea

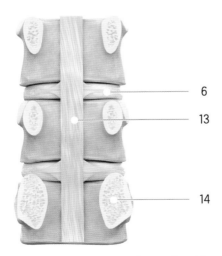

椎体后面观 Posterior view of vertebral body

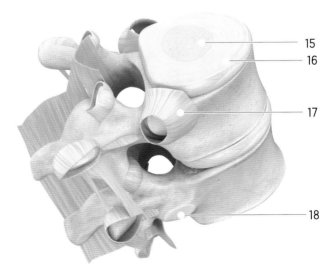

上外侧面观 Superior lateral view

图 2-3　椎骨间连结
Intervertebral joints

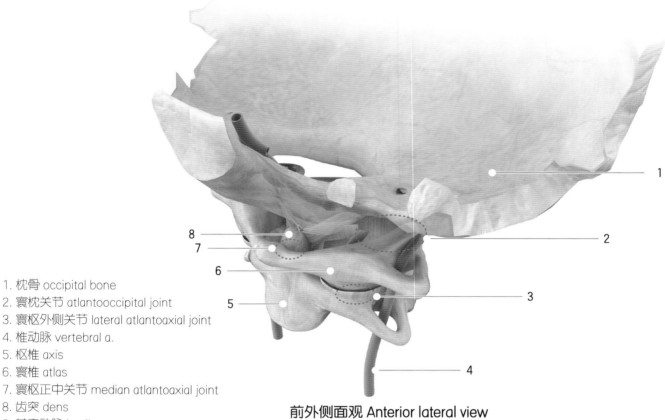

1. 枕骨 occipital bone
2. 寰枕关节 atlantooccipital joint
3. 寰枢外侧关节 lateral atlantoaxial joint
4. 椎动脉 vertebral a.
5. 枢椎 axis
6. 寰椎 atlas
7. 寰枢正中关节 median atlantoaxial joint
8. 齿突 dens
9. 基底动脉 basilar a.
10. 翼状韧带 alar lig.
11. 寰椎横韧带 transverse lig. of atlas
12. 十字韧带 cruciform lig. of atlas

前外侧面观 Anterior lateral view

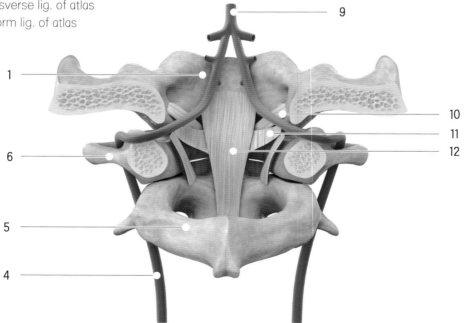

后面观 Posterior view

图 2-4 寰枕、寰枢关节
Atlantooccipital and atlantoaxial joints

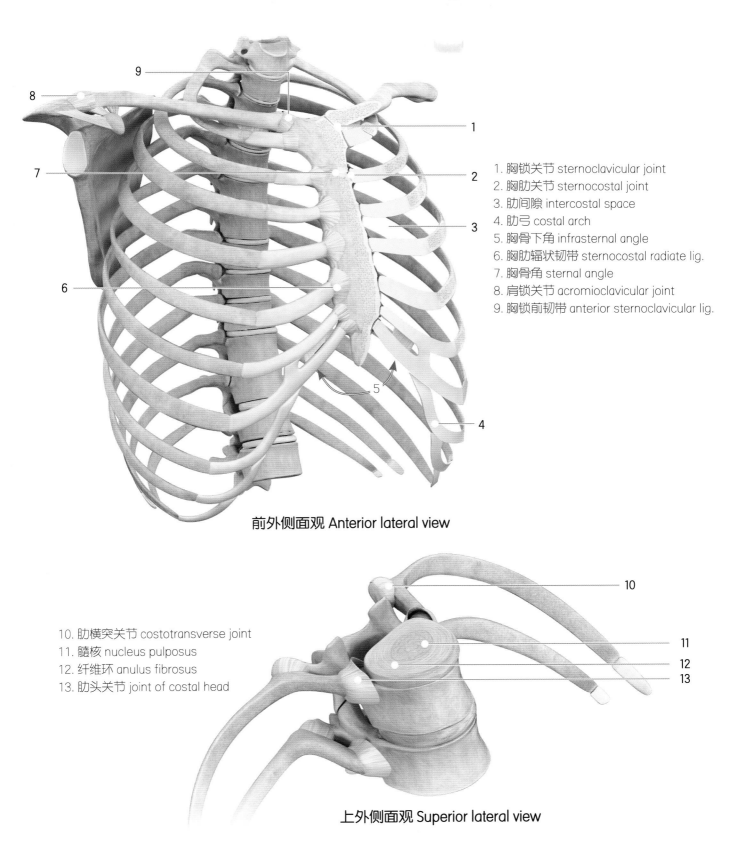

前外侧面观 Anterior lateral view

1. 胸锁关节 sternoclavicular joint
2. 胸肋关节 sternocostal joint
3. 肋间隙 intercostal space
4. 肋弓 costal arch
5. 胸骨下角 infrasternal angle
6. 胸肋辐状韧带 sternocostal radiate lig.
7. 胸骨角 sternal angle
8. 肩锁关节 acromioclavicular joint
9. 胸锁前韧带 anterior sternoclavicular lig.

10. 肋横突关节 costotransverse joint
11. 髓核 nucleus pulposus
12. 纤维环 anulus fibrosus
13. 肋头关节 joint of costal head

上外侧面观 Superior lateral view

图 2-5　胸廓
Thorax

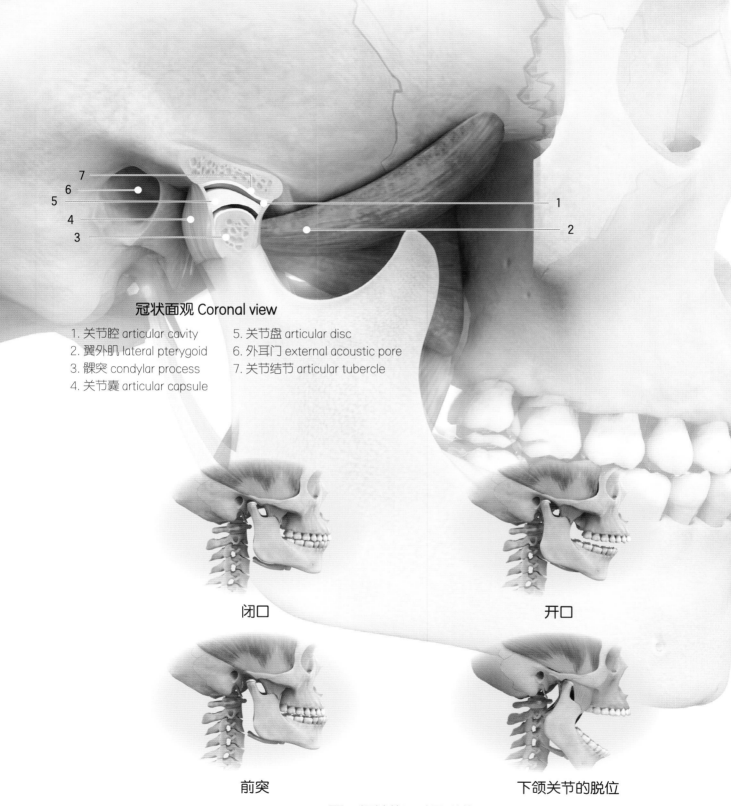

冠状面观 Coronal view

1. 关节腔 articular cavity　　5. 关节盘 articular disc
2. 翼外肌 lateral pterygoid　　6. 外耳门 external acoustic pore
3. 髁突 condylar process　　　7. 关节结节 articular tubercle
4. 关节囊 articular capsule

闭口　　　　　　　　　　　开口

前突　　　　　　　　　　　下颌关节的脱位

颞下颌关节运动及脱位
Motion of temporomandibular joint and its dislocation

图 2-6　颞下颌关节及运动
Temporomandibular joint and its motion

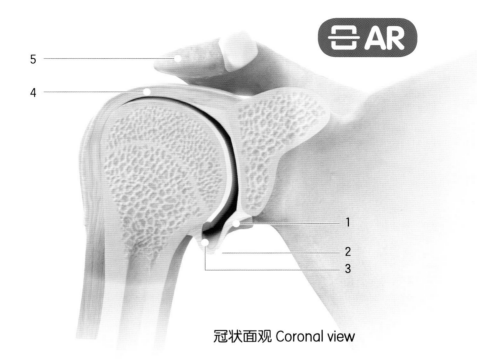

冠状面观 Coronal view

1. 盂唇 glenoid labrum
2. 关节囊 articular capsule
3. 关节腔 articular cavity
4. 肱二头肌长头腱 tendon of long head of biceps brachii
5. 肩峰 acromion
6. 锥状韧带 conoid lig.
7. 斜方韧带 trapezoid lig.
8. 喙突 coracoid process
9. 关节盂 glenoid cavity
10. 喙肩韧带 coracoacromial lig.
11. 肩锁韧带 acromioclavicular lig.

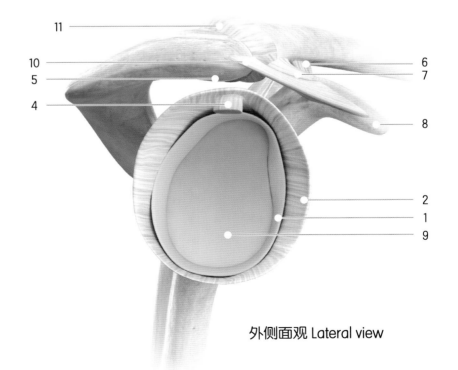

外侧面观 Lateral view

图 2-7　肩关节
Shoulder joint

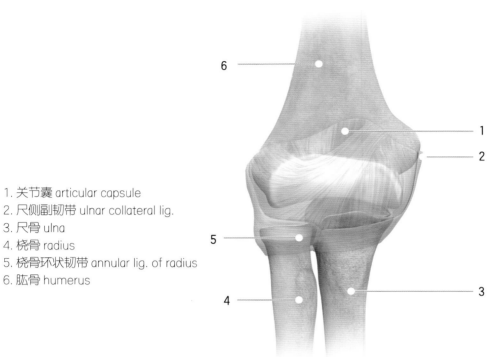

1. 关节囊 articular capsule
2. 尺侧副韧带 ulnar collateral lig.
3. 尺骨 ulna
4. 桡骨 radius
5. 桡骨环状韧带 annular lig. of radius
6. 肱骨 humerus

前面观 Anterior view

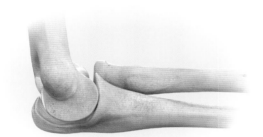

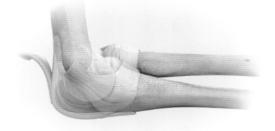

内面观 Internal view

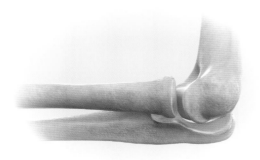

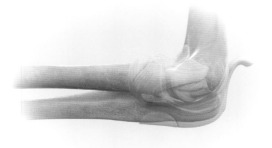

外侧面观 Lateral view

图 2-8   肘关节
Elbow joint

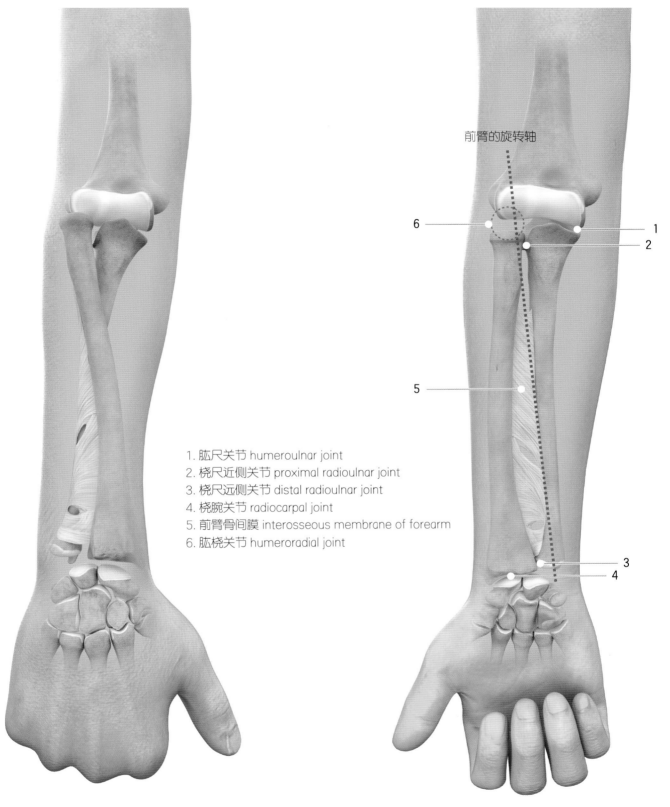

前臂的旋转轴

6
1
2
5
3
4

1. 肱尺关节 humeroulnar joint
2. 桡尺近侧关节 proximal radioulnar joint
3. 桡尺远侧关节 distal radioulnar joint
4. 桡腕关节 radiocarpal joint
5. 前臂骨间膜 interosseous membrane of forearm
6. 肱桡关节 humeroradial joint

前臂旋前 Pronation of forearm   前臂旋后 Supination of forearm

图 2-9 前臂骨的连结及运动
Joints and movements of the forearm

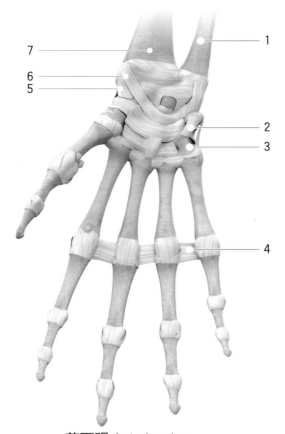

前面观 Anterior view

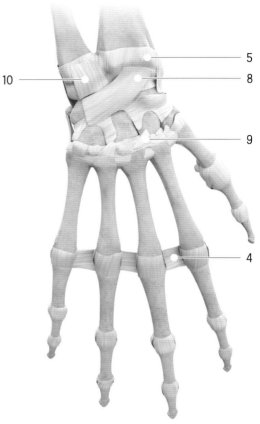

后面观 Posterior view

1. 尺骨 ulna
2. 豆掌韧带 pisometacarpal lig.
3. 掌骨骨间韧带 interosseous metacarpal lig.
4. 掌骨深横韧带 deep transverse metacarpal lig.
5. 腕桡侧副韧带 radial carpal collateral lig.

6. 桡腕掌侧韧带 palmar radiocarpal lig.
7. 桡骨 radius
8. 桡腕背侧韧带 dorsal radiocarpal lig.
9. 腕掌背侧韧带 dorsal carpometacarpal lig.
10. 腕尺侧副韧带 ulnar carpal collateral lig.

图 2-10　手的连结
Joints of the hand

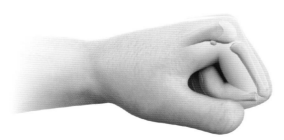

掌指关节和指间关节屈曲
Flexion of metacarpophalangeal
and interphalangeal joints

掌指关节伸展和指间关节屈曲
Extension of metacarpophalangeal joint
and flexion of interphalangeal joint

图 2-11　手指的运动 1
Motion of the fingers 1

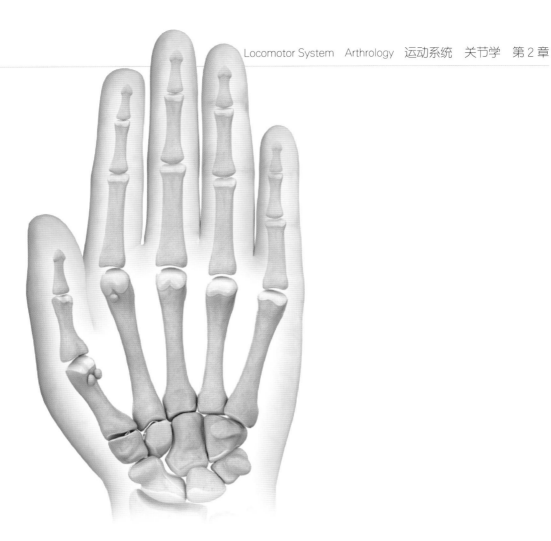

未运动状态 Steady state

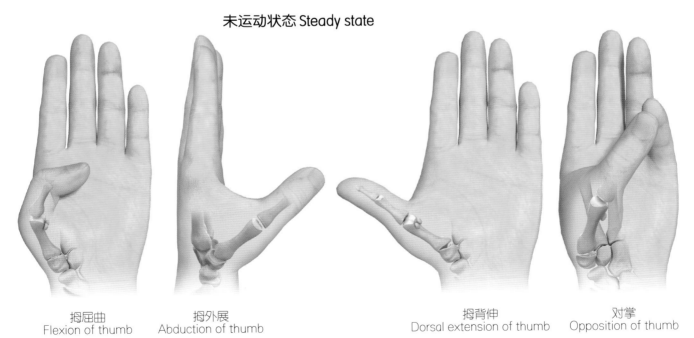

拇屈曲
Flexion of thumb

拇外展
Abduction of thumb

拇背伸
Dorsal extension of thumb

对掌
Opposition of thumb

拇指的运动 Motion of thumb

图 2-12　手指的运动 2
Motion of the fingers 2

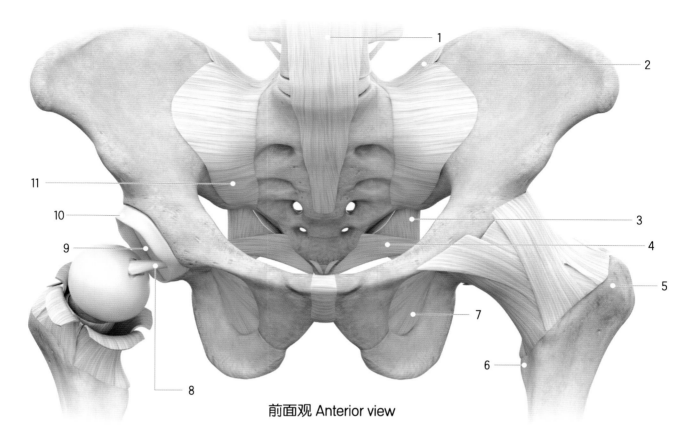

前面观 Anterior view

1. 前纵韧带 anterior longitudinal lig.
2. 髂腰韧带 iliolumbar lig.
3. 骶结节韧带 sacrotuberous lig.
4. 骶棘韧带 sacrospinous lig.
5. 股骨大转子 greater trochanter of femur
6. 股骨小转子 lesser trochanter of femur
7. 闭孔膜 obturator membrane
8. 股骨头韧带 ligament of head of femur
9. 髋臼 acetabulum
10. 髋臼唇 acetabular labrum
11. 髂骶腹侧韧带 sacroiliac ventral lig.

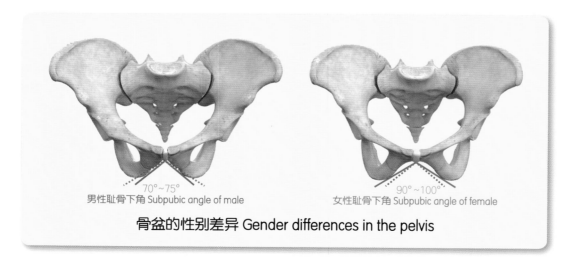

男性耻骨下角 Subpubic angle of male   70°~75°

女性耻骨下角 Subpubic angle of female   90°~100°

骨盆的性别差异 Gender differences in the pelvis

图 2-13   骨盆 1
Pelvis 1

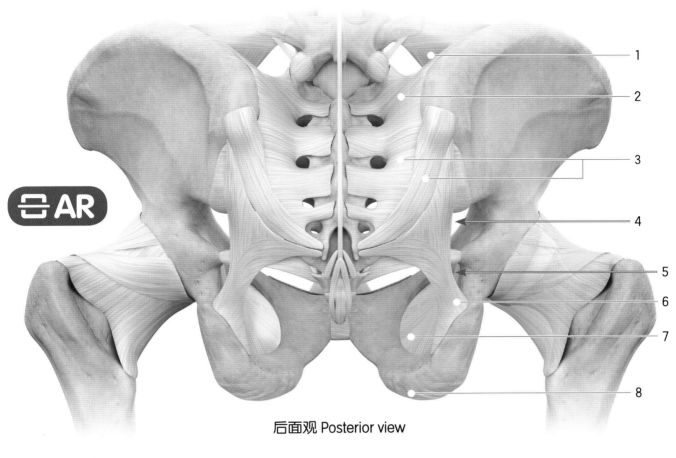

后面观 Posterior view

1. 髂腰韧带 iliolumbar lig.
2. 骶髂骨间韧带 interosseous sacroiliac lig.
3. 骶髂背侧韧带 dorsal sacroiliac lig.
4. 坐骨大孔 greater sciatic foramen
5. 坐骨小孔 lesser sciatic foramen
6. 骶结节韧带 sacrotuberous lig.
7. 闭孔膜 obturator membrane
8. 坐骨结节 ischial tuberosity

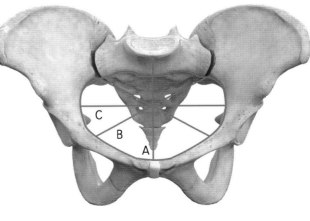

骨盆径线 Pelvic diameter

A. 真结合径（前后径）true conjugate
B. 斜径 oblique diameter
C. 横径 transverse diameter

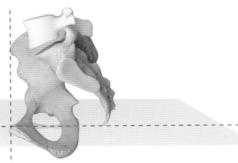

骨盆的解剖学位置 Anatomical position of the pelvis

图 2-14　骨盆 2
Pelvis 2

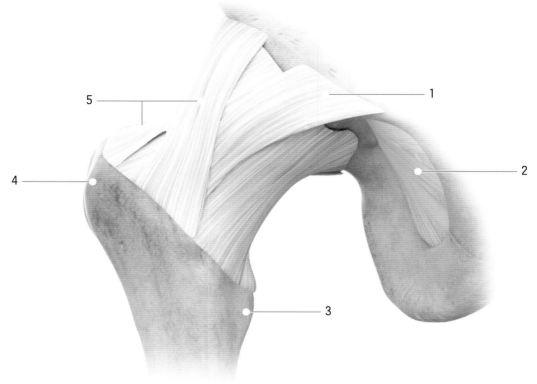

前面观 Anterior view

1. 耻股韧带 pubofemoral lig.
2. 闭孔膜 obturator membrane
3. 股骨小转子 lesser trochanter of femur
4. 股骨大转子 greater trochanter of femur
5. 髂股韧带 iliofemoral lig.
6. 髋臼唇 acetabular labrum
7. 股骨头韧带 ligament of head of femur
8. 股骨颈 neck of femur
9. 髂股韧带 iliofemoral lig.
10. 股骨头 femoral head
11. 月状面 lunate surface

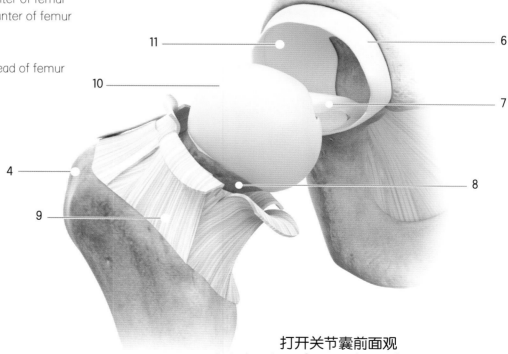

打开关节囊前面观
Anterior view of opened articular capsure

图 2-15　髋关节 1
Hip joint 1

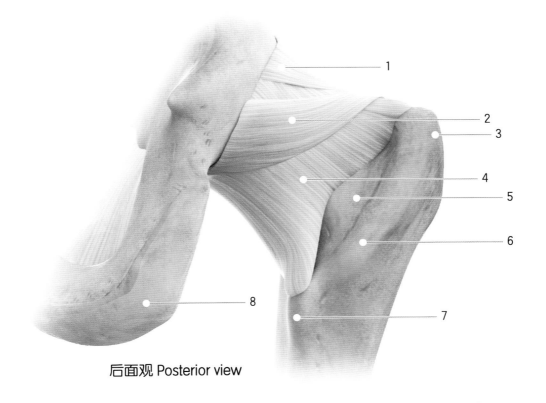

后面观 Posterior view

1. 髂股韧带 iliofemoral lig.
2. 坐股韧带 ischiofemoral lig.
3. 股骨大转子 greater trochanter of femur
4. 坐股关节囊 ischiofemoral articular capsule
5. 股骨颈 neck of femur
6. 转子间嵴 intertrochanteric crest
7. 股骨小转子 lesser trochanter of femur
8. 坐骨结节 ischial tuberosity
9. 轮匝带 zona orbicularis

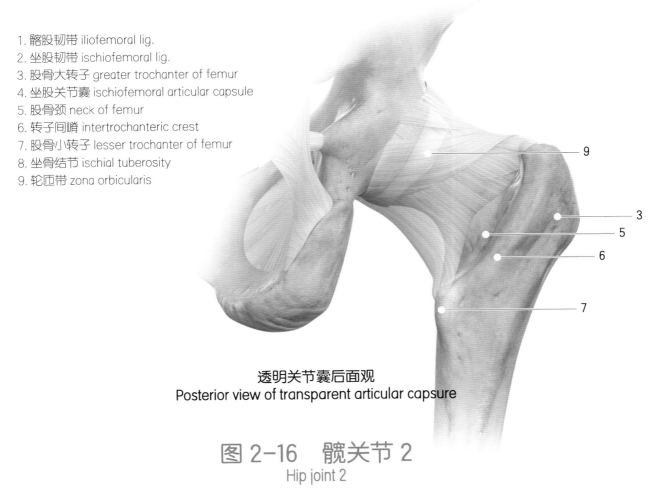

透明关节囊后面观
Posterior view of transparent articular capsure

图 2-16　髋关节 2
Hip joint 2

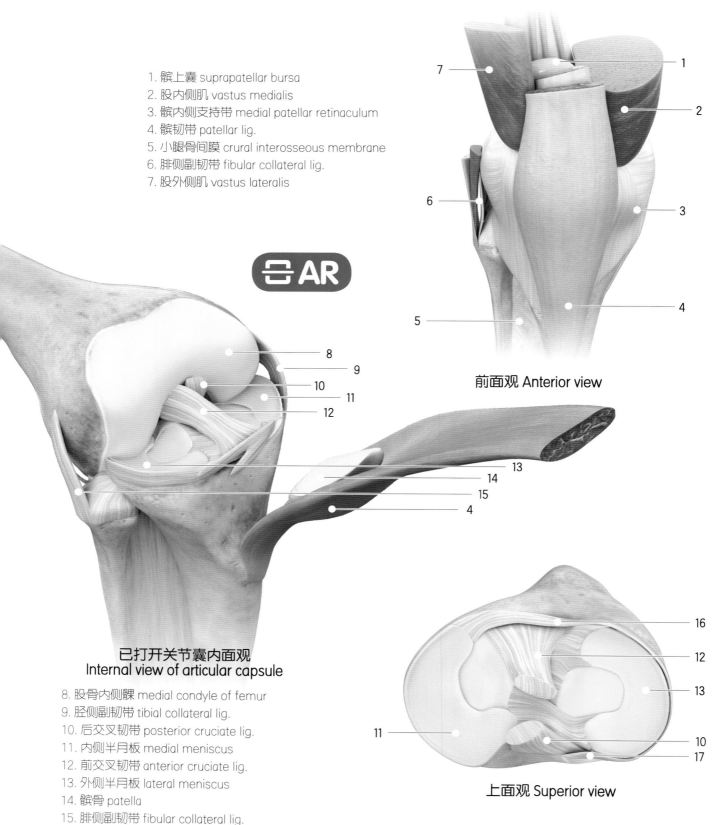

1. 髌上囊 suprapatellar bursa
2. 股内侧肌 vastus medialis
3. 髌内侧支持带 medial patellar retinaculum
4. 髌韧带 patellar lig.
5. 小腿骨间膜 crural interosseous membrane
6. 腓侧副韧带 fibular collateral lig.
7. 股外侧肌 vastus lateralis

前面观 Anterior view

已打开关节囊内面观
Internal view of articular capsule

8. 股骨内侧髁 medial condyle of femur
9. 胫侧副韧带 tibial collateral lig.
10. 后交叉韧带 posterior cruciate lig.
11. 内侧半月板 medial meniscus
12. 前交叉韧带 anterior cruciate lig.
13. 外侧半月板 lateral meniscus
14. 髌骨 patella
15. 腓侧副韧带 fibular collateral lig.
16. 膝横韧带 transverse lig. of the knee
17. 板股后韧带 posterior meniscofemoral lig.

上面观 Superior view

图 2-17 膝关节
Knee joint

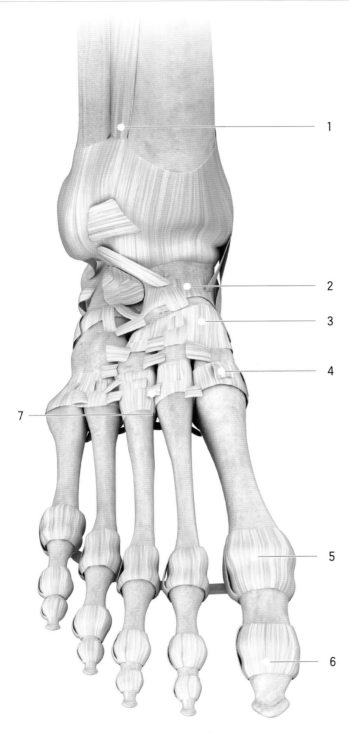

上面观 Superior view

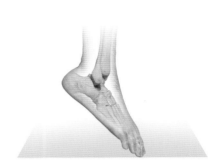

跖屈 plantar flexion

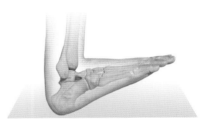

背屈 dorsiflexion

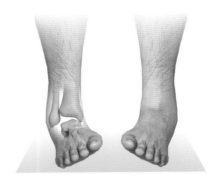

内翻 inversion

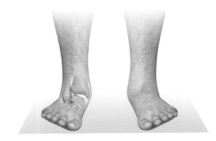

外翻 ectropium

足的运动 Motion of the foot

1. 胫腓韧带 tibiofibular lig.
2. 距舟关节 talonavicular joint
3. 楔舟关节 cuneonavicular joint
4. 跗跖关节 tarsometatarsal joint
5. 跖趾关节 metatarsophalangeal joint
6. 趾骨间关节 interphalangeal joint
7. 跖骨间关节 intermetatarsal joint

图 2-18 足关节及运动
Foot joints and their motion

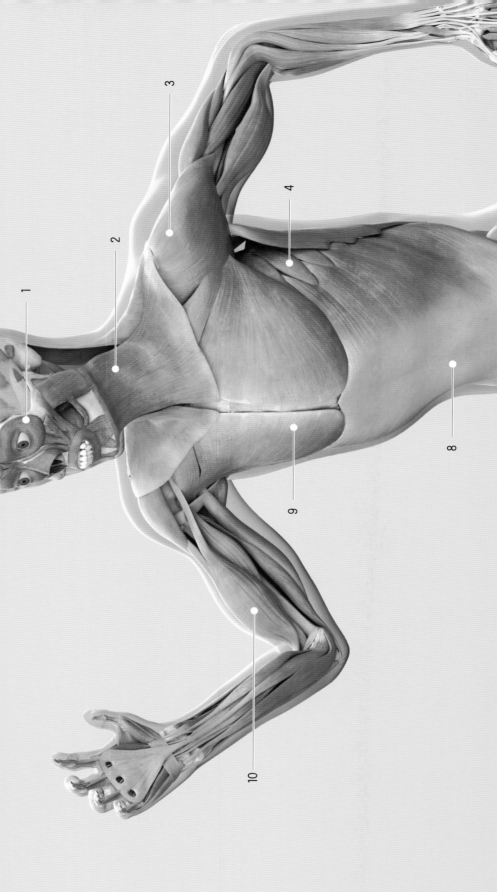

第3章 运动系统 Locomotor System

肌学 Myology

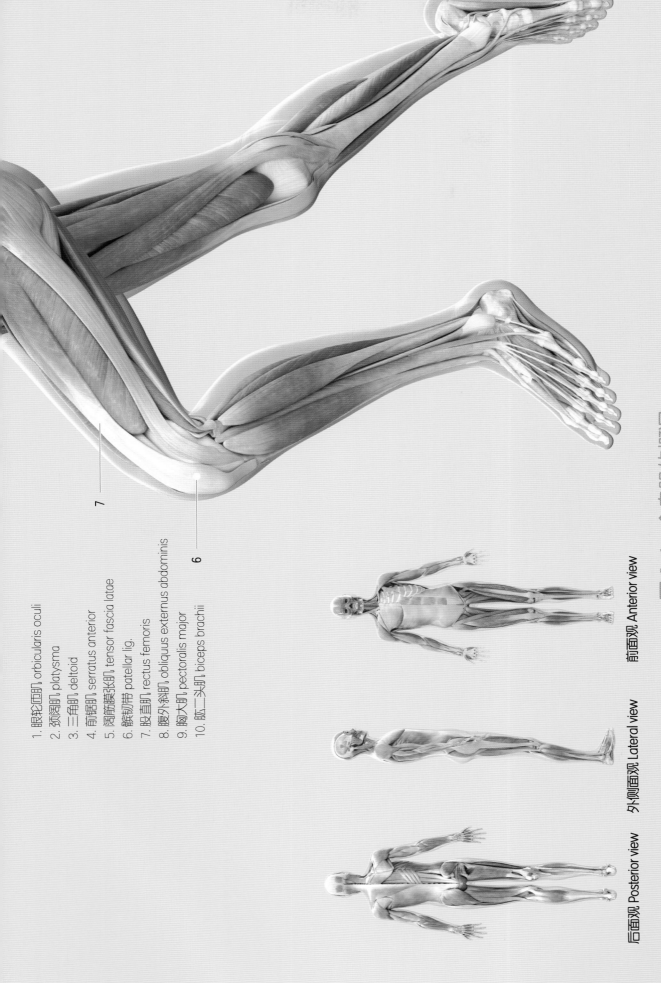

1. 眼轮匝肌 orbicularis oculi
2. 颈阔肌 platysma
3. 三角肌 deltoid
4. 前锯肌 serratus anterior
5. 阔筋膜张肌 tensor fascia latae
6. 髌韧带 patellar lig.
7. 股直肌 rectus femoris
8. 腹外斜肌 obliquus externus abdominis
9. 胸大肌 pectoralis major
10. 肱二头肌 biceps brachii

后面观 Posterior view   外侧面观 Lateral view   前面观 Anterior view

图 3-1　全身肌的概况
Overview of the muscular system

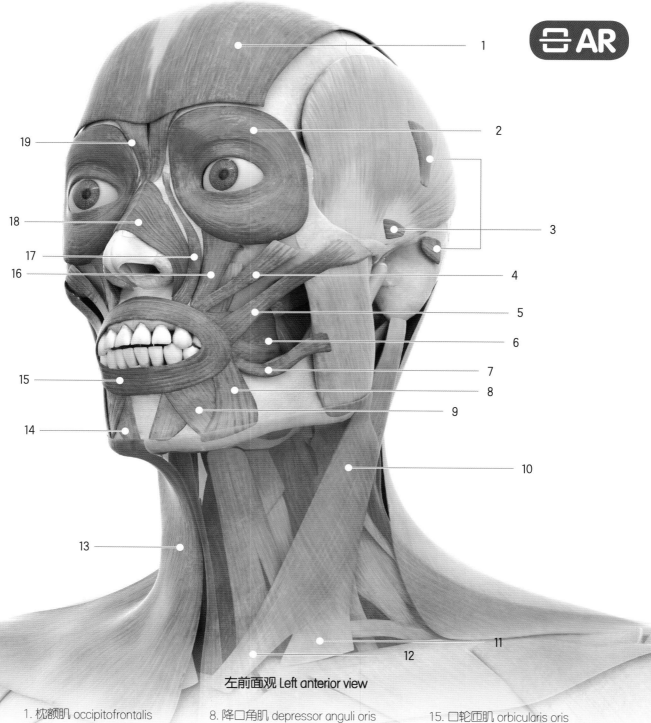

左前面观 Left anterior view

1. 枕额肌 occipitofrontalis
2. 眼轮匝肌 orbicularis oculi
3. 耳肌 auricularis muscle
4. 颧小肌 zygomaticus minor
5. 颧大肌 zygomaticus major
6. 颊肌 buccinator
7. 笑肌 risorius

8. 降口角肌 depressor anguli oris
9. 降下唇肌 depressor labii inferioris
10. 胸锁乳突肌 sternocleidomastoid
11. 锁骨端 clavicle end
12. 胸骨端 sternal end
13. 颈阔肌 platysma
14. 颏肌 mentalis

15. 口轮匝肌 orbicularis oris
16. 提上唇肌外侧部 lateral part of levator labii superioris
17. 提上唇肌内侧部 medial part of levator labii superioris
18. 鼻肌 nasalis
19. 降眉间肌 procerus

图 3-2 面肌
Facial muscles

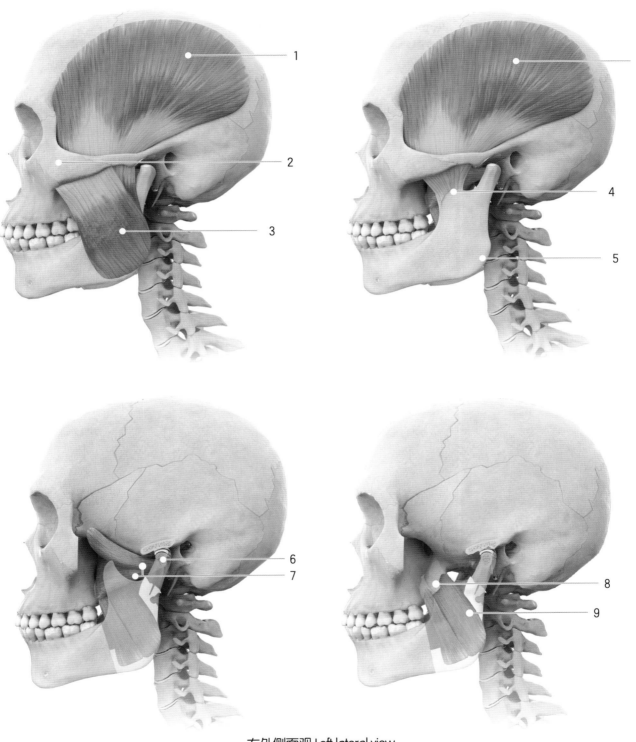

左外侧面观 Left lateral view

1. 颞肌 temporalis
2. 颧弓 zygomatic arch
3. 咬肌 masseter
4. 下颌骨冠突 coronoid process of the mandible
5. 下颌角 angle of mandible
6. 下颌头 head of mandible
7. 翼外肌 lateral pterygoid
8. 翼突外侧板 lateral pterygoid plate
9. 翼内肌 medial pterygoid

图 3-3　咀嚼肌
Masticatory muscles

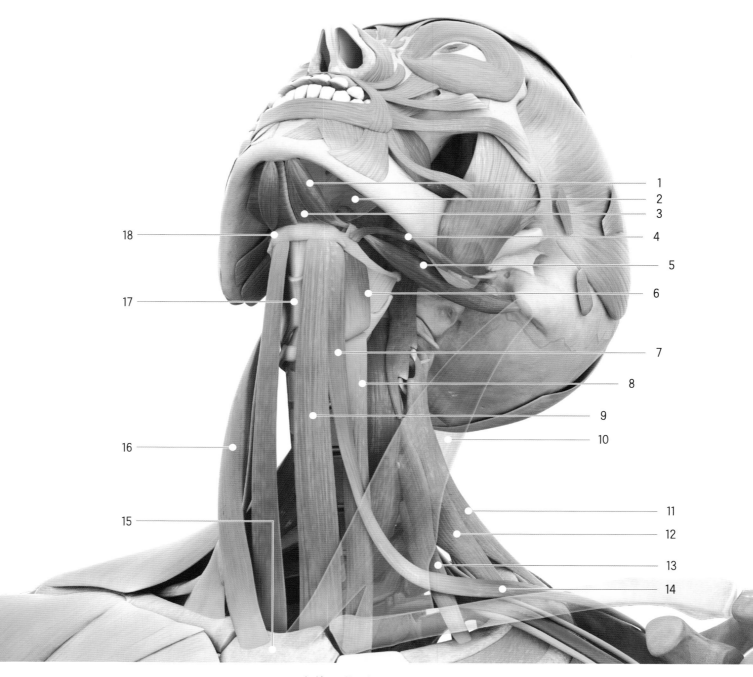

1
2
3
4
5
6
7
8
9
10
11
12
13
14
15
16
17
18

左前面观 Left anterior view

1. 二腹肌前腹 anterior belly of digastric
2. 下颌舌骨肌 mylohyoid
3. 颏舌骨肌 geniohyoid
4. 茎突舌骨肌 stylohyoid
5. 二腹肌后腹 posterior belly of digastric
6. 甲状舌骨肌 thyrohyoid

7. 肩胛舌骨肌上腹 superior belly of omohyoid
8. 胸骨甲状肌 sternothyroid
9. 胸骨舌骨肌 sternohyoid
10. 胸锁乳突肌 sternocleidomastoid
11. 后斜角肌 scalenus posterior
12. 中斜角肌 scalenus medius

13. 前斜角肌 scalenus anterior
14. 肩胛舌骨肌下腹 inferior belly of omohyoid
15. 胸骨柄 manubrium sterni
16. 胸锁乳突肌 sternocleidomastoid
17. 甲状软骨 thyroid cartilage
18. 舌骨 hyoid bone

图 3-4 颈肌
Neck muscles

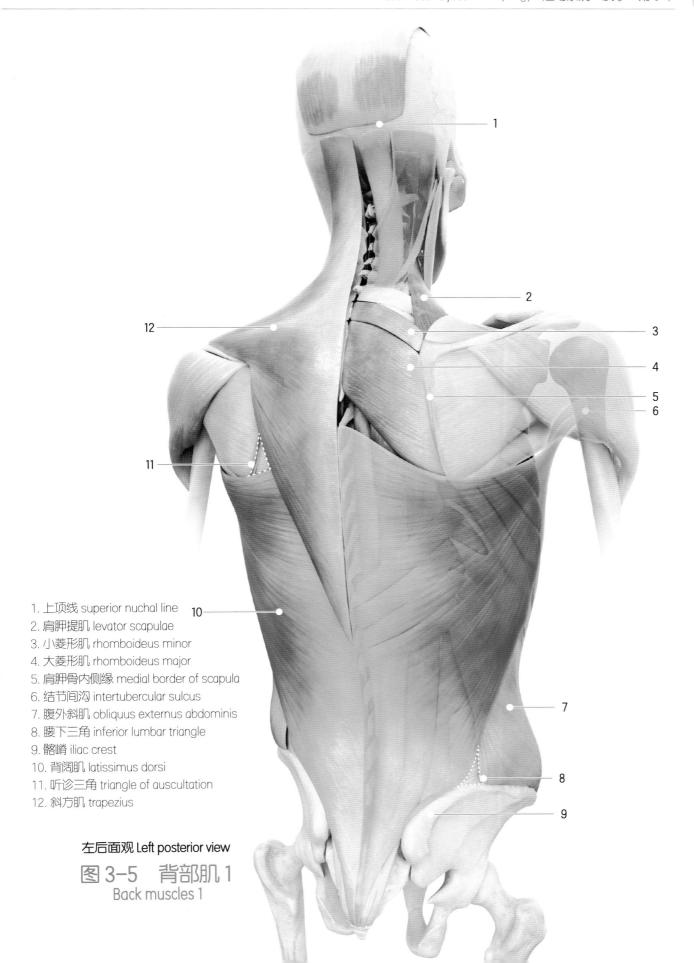

1. 上项线 superior nuchal line
2. 肩胛提肌 levator scapulae
3. 小菱形肌 rhomboideus minor
4. 大菱形肌 rhomboideus major
5. 肩胛骨内侧缘 medial border of scapula
6. 结节间沟 intertubercular sulcus
7. 腹外斜肌 obliquus externus abdominis
8. 腰下三角 inferior lumbar triangle
9. 髂嵴 iliac crest
10. 背阔肌 latissimus dorsi
11. 听诊三角 triangle of auscultation
12. 斜方肌 trapezius

左后面观 Left posterior view

图 3-5　背部肌 1
Back muscles 1

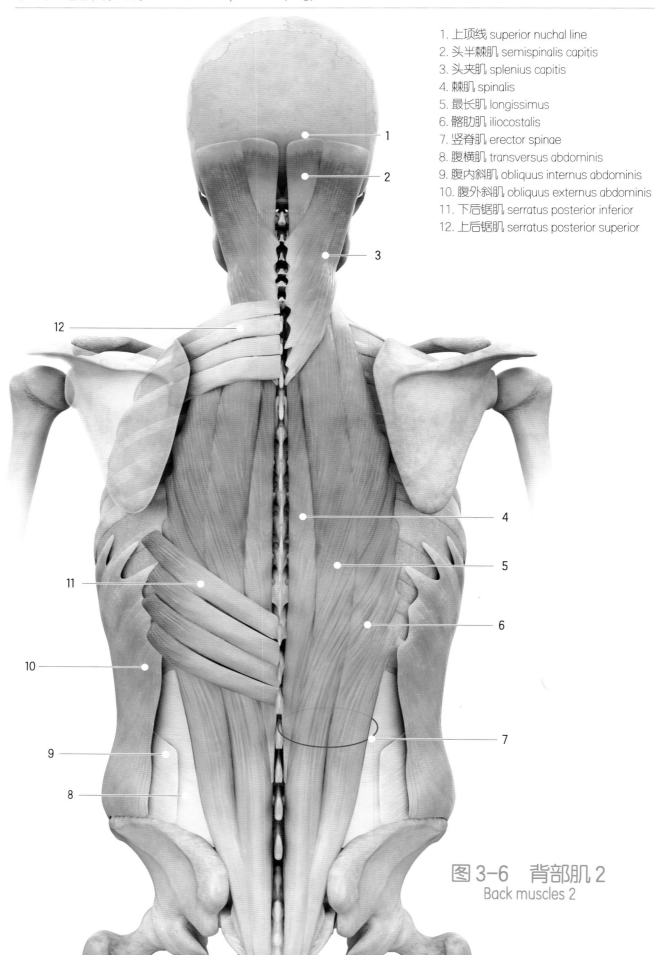

1. 上项线 superior nuchal line
2. 头半棘肌 semispinalis capitis
3. 头夹肌 splenius capitis
4. 棘肌 spinalis
5. 最长肌 longissimus
6. 髂肋肌 iliocostalis
7. 竖脊肌 erector spinae
8. 腹横肌 transversus abdominis
9. 腹内斜肌 obliquus internus abdominis
10. 腹外斜肌 obliquus externus abdominis
11. 下后锯肌 serratus posterior inferior
12. 上后锯肌 serratus posterior superior

图 3-6 背部肌 2
Back muscles 2

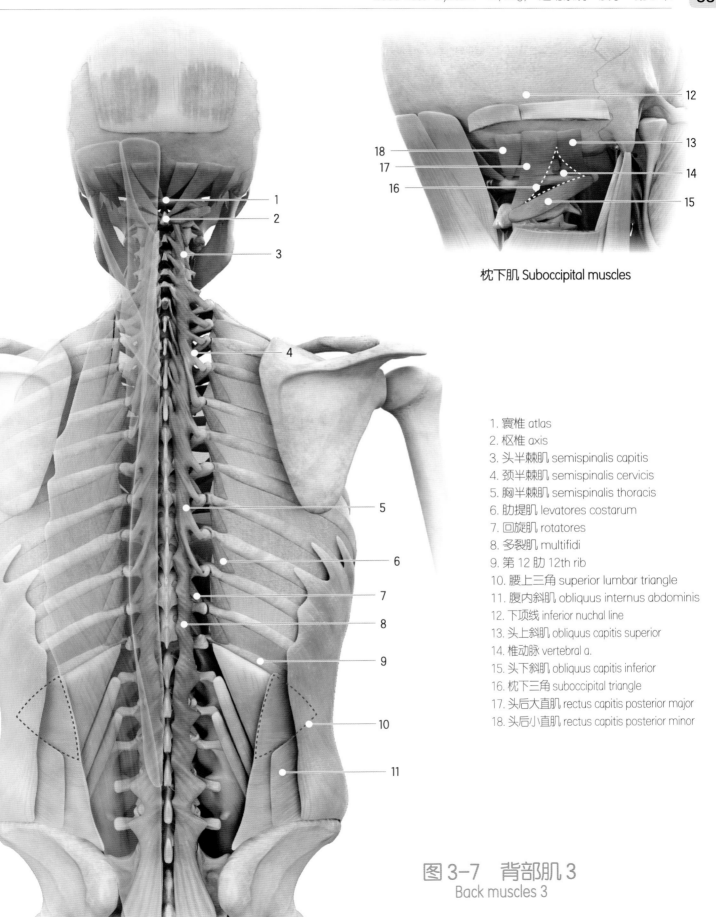

枕下肌 Suboccipital muscles

1. 寰椎 atlas
2. 枢椎 axis
3. 头半棘肌 semispinalis capitis
4. 颈半棘肌 semispinalis cervicis
5. 胸半棘肌 semispinalis thoracis
6. 肋提肌 levatores costarum
7. 回旋肌 rotatores
8. 多裂肌 multifidi
9. 第 12 肋 12th rib
10. 腰上三角 superior lumbar triangle
11. 腹内斜肌 obliquus internus abdominis
12. 下项线 inferior nuchal line
13. 头上斜肌 obliquus capitis superior
14. 椎动脉 vertebral a.
15. 头下斜肌 obliquus capitis inferior
16. 枕下三角 suboccipital triangle
17. 头后大直肌 rectus capitis posterior major
18. 头后小直肌 rectus capitis posterior minor

图 3-7　背部肌 3
Back muscles 3

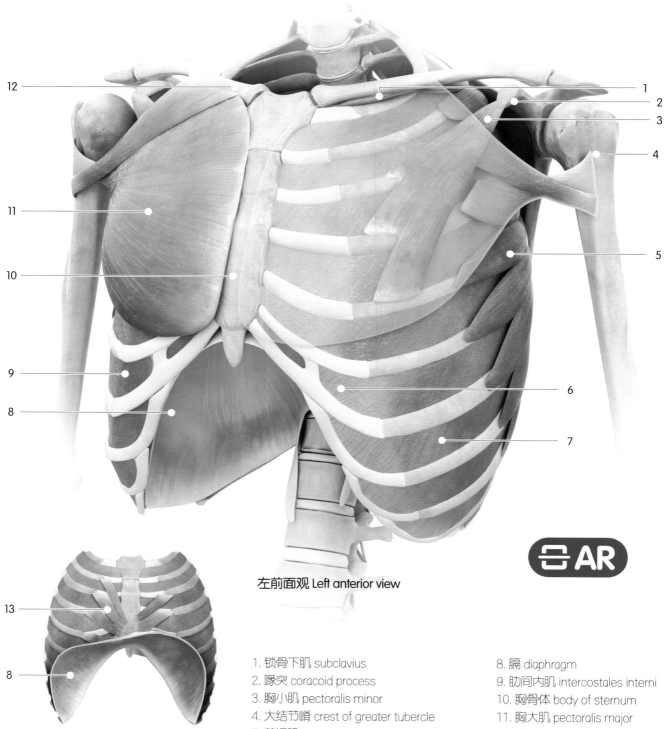

左前面观 Left anterior view

内侧面观 Medial view

1. 锁骨下肌 subclavius
2. 喙突 coracoid process
3. 胸小肌 pectoralis minor
4. 大结节嵴 crest of greater tubercle
5. 前锯肌 serratus anterior
6. 肋间外膜 external intercostal membrane
7. 肋间外肌 intercostales externi
8. 膈 diaphragm
9. 肋间内肌 intercostales interni
10. 胸骨体 body of sternum
11. 胸大肌 pectoralis major
12. 锁骨 clavicle
13. 胸横肌 transversus thoracis

图 3-8　胸部肌 1
Thoracic muscles 1

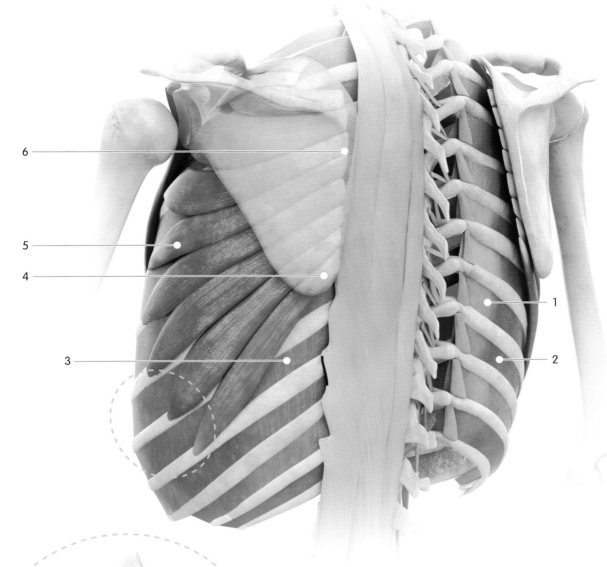

左后面观 Left posterior view

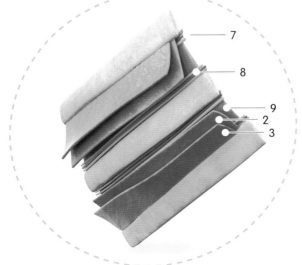

肋间肌的层次 Intercostal muscle layer

1. 肋间内膜 internal intercostal membrane
2. 肋间内肌 intercostales interni
3. 肋间外肌 intercostales externi
4. 肩胛下角 inferior angle of scapula
5. 前锯肌 serratus anterior
6. 肩胛骨内侧缘 medial border of scapula
7. 肋间后动、静脉和肋间神经上支
   posterior intercostal vessels and superior branch of intercostal nerve
8. 肋间后动、静脉和肋间神经上支
   posterior intercostal vessels and inferior branch of intercostal nerve
9. 肋间最内肌 intercostales intimi

图 3-9　胸部肌 2
Thoracic muscles 2

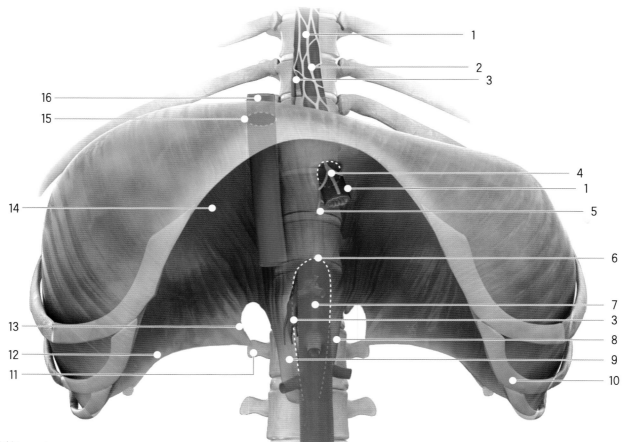

前面观 Anterior view

1. 食管 esophagus
2. 迷走神经食管丛 esophageal plexus of vagus nerve
3. 胸导管 thoracic duct
4. 迷走神经前干 anterior vagal trunk
5. 迷走神经后干 posterior vagal trunk
6. 主动脉裂孔 aortic hiatus
7. 腹主动脉 abdominal aorta
8. 左膈脚 left crus of diaphragm
9. 右膈脚 right crus of diaphragm
10. 肋弓 costal arch
11. 第 1 腰椎横突 transverse process of 1st lumbar vertebrae
12. 外侧弓状韧带 lateral arcuate lig.
13. 内侧弓状韧带 medial arcuate lig.
14. 中心腱 central tendon of diaphragm
15. 腔静脉孔 vena caval foramen
16. 下腔静脉 inferior vena cava
17. 肋间内肌 intercostales interni
18. 腹外斜肌 obliquus externus abdominis
19. 腹直肌 rectus abdominis
20. 腹横肌 transversus abdominis
21. 腹内斜肌 obliquus internus abdominis
22. 肋间外肌 intercostales externi
23. 前斜角肌 scalenus anterior
24. 胸锁乳突肌 sternocleidomastoid

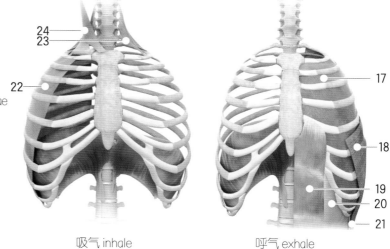

吸气 inhale　　呼气 exhale

膈肌的运动 Movement of diaphragm during respiration

图 3-10 膈
Diaphragm

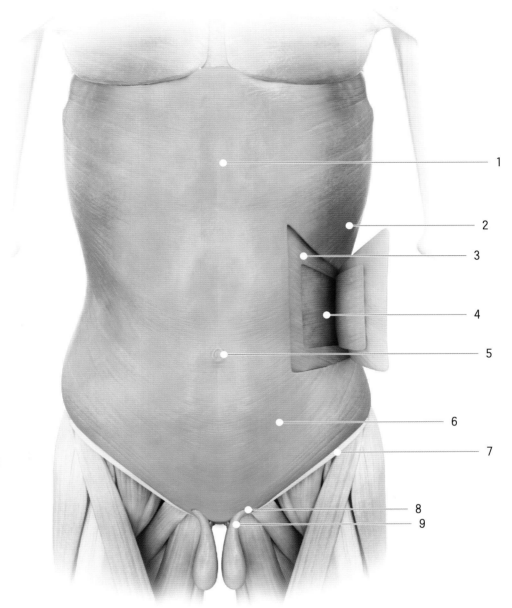

前面观 Anterior view

1. 白线 linea alba
2. 腹外斜肌 obliquus externus abdominis
3. 腹内斜肌 obliquus internus abdominis
4. 腹横肌 transversus abdominis
5. 脐 umbilicus
6. 腹外斜肌腱膜 external oblique aponeurosis
7. 腹股沟韧带 inguinal lig.
8. 腹股沟管浅环 superficial inguinal ring
9. 精索外筋膜 external spermatic fascia
10. 腔隙韧带 lacunar lig.
11. 耻骨梳韧带 pectineal lig.
12. 髂前上棘 anterior superior iliac spine

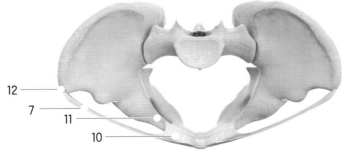

腹外斜肌腱膜形成的结构
Structures formed by external oblique aponeurosis

图 3-11　腹前外侧肌 1
Anterolateral abdominal muscles 1

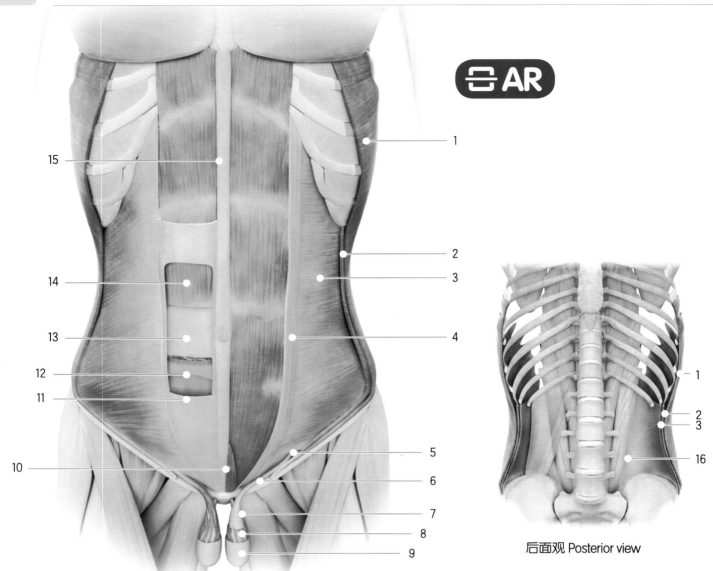

前面观 Anterior view

后面观 Posterior view

图 3-12 腹前外侧肌 2
Anterolateral abdominal muscles 2

1. 腹外斜肌 obliquus externus abdominis
2. 腹内斜肌 obliquus internus abdominis
3. 腹横肌 transversus abdominis
4. 半月线 semilunar line
5. 腹股沟管深环 deep inguinal ring
6. 精索 spermatic cord
7. 精索内筋膜 internal spermatic fascia
8. 提睾肌 cremaster

9. 精索外筋膜 external spermatic fascia
10. 锥状肌 pyramidalis
11. 腹直肌鞘前层 anterior layer of sheath of rectus abdominis
12. 弓状线 arcuate line
13. 腹直肌鞘后层 posterior layer of sheath of rectus abdominis
14. 腹直肌 rectus abdominis
15. 白线 linea alba
16. 髂肋肌 iliocostalis

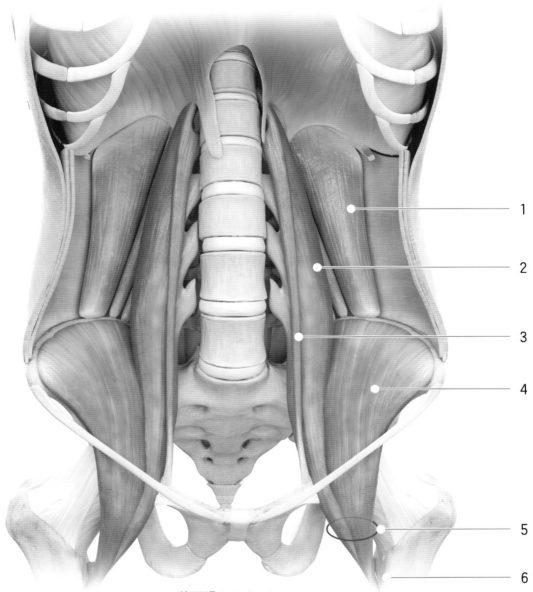

前面观 Anterior view

1. 腰方肌 quadratus lumborum
2. 腰大肌 psoas major
3. 腰小肌 psoas minor
4. 髂肌 iliacus
5. 髂腰肌 iliopsoas
6. 股骨小转子 lesser trochanter of femur
7. 第 1 腰椎 1st lumbar vertebrae
8. 胸腰筋膜前层 anterior layer of thoracolumbar fascia
9. 胸腰筋膜中层 middle layer of thoracolumbar fascia
10. 竖脊肌 erector spinae
11. 胸腰筋膜后层 posterior layer of thoracolumbar fascia

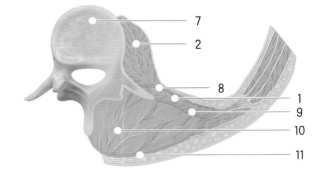

腹后壁肌横切面
Transverse section of abdominal posterior wall muscles

图 3-13　腹后壁的肌
Muscles of the posterior abdominal wall

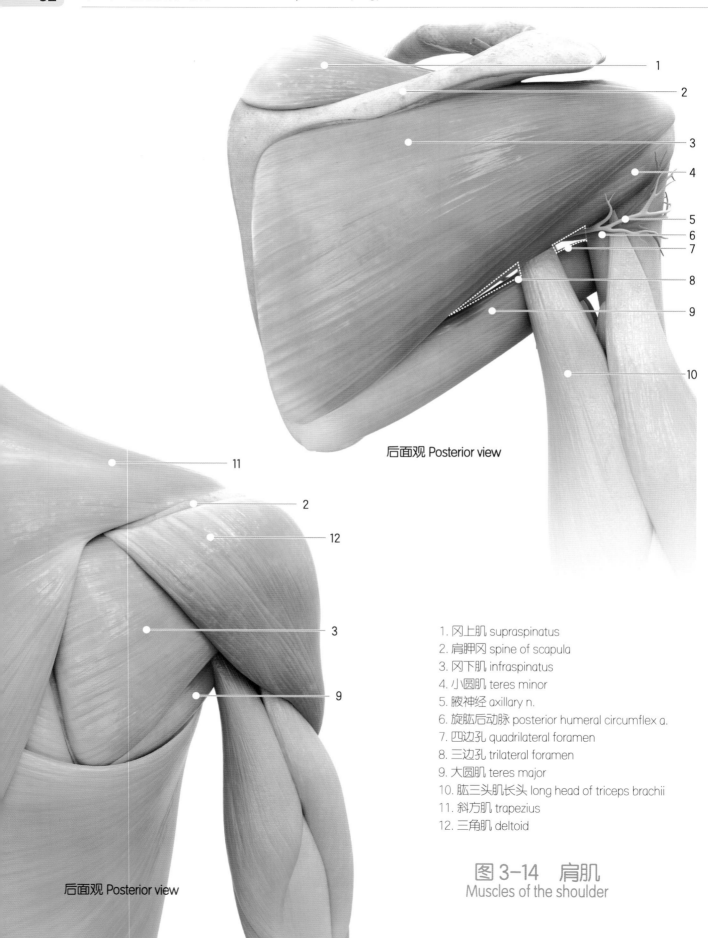

后面观 Posterior view

后面观 Posterior view

1. 冈上肌 supraspinatus
2. 肩胛冈 spine of scapula
3. 冈下肌 infraspinatus
4. 小圆肌 teres minor
5. 腋神经 axillary n.
6. 旋肱后动脉 posterior humeral circumflex a.
7. 四边孔 quadrilateral foramen
8. 三边孔 trilateral foramen
9. 大圆肌 teres major
10. 肱三头肌长头 long head of triceps brachii
11. 斜方肌 trapezius
12. 三角肌 deltoid

图 3-14   肩肌
Muscles of the shoulder

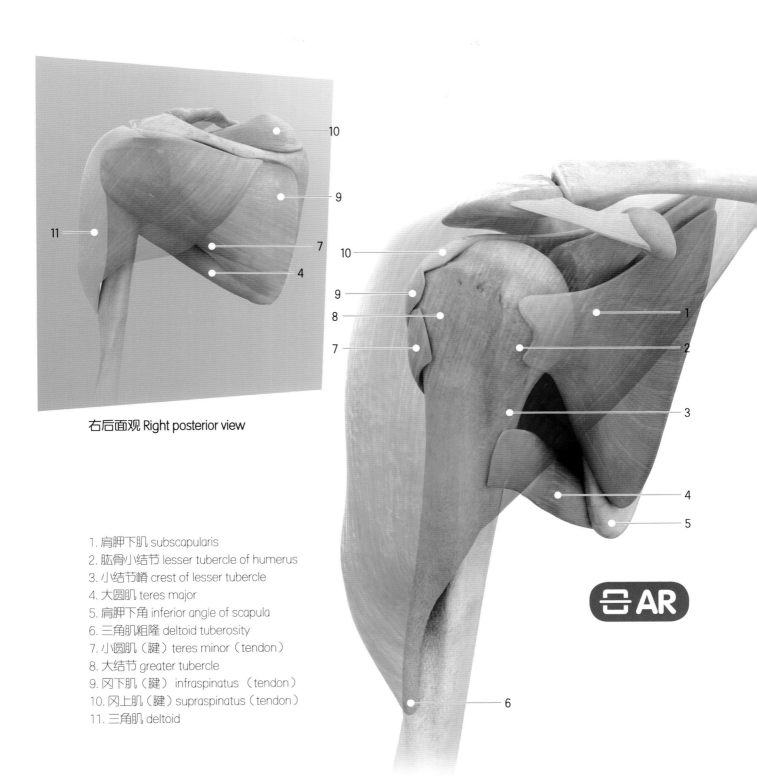

右后面观 Right posterior view

右外侧面观 Right lateral view

1. 肩胛下肌 subscapularis
2. 肱骨小结节 lesser tubercle of humerus
3. 小结节嵴 crest of lesser tubercle
4. 大圆肌 teres major
5. 肩胛下角 inferior angle of scapula
6. 三角肌粗隆 deltoid tuberosity
7. 小圆肌（腱）teres minor（tendon）
8. 大结节 greater tubercle
9. 冈下肌（腱）infraspinatus（tendon）
10. 冈上肌（腱）supraspinatus（tendon）
11. 三角肌 deltoid

图 3-15　肩袖肌
Rotator cuff muscles

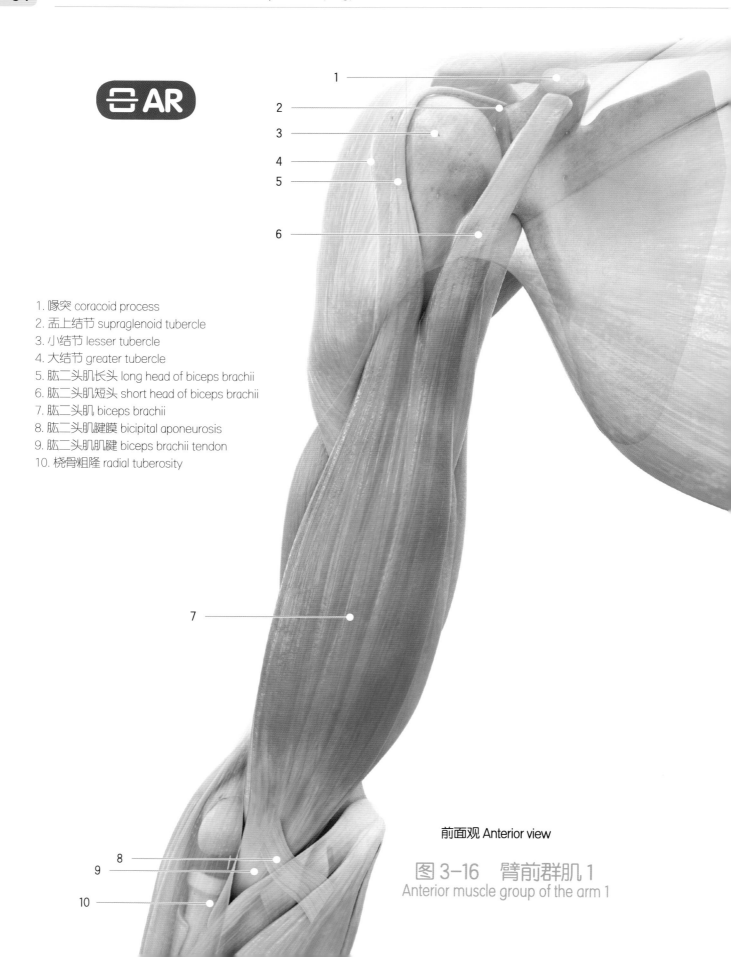

1. 喙突 coracoid process
2. 盂上结节 supraglenoid tubercle
3. 小结节 lesser tubercle
4. 大结节 greater tubercle
5. 肱二头肌长头 long head of biceps brachii
6. 肱二头肌短头 short head of biceps brachii
7. 肱二头肌 biceps brachii
8. 肱二头肌腱膜 bicipital aponeurosis
9. 肱二头肌肌腱 biceps brachii tendon
10. 桡骨粗隆 radial tuberosity

前面观 Anterior view

图 3-16　臂前群肌 1
Anterior muscle group of the arm 1

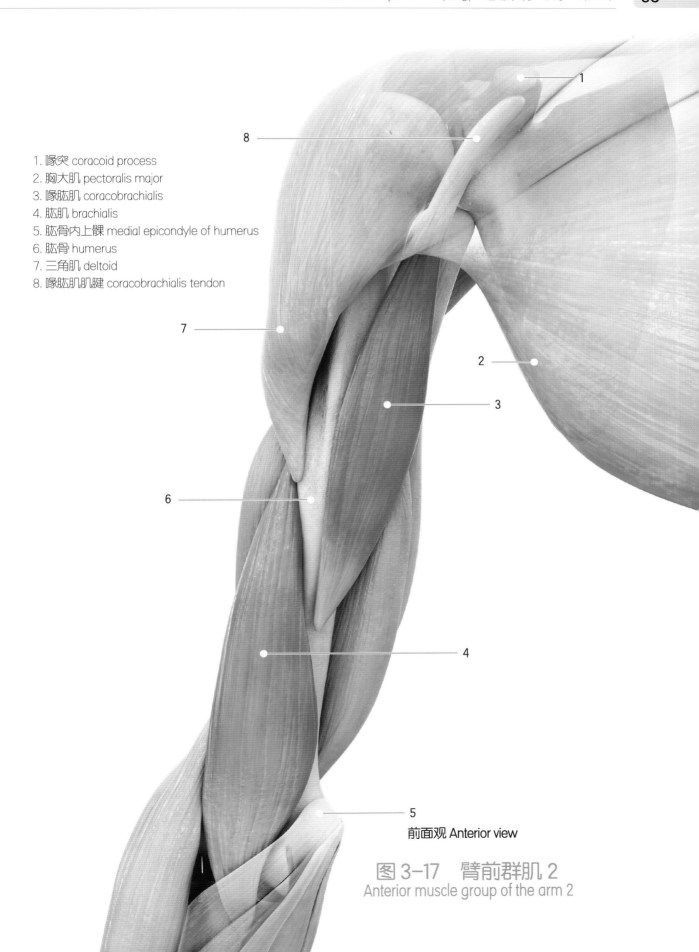

1. 喙突 coracoid process
2. 胸大肌 pectoralis major
3. 喙肱肌 coracobrachialis
4. 肱肌 brachialis
5. 肱骨内上髁 medial epicondyle of humerus
6. 肱骨 humerus
7. 三角肌 deltoid
8. 喙肱肌肌腱 coracobrachialis tendon

前面观 Anterior view

图 3-17　臂前群肌 2
Anterior muscle group of the arm 2

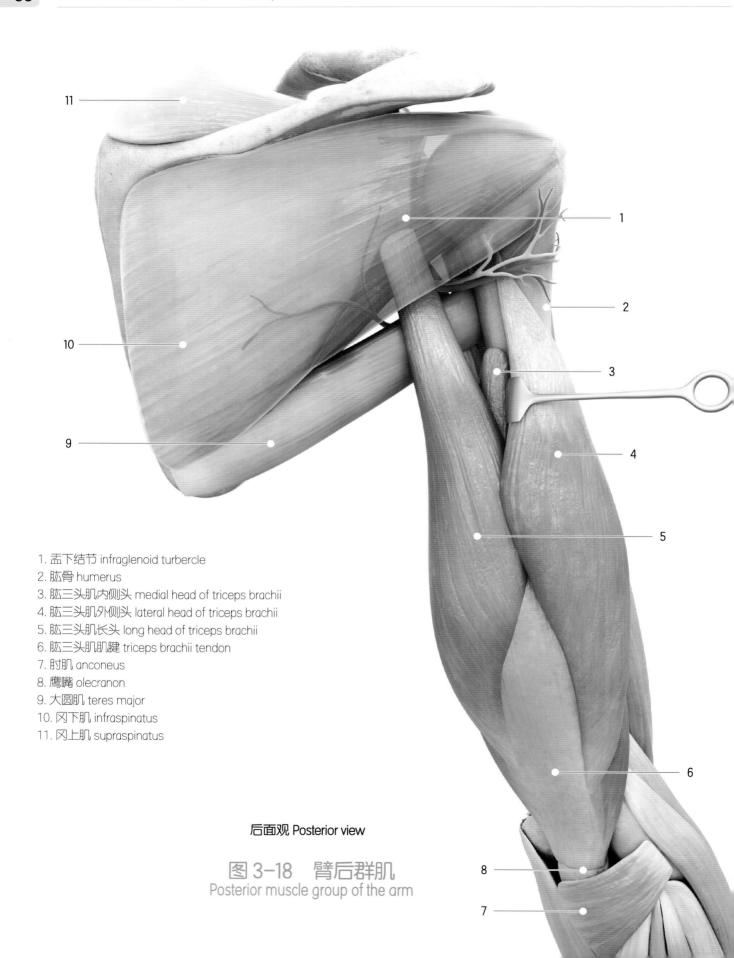

1. 盂下结节 infraglenoid turbercle
2. 肱骨 humerus
3. 肱三头肌内侧头 medial head of triceps brachii
4. 肱三头肌外侧头 lateral head of triceps brachii
5. 肱三头肌长头 long head of triceps brachii
6. 肱三头肌肌腱 triceps brachii tendon
7. 肘肌 anconeus
8. 鹰嘴 olecranon
9. 大圆肌 teres major
10. 冈下肌 infraspinatus
11. 冈上肌 supraspinatus

后面观 Posterior view

图 3-18 臂后群肌
Posterior muscle group of the arm

1. 肱骨内上髁 medial epicondyle of humerus
2. 肱二头肌腱膜 bicipital aponeurosis
3. 旋前圆肌 pronator teres
4. 桡侧腕屈肌 flexor carpi radialis
5. 掌长肌 palmaris longus
6. 尺侧腕屈肌 flexor carpi ulnaris
7. 豌豆骨 pisiform bone
8. 第 5 掌骨 5th metacarpal bone
9. 掌腱膜 palmar aponeurosis
10. 第 1 掌骨 1st metacarpal bone
11. 桡骨茎突 styloid process of radius
12. 肱桡肌 brachioradialis
13. 肱二头肌 biceps brachii
14. 指浅屈肌 flexor digitorum superficialis
15. 指浅屈肌腱 flexor digitorum superficialis tendon
16. 拇长屈肌 flexor pollicis longus

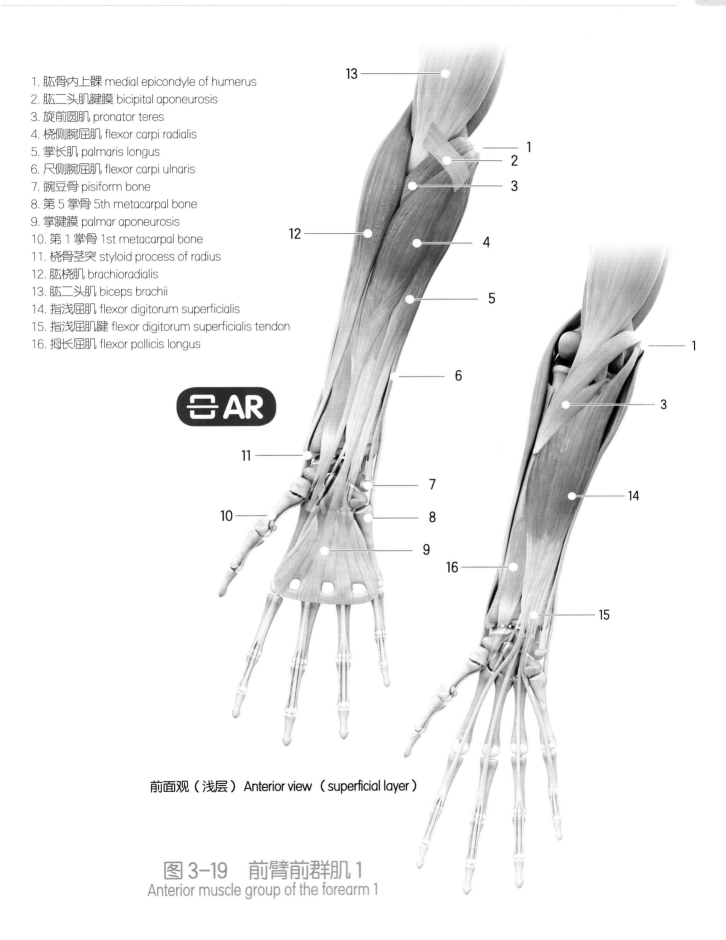

前面观（浅层）Anterior view（superficial layer）

图 3-19　前臂前群肌 1
Anterior muscle group of the forearm 1

1. 肱骨内上髁 medial epicondyle of humerus
2. 尺骨 ulna
3. 桡骨 radius
4. 骨间膜 interosseous membrane
5. 指深屈肌 flexor digitorum profundus
6. 指深屈肌腱 flexor digitorum profundus tendon
7. 拇长屈肌 flexor pollicis longus
8. 尺骨冠突 coronoid process of ulna
9. 旋前圆肌 pronator teres
10. 旋前方肌 pronator quadratus
11. 指浅屈肌腱 flexor digitorum superficialis tendon

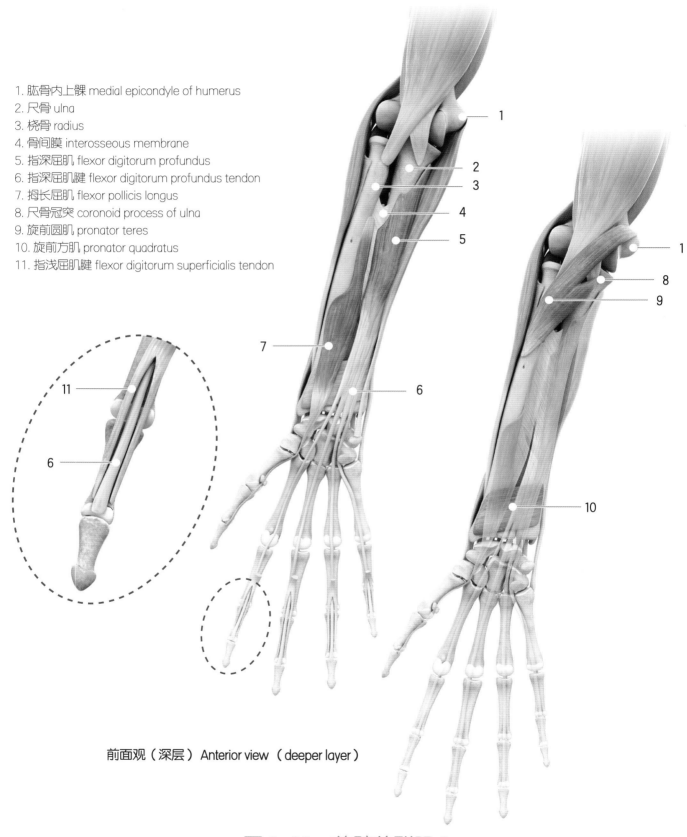

前面观（深层）Anterior view（deeper layer）

图 3-20　前臂前群肌 2
Anterior muscle group of the forearm 2

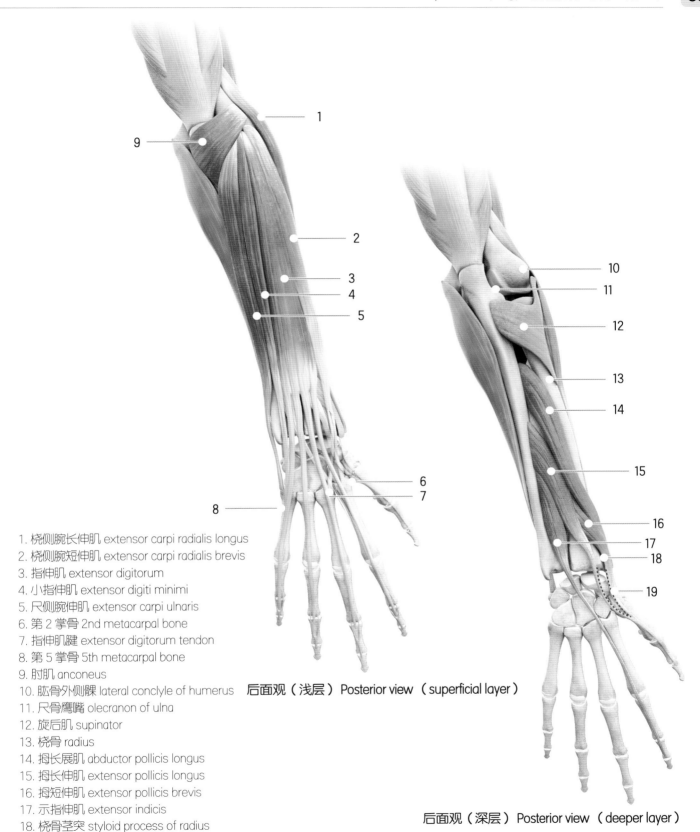

1. 桡侧腕长伸肌 extensor carpi radialis longus
2. 桡侧腕短伸肌 extensor carpi radialis brevis
3. 指伸肌 extensor digitorum
4. 小指伸肌 extensor digiti minimi
5. 尺侧腕伸肌 extensor carpi ulnaris
6. 第 2 掌骨 2nd metacarpal bone
7. 指伸肌腱 extensor digitorum tendon
8. 第 5 掌骨 5th metacarpal bone
9. 肘肌 anconeus
10. 肱骨外侧髁 lateral conclyle of humerus
11. 尺骨鹰嘴 olecranon of ulna
12. 旋后肌 supinator
13. 桡骨 radius
14. 拇长展肌 abductor pollicis longus
15. 拇长伸肌 extensor pollicis longus
16. 拇短伸肌 extensor pollicis brevis
17. 示指伸肌 extensor indicis
18. 桡骨茎突 styloid process of radius
19. 鼻烟窝 anatomical snuff box

后面观（浅层）Posterior view（superficial layer）

后面观（深层）Posterior view（deeper layer）

图 3-21　前臂后群肌
Posterior muscle group of the forearm

1. 指深屈肌腱 flexor digitorum profundus tendon
2. 豌豆骨 pisiform bone
3. 钩骨 hamate bone
4. 小指展肌 abductor digiti minimi
5. 小指短屈肌 flexor digiti minimi brevis
6. 蚓状肌 lumbricalis
7. 拇收肌 adductor pollicis
8. 拇短屈肌 flexor pollicis brevis
9. 拇短展肌 abductor pollicis brevis

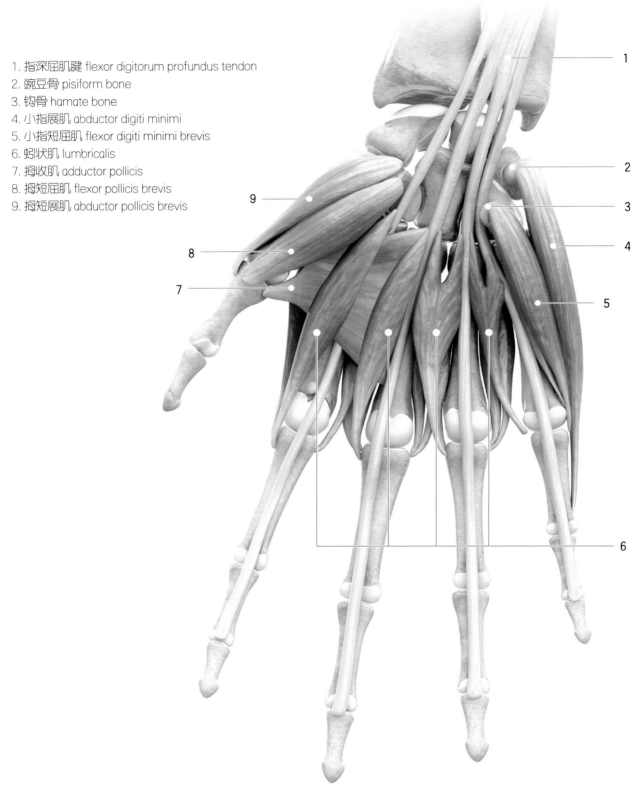

前面观（浅层）Anterior view（superficial layer）

图 3-22　手肌 1
Muscles of the hand 1

1. 骨间背侧肌 dorsal interossei
2. 小指对掌肌 opponens digiti minimi
3. 第5掌骨 5th metacarpal bone
4. 骨间掌侧肌 palmar interossei
5. 近节指骨 proximal phalanx
6. 第1掌骨 1st metacarpal bone
7. 拇对掌肌 opponens pollicis
8. 大多角骨 trapezium bone

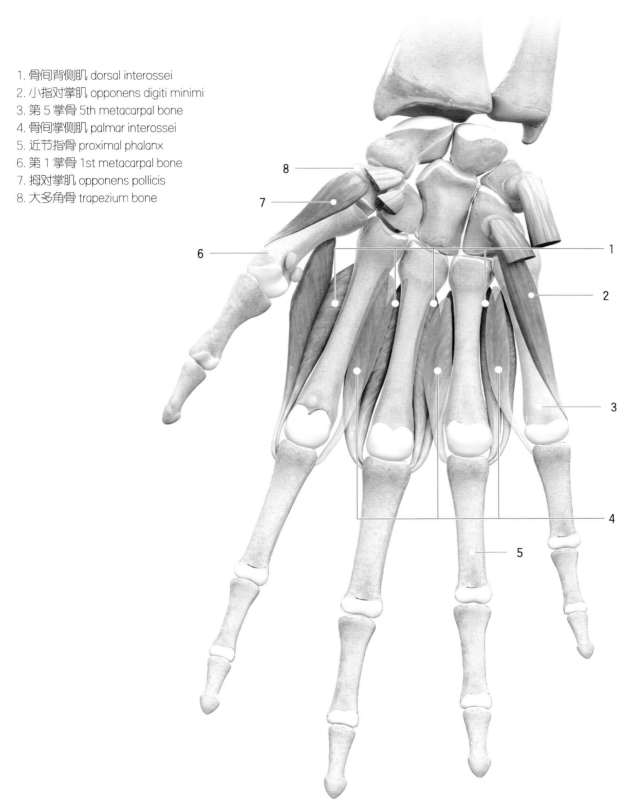

前面观（深层） Anterior view （deeper layer）

图 3-23　手肌 2
Muscles of the hand 2

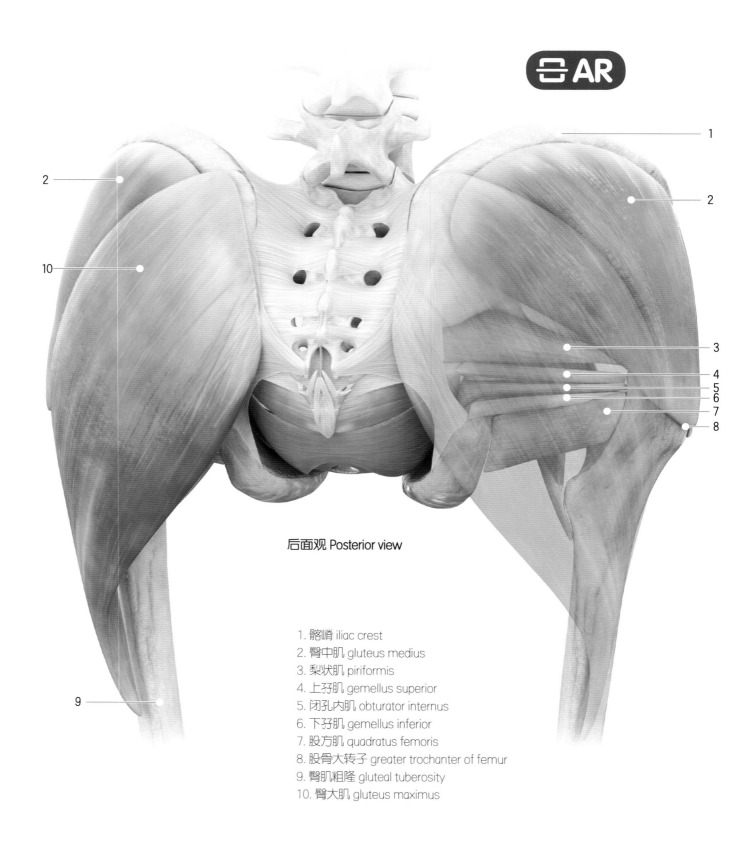

后面观 Posterior view

1. 髂嵴 iliac crest
2. 臀中肌 gluteus medius
3. 梨状肌 piriformis
4. 上孖肌 gemellus superior
5. 闭孔内肌 obturator internus
6. 下孖肌 gemellus inferior
7. 股方肌 quadratus femoris
8. 股骨大转子 greater trochanter of femur
9. 臀肌粗隆 gluteal tuberosity
10. 臀大肌 gluteus maximus

图 3-24　臀肌 1
Gluteal muscles 1

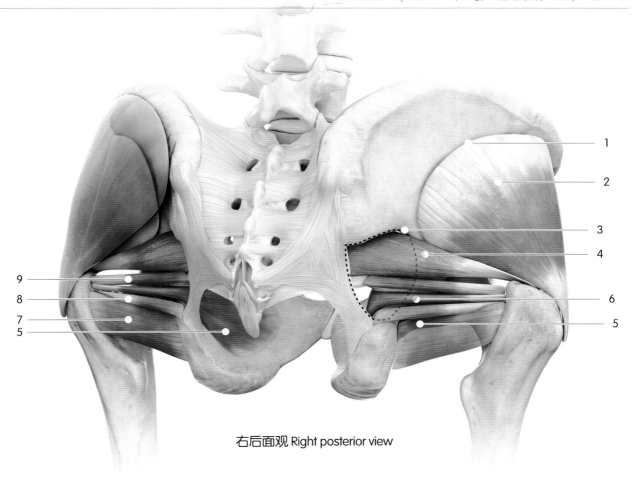

右后面观 Right posterior view

1. 臀前线 anterior gluteal line
2. 臀小肌 gluteus minimus
3. 坐骨大孔 greater sciatic foramen
4. 梨状肌 piriformis
5. 闭孔内肌 obturator internus
6. 闭孔外肌 obturator externus
7. 股方肌 quadratus femoris
8. 下孖肌 gemellus inferior
9. 上孖肌 gemellus superior
10. 股骨大转子 greater trochanter of femur
11. 转子窝 trochanteric fossa

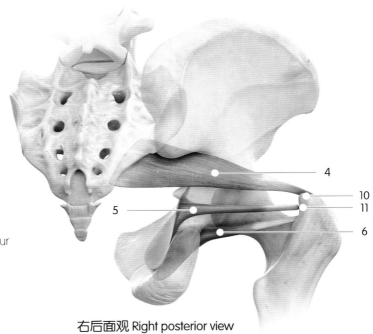

右后面观 Right posterior view

图 3-25　臀肌 2
Gluteal muscles 2

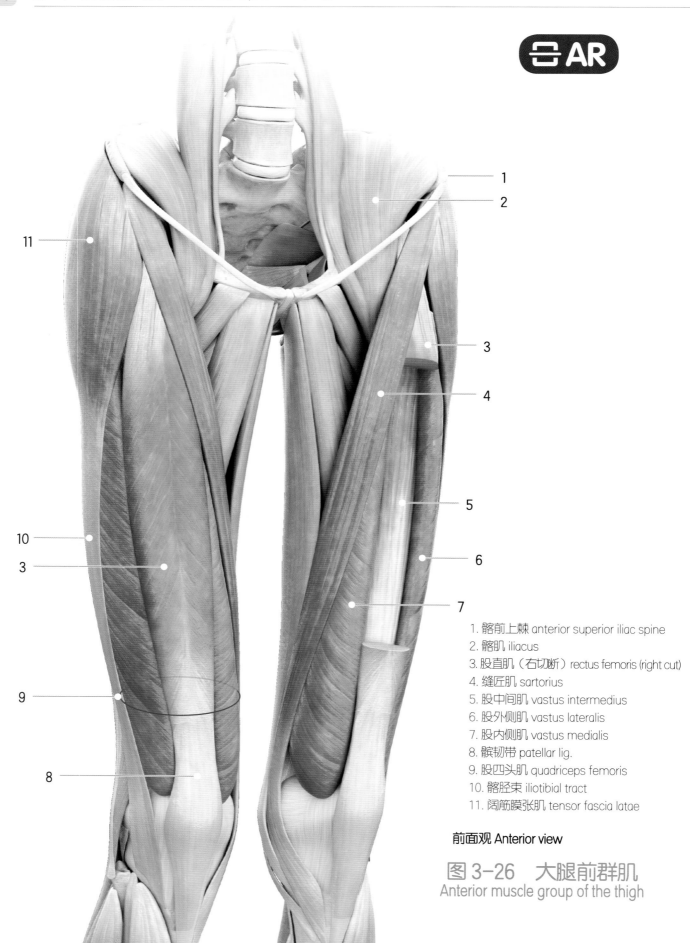

1. 髂前上棘 anterior superior iliac spine
2. 髂肌 iliacus
3. 股直肌（右切断）rectus femoris (right cut)
4. 缝匠肌 sartorius
5. 股中间肌 vastus intermedius
6. 股外侧肌 vastus lateralis
7. 股内侧肌 vastus medialis
8. 髌韧带 patellar lig.
9. 股四头肌 quadriceps femoris
10. 髂胫束 iliotibial tract
11. 阔筋膜张肌 tensor fascia latae

前面观 Anterior view

图 3-26　大腿前群肌
Anterior muscle group of the thigh

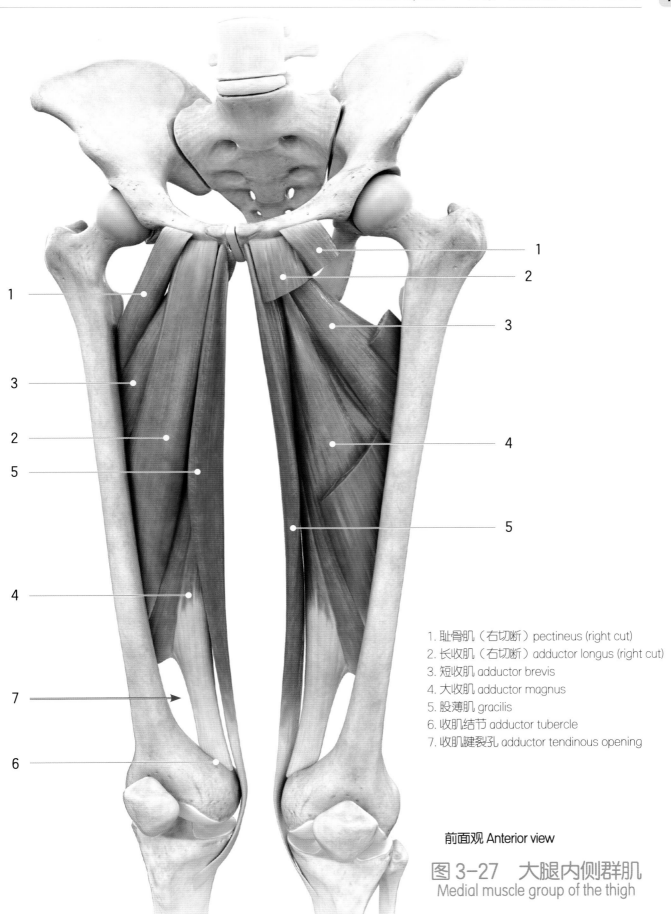

1. 耻骨肌（右切断）pectineus (right cut)
2. 长收肌（右切断）adductor longus (right cut)
3. 短收肌 adductor brevis
4. 大收肌 adductor magnus
5. 股薄肌 gracilis
6. 收肌结节 adductor tubercle
7. 收肌腱裂孔 adductor tendinous opening

前面观 Anterior view

图 3-27　大腿内侧群肌
Medial muscle group of the thigh

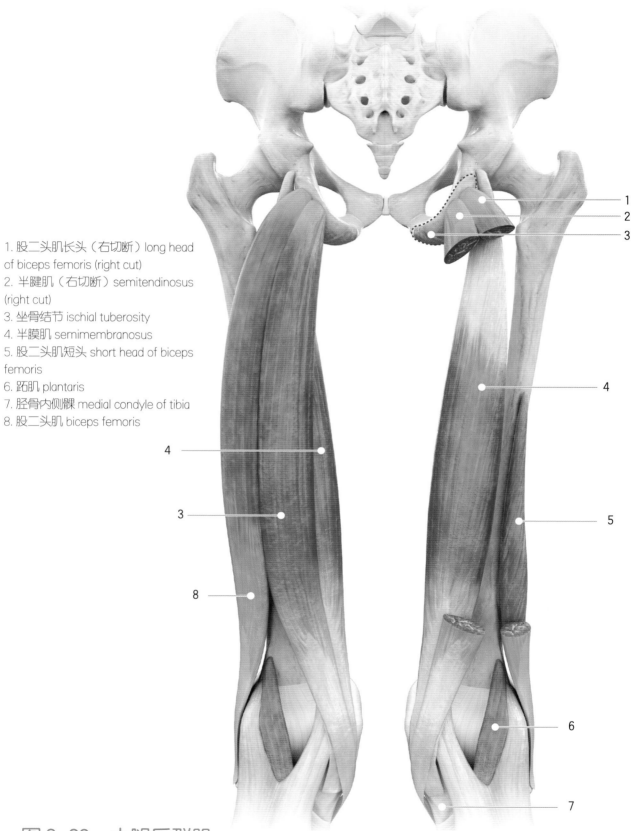

1. 股二头肌长头（右切断）long head of biceps femoris (right cut)
2. 半腱肌（右切断）semitendinosus (right cut)
3. 坐骨结节 ischial tuberosity
4. 半膜肌 semimembranosus
5. 股二头肌短头 short head of biceps femoris
6. 跖肌 plantaris
7. 胫骨内侧髁 medial condyle of tibia
8. 股二头肌 biceps femoris

图 3-28　大腿后群肌
Posterior muscle group of the thigh

后面观 Posterior view

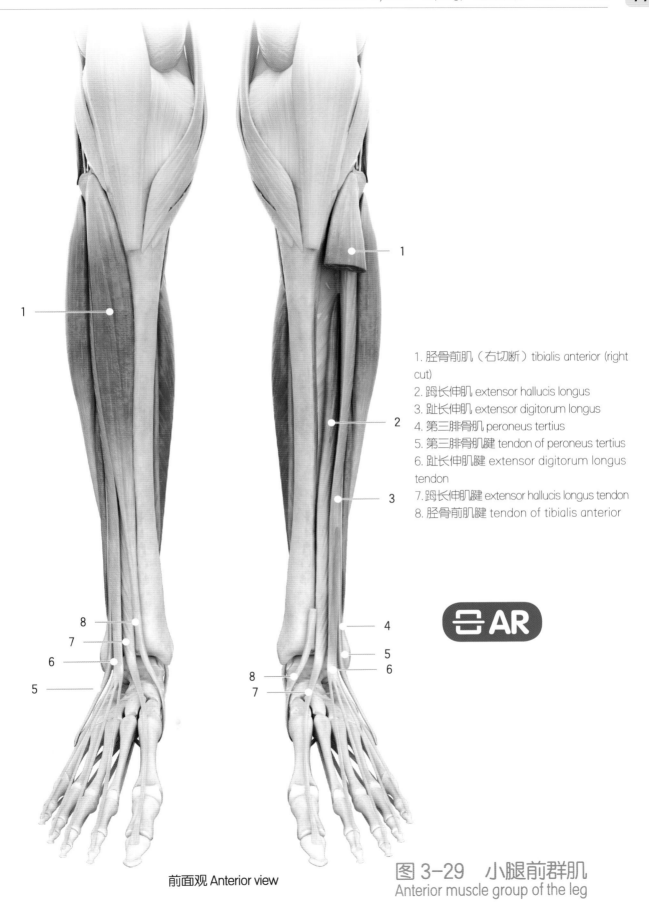

1. 胫骨前肌（右切断）tibialis anterior (right cut)
2. 踇长伸肌 extensor hallucis longus
3. 趾长伸肌 extensor digitorum longus
4. 第三腓骨肌 peroneus tertius
5. 第三腓骨肌腱 tendon of peroneus tertius
6. 趾长伸肌腱 extensor digitorum longus tendon
7. 踇长伸肌腱 extensor hallucis longus tendon
8. 胫骨前肌腱 tendon of tibialis anterior

前面观 Anterior view

图 3-29　小腿前群肌
Anterior muscle group of the leg

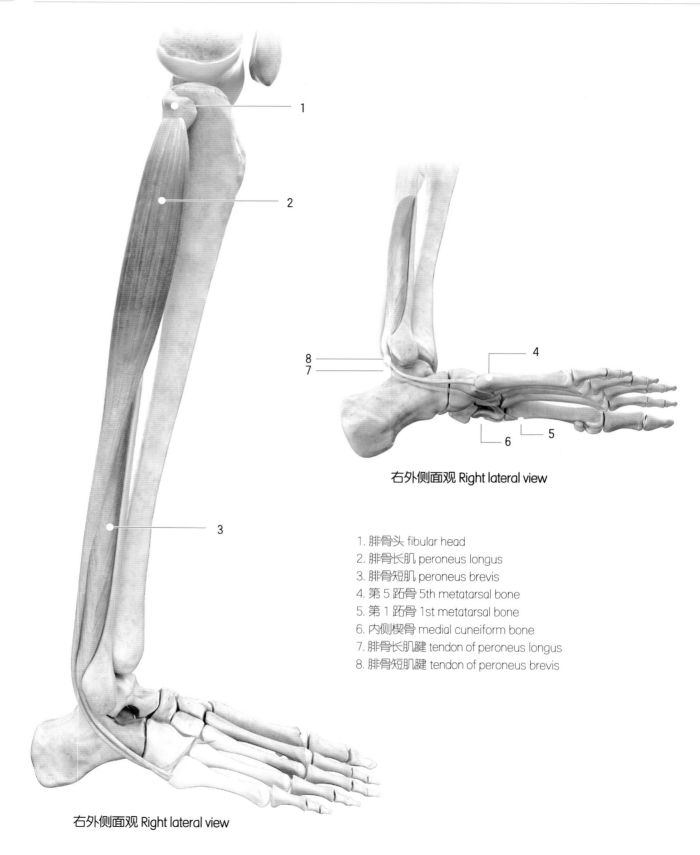

右外侧面观 Right lateral view

右外侧面观 Right lateral view

1. 腓骨头 fibular head
2. 腓骨长肌 peroneus longus
3. 腓骨短肌 peroneus brevis
4. 第 5 跖骨 5th metatarsal bone
5. 第 1 跖骨 1st metatarsal bone
6. 内侧楔骨 medial cuneiform bone
7. 腓骨长肌腱 tendon of peroneus longus
8. 腓骨短肌腱 tendon of peroneus brevis

图 3-30 小腿外侧群肌
Lateral muscle group of the leg

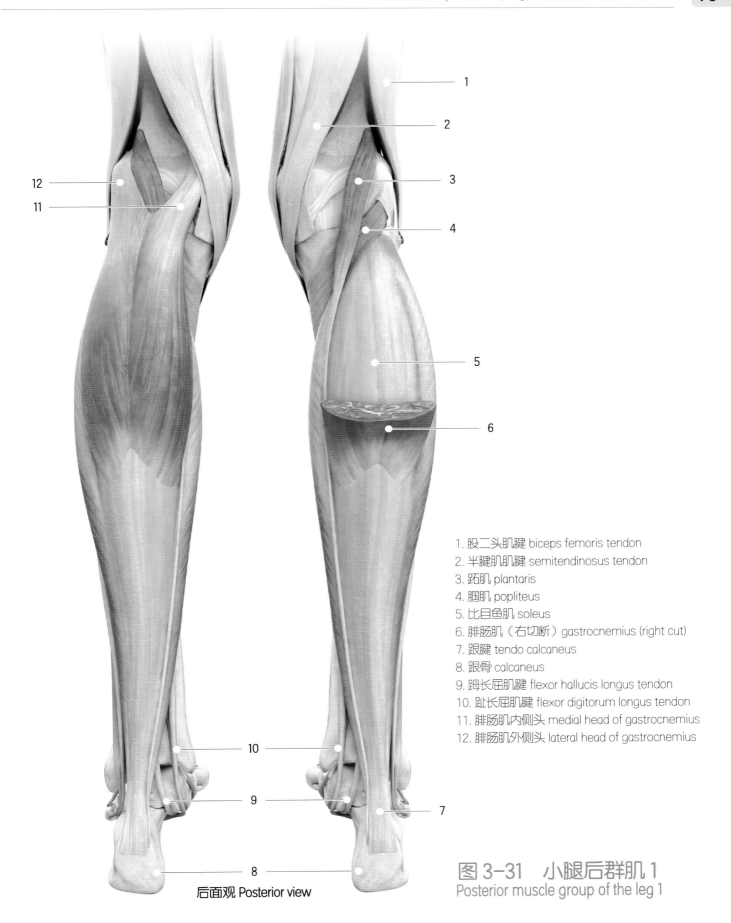

1. 股二头肌腱 biceps femoris tendon
2. 半腱肌肌腱 semitendinosus tendon
3. 跖肌 plantaris
4. 腘肌 popliteus
5. 比目鱼肌 soleus
6. 腓肠肌（右切断）gastrocnemius (right cut)
7. 跟腱 tendo calcaneus
8. 跟骨 calcaneus
9. 踇长屈肌腱 flexor hallucis longus tendon
10. 趾长屈肌腱 flexor digitorum longus tendon
11. 腓肠肌内侧头 medial head of gastrocnemius
12. 腓肠肌外侧头 lateral head of gastrocnemius

后面观 Posterior view

图 3-31　小腿后群肌 1
Posterior muscle group of the leg 1

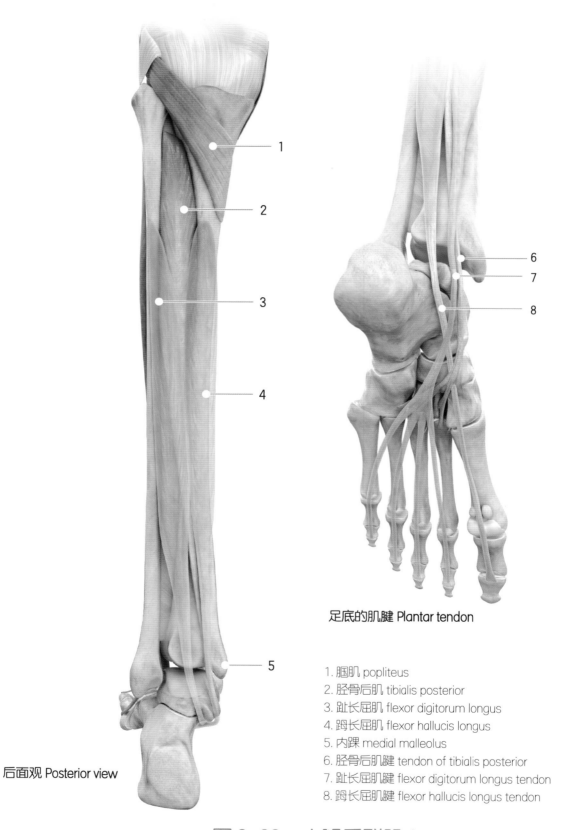

足底的肌腱 Plantar tendon

后面观 Posterior view

1. 腘肌 popliteus
2. 胫骨后肌 tibialis posterior
3. 趾长屈肌 flexor digitorum longus
4. 蹈长屈肌 flexor hallucis longus
5. 内踝 medial malleolus
6. 胫骨后肌腱 tendon of tibialis posterior
7. 趾长屈肌腱 flexor digitorum longus tendon
8. 蹈长屈肌腱 flexor hallucis longus tendon

图 3-32 小腿后群肌 2
Posterior muscle group of the leg 2

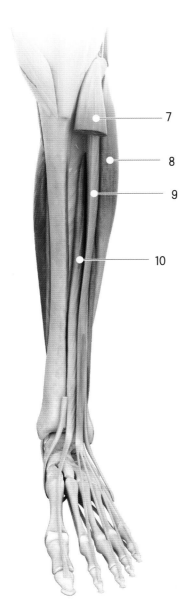

前面观 Anterior view

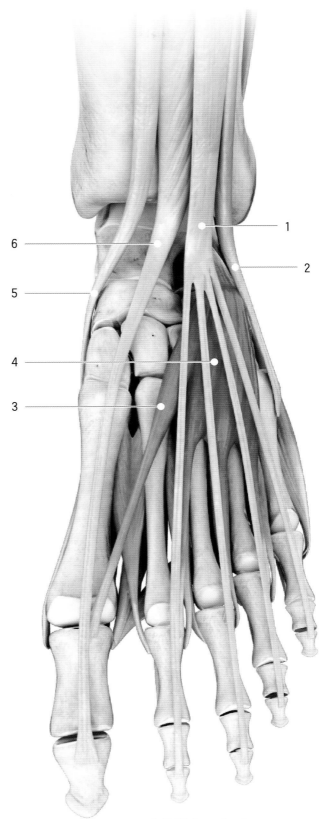

上面观 Superior view

1. 趾长伸肌腱 extensor digitorum longus tendon
2. 第三腓骨肌腱 tendon of peroneus tertius
3. 踇短伸肌 extensor hallucis brevis
4. 趾短伸肌 extensor digitorum brevis
5. 胫骨前肌腱 tendon of tibialis anterior
6. 踇长伸肌腱 extensor hallucis longus tendon
7. 胫骨前肌 tibialis anterior
8. 腓骨长肌 peroneus longus
9. 趾长伸肌 extensor digitorum longus
10. 踇长伸肌 extensor hallucis longus

图 3-33　足背肌
Dorsal muscles of foot

1. 跨收肌, adductor hallucis
2. 跨短屈肌, flexor hallucis brevis
3. 跨展肌, abductor hallucis
4. 趾短屈肌, flexor digitorum brevis
5. 小趾展肌, abductor digiti minimi
6. 小趾短屈肌, flexor digiti minimi brevis
7. 跨收肌横头, transverse head of adductor hallucis
8. 跨收肌斜头, oblique head of adductor hallucis
9. 蚓状肌, lumbricalis
10. 趾长屈肌腱, flexor digitorum longus tendon
11. 足底方肌, quadratus plantae
12. 近节趾骨, proximal phalanx
13. 骨间背侧肌, dorsal interossei
14. 骨间掌侧肌, palmar interossei
15. 骰骨, cuboid bone
16. 跖骨, metatarsal bone

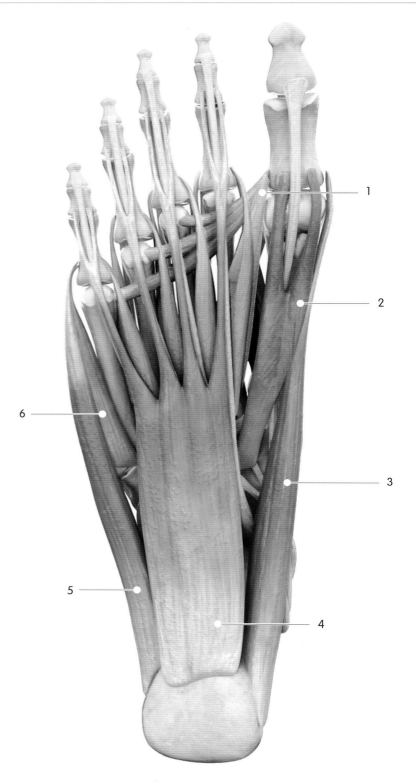

浅层 Superficial layer

图 3-34   足底肌
Plantar muscles

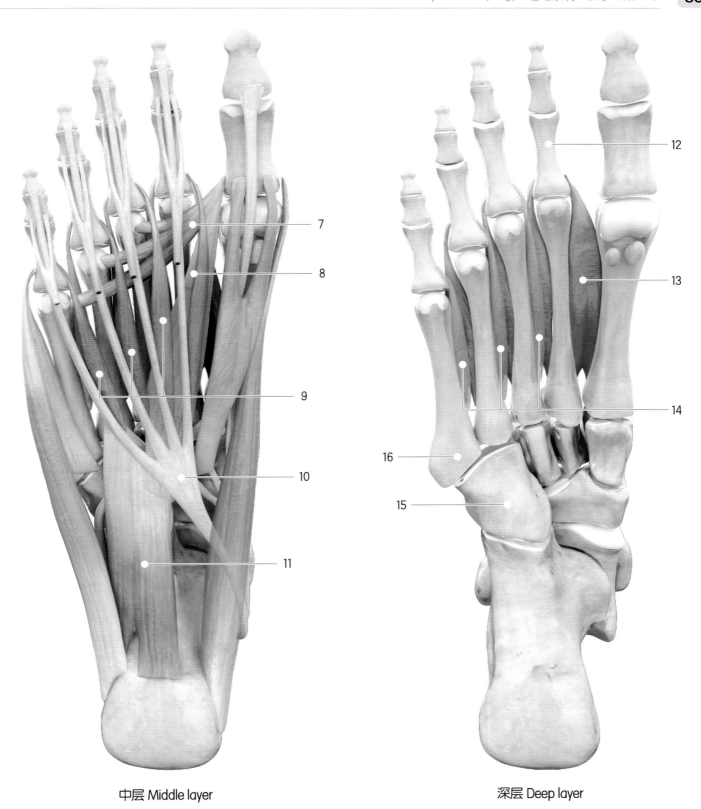

中层 Middle layer

深层 Deep layer

图 3-34　足底肌（续）
Plantar muscles

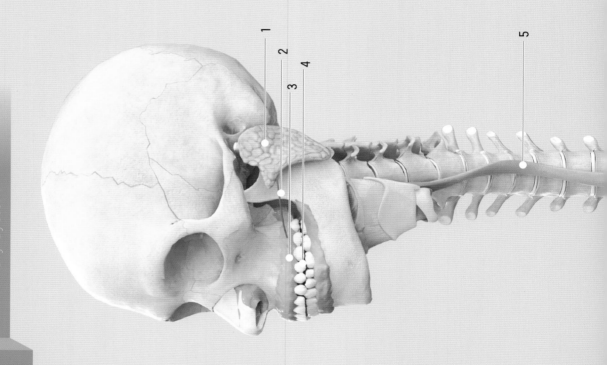

第4章 内脏学 Splanchnology

消化系统 Alimentary System

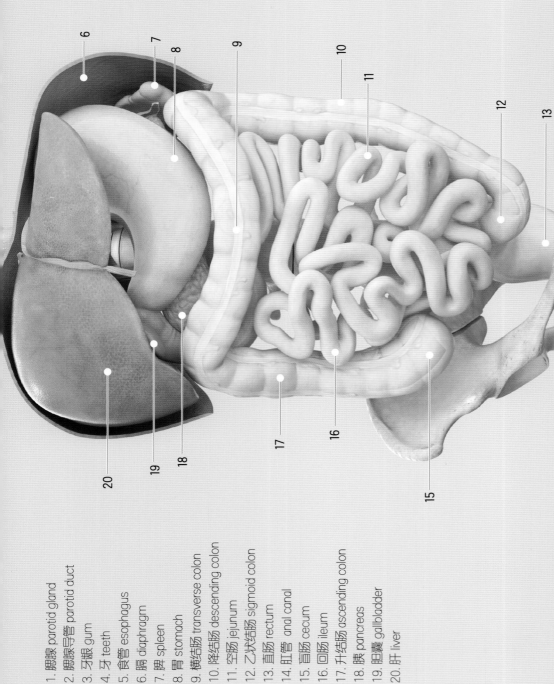

1. 腮腺 parotid gland
2. 腮腺导管 parotid duct
3. 牙龈 gum
4. 牙 teeth
5. 食管 esophagus
6. 膈 diaphragm
7. 脾 spleen
8. 胃 stomach
9. 横结肠 transverse colon
10. 降结肠 descending colon
11. 空肠 jejunum
12. 乙状结肠 sigmoid colon
13. 直肠 rectum
14. 肛管 anal canal
15. 盲肠 cecum
16. 回肠 ileum
17. 升结肠 ascending colon
18. 胰 pancreas
19. 胆囊 gallbladder
20. 肝 liver

图 4-1　消化系统概观
Overview of the alimentary system

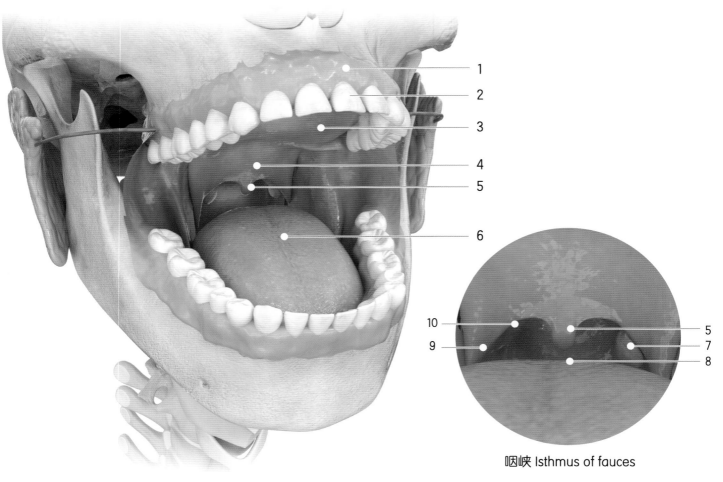

咽峡 Isthmus of fauces

口腔前外侧面观 Oral cavity (anterolateral view)

1. 牙龈 gum
2. 牙 teeth
3. 硬腭 hard palate
4. 软腭 soft palate
5. 腭垂 uvula
6. 舌 tongue
7. 腭扁桃体 palatine tonsil
8. 舌根 root of tongue
9. 腭舌弓 palatoglossal arch
10. 腭咽弓 palatopharyngeal arch
11. 舌体 body of tongue
12. 轮廓乳头 vallate papillae
13. 舌盲孔 foramen cecum of tongue
14. 叶状乳头 foliate papillae
15. 菌状乳头 fungiform papillae
16. 舌尖 apex of tongue

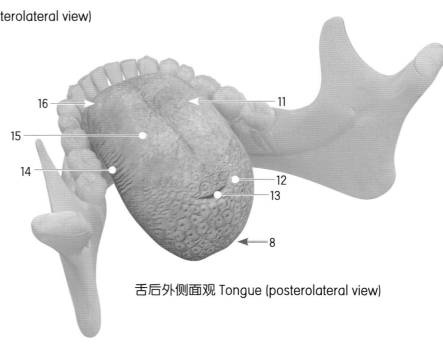

舌后外侧面观 Tongue (posterolateral view)

图 4-2 口腔、咽峡及舌
Oral cavity, isthmus of fauces and tongue

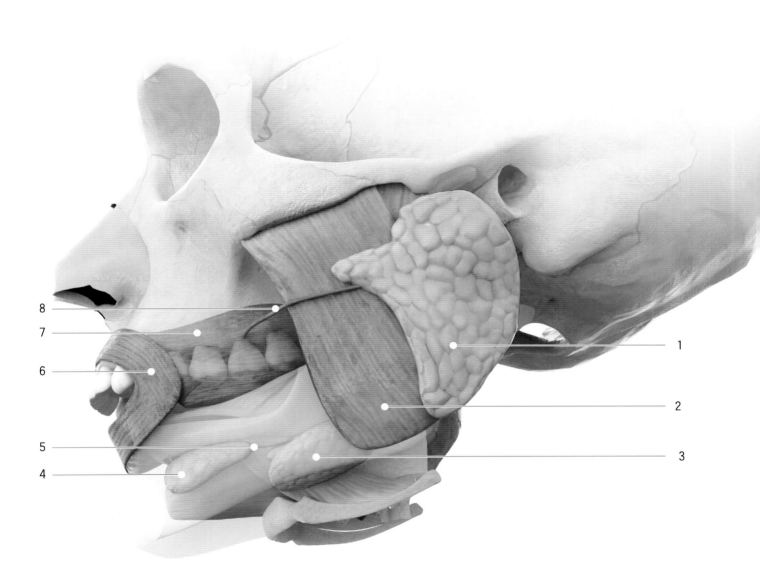

外侧面观 Lateral view

1. 腮腺 parotid gland
2. 咬肌 masseter
3. 下颌下腺 submandibular gland
4. 舌下腺 sublingual gland

5. 下颌下腺导管 submandibular duct
6. 口轮匝肌 orbicularis oris
7. 颊肌 buccinator
8. 腮腺导管 parotid duct

图 4-3　大唾液腺
Major salivary glands

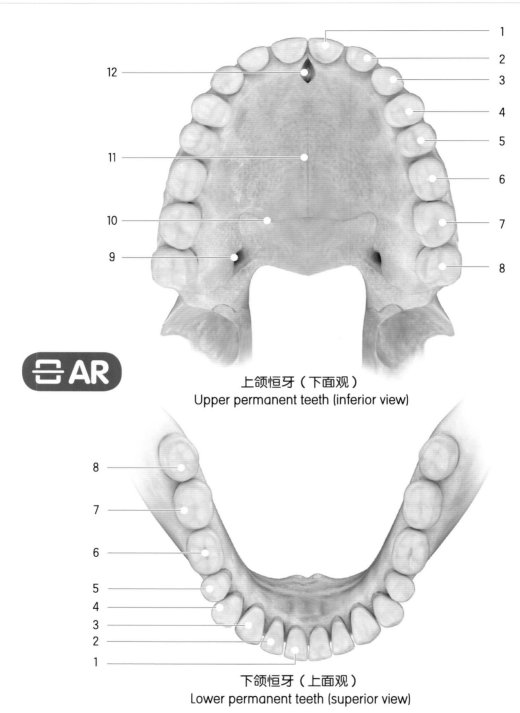

上颌恒牙（下面观）
Upper permanent teeth (inferior view)

下颌恒牙（上面观）
Lower permanent teeth (superior view)

1. 中切牙 medial incisor
2. 侧切牙 lateral incisor
3. 尖牙 canine tooth
4. 第一前磨牙 1st premolar
5. 第二前磨牙 2nd premolar
6. 第一磨牙 1st molar
7. 第二磨牙 2nd molar
8. 第三磨牙 3rd molar
9. 腭大孔 greater palatine foramen
10. 腭横缝 transverse palatine suture
11. 腭正中缝 median palatine suture
12. 切牙孔 incisive foramen

图 4-4 恒牙
Permanent teeth

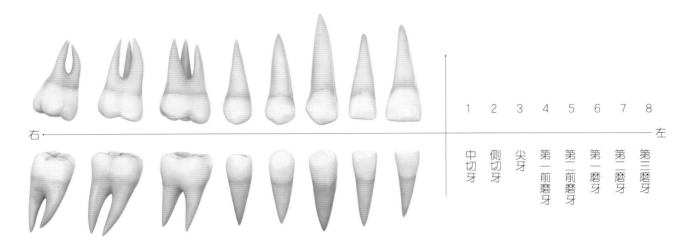

	1	2	3	4	5	6	7	8
	中切牙	侧切牙	尖牙	第一前磨牙	第二前磨牙	第一磨牙	第二磨牙	第三磨牙

右 —— 左

图 4-5　恒牙的名称及符号
Names and symbols of the permanent teeth

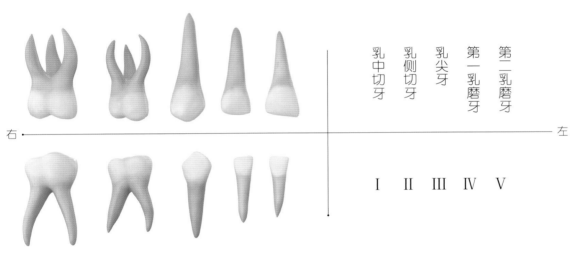

乳中切牙	乳侧切牙	乳尖牙	第一乳磨牙	第二乳磨牙
I	II	III	IV	V

右 —— 左

图 4-6　乳牙的名称及符号
Names and symbols of the deciduous teeth

1. 牙釉质 enamel
2. 牙质 dentine of tooth
3. 牙腔 dental cavity
4. 牙髓 dental pulp
5. 牙根管 root canal
6. 根尖孔 apical foramen
7. 牙根 root of tooth
8. 牙颈 neck of tooth
9. 牙冠 crown of tooth

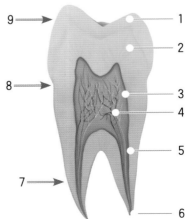

图 4-7　牙的构造模式图（矢状断面）
Diagram of the structure of the teeth (sagittal section)

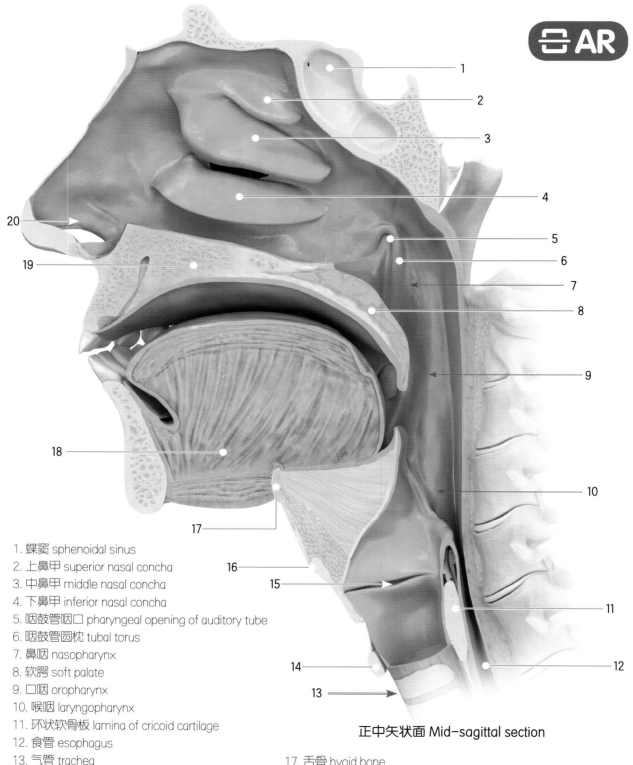

1. 蝶窦 sphenoidal sinus
2. 上鼻甲 superior nasal concha
3. 中鼻甲 middle nasal concha
4. 下鼻甲 inferior nasal concha
5. 咽鼓管咽口 pharyngeal opening of auditory tube
6. 咽鼓管圆枕 tubal torus
7. 鼻咽 nasopharynx
8. 软腭 soft palate
9. 口咽 oropharynx
10. 喉咽 laryngopharynx
11. 环状软骨板 lamina of cricoid cartilage
12. 食管 esophagus
13. 气管 trachea
14. 环状软骨弓 arch of cricoid cartilage
15. 喉室 ventricle of larynx
16. 甲状软骨 thyroid cartilage

17. 舌骨 hyoid bone
18. 颏舌肌 genioglossus
19. 硬腭 hard palate
20. 鼻阈 nasal limen

正中矢状面 Mid-sagittal section

图 4-8 鼻、咽和喉
Nose, pharynx and larynx

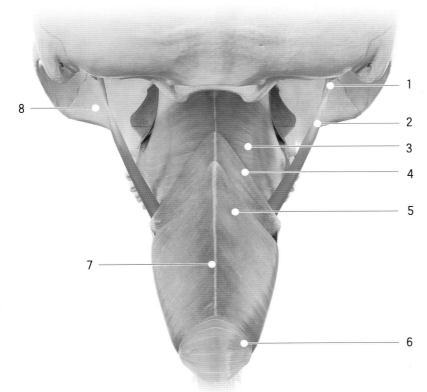

1. 茎突 styloid process
2. 茎突舌骨肌 stylohyoid
3. 咽上缩肌 superior constrictor of pharynx
4. 咽中缩肌 middle constrictor of pharynx
5. 咽下缩肌 inferior constrictor of pharynx
6. 环咽肌 cricopharyngeal muscle
7. 咽缝 raphe of pharynx
8. 上颌骨 maxilla

后面观 Posterior view

图 4-9　咽肌
Muscles of pharynx

1. 会厌 epiglottis
2. 杓状会厌襞 aryepiglottic fold
3. 喉口 aperture of larynx
4. 楔状结节 cuneiform tubercle
5. 小角结节 corniculate tubercle
6. 梨状隐窝 piriform recess
7. 喉咽 laryngopharynx
8. 口咽 oropharynx
9. 舌根 root of tongue
10. 腭垂 uvula
11. 鼻咽 nasopharynx

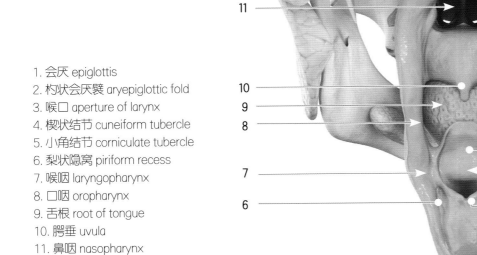

切开咽后壁 Incision of posterior wall of pharynx

图 4-10　咽腔
Pharyngeal cavity

1. 第 6 颈椎 6th cervical vertebra
2. 食管颈部 cervical part of esophagus
3. 气管 trachea
4. 主动脉弓 aortic arch
5. 左主支气管 left principal bronchus
6. 胸主动脉 thoracic aorta
7. 食管胸部 thoracic part of esophagus
8. 食管腹部 abdominal part of esophagus
9. 膈 diaphragm
10. 胃 stomach
11. 下腔静脉 inferior vena cava
12. 第 10 胸椎 10th thoracic vertebrae
13. 右主支气管 right principal bronchus

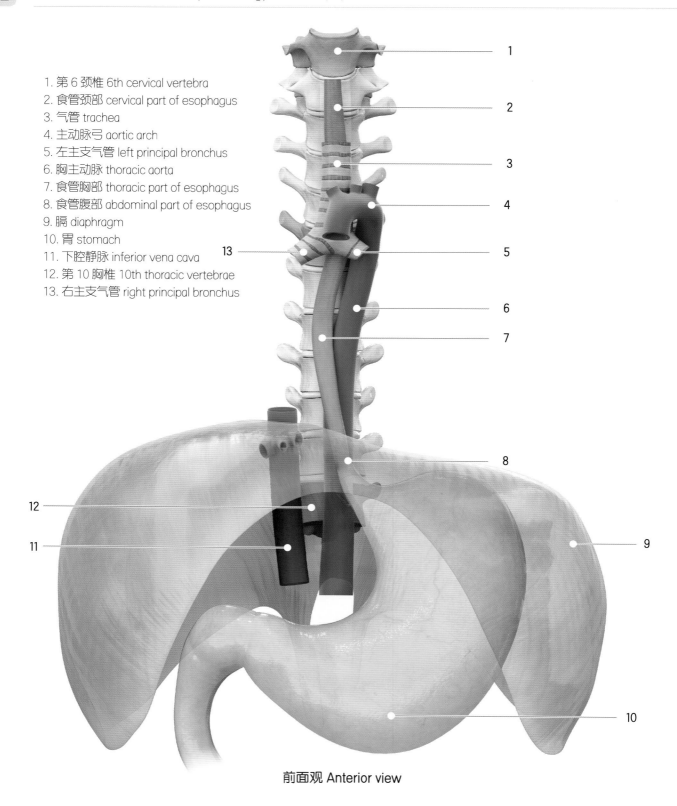

前面观 Anterior view

图 4-11 食管
Esophagus

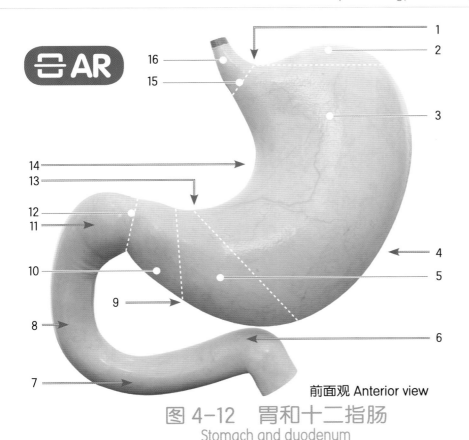

1. 贲门切迹 cardiac incisure
2. 胃底 fundus of stomach
3. 胃体 body of stomach
4. 胃大弯 greater curvature of stomach
5. 幽门窦 pyloric antrum
6. 十二指肠升部 ascending part of duodenum
7. 十二指肠水平部 horizontal part of duodenum
8. 十二指肠降部 descending part of duodenum
9. 中间沟 intermediate sulcus
10. 幽门管 pyloric canal
11. 十二指肠上部 superior part of duodenum
12. 幽门 pylorus
13. 角切迹 angular incisure
14. 胃小弯 lesser curvature of stomach
15. 贲门 cardia
16. 食管腹部 abdominal part of esophagus

前面观 Anterior view

图 4-12　胃和十二指肠
Stomach and duodenum

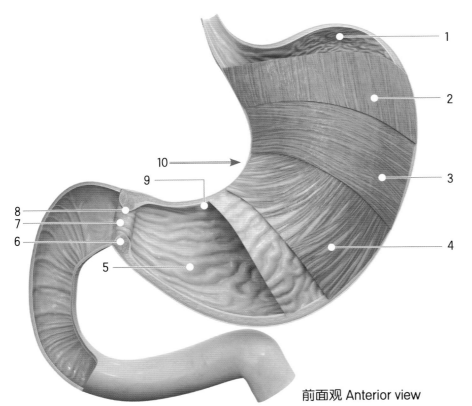

1. 胃底 fundus of stomach
2. 外纵肌层 longitudinal muscular layer
3. 中环肌层 circular muscular layer
4. 内斜肌层 oblique muscular layer
5. 幽门窦 pyloric antrum
6. 幽门括约肌 sphincter of pylorus
7. 幽门 pylorus
8. 幽门瓣 pyloric valve
9. 胃管 gastric canal
10. 胃小弯 lesser curvature of stomach

前面观 Anterior view

图 4-13　胃和十二指肠的肌层与黏膜
Muscular and mucous membranes of the stomach and duodenum

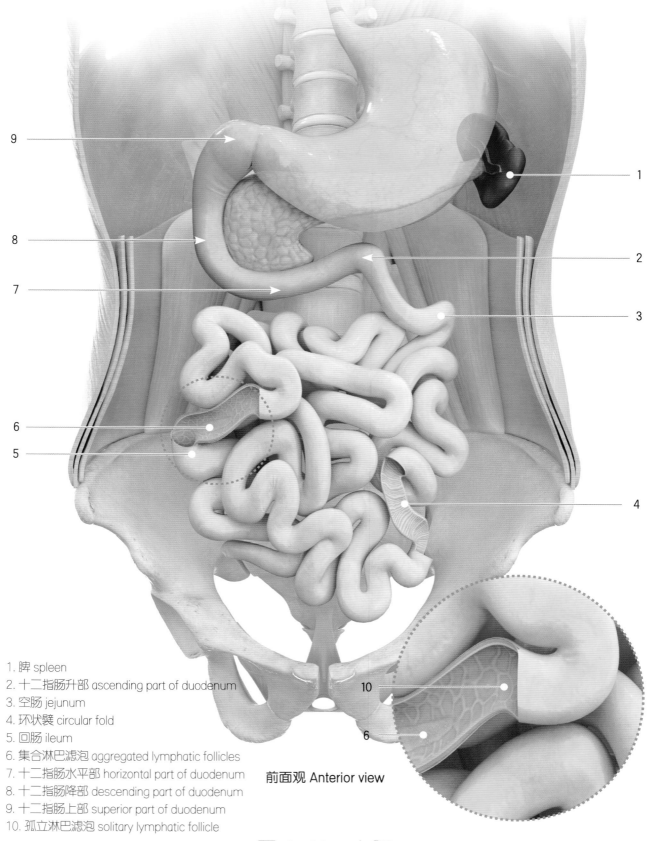

1. 脾 spleen
2. 十二指肠升部 ascending part of duodenum
3. 空肠 jejunum
4. 环状襞 circular fold
5. 回肠 ileum
6. 集合淋巴滤泡 aggregated lymphatic follicles
7. 十二指肠水平部 horizontal part of duodenum
8. 十二指肠降部 descending part of duodenum
9. 十二指肠上部 superior part of duodenum
10. 孤立淋巴滤泡 solitary lymphatic follicle

前面观 Anterior view

图 4-14   小肠
Small intestine

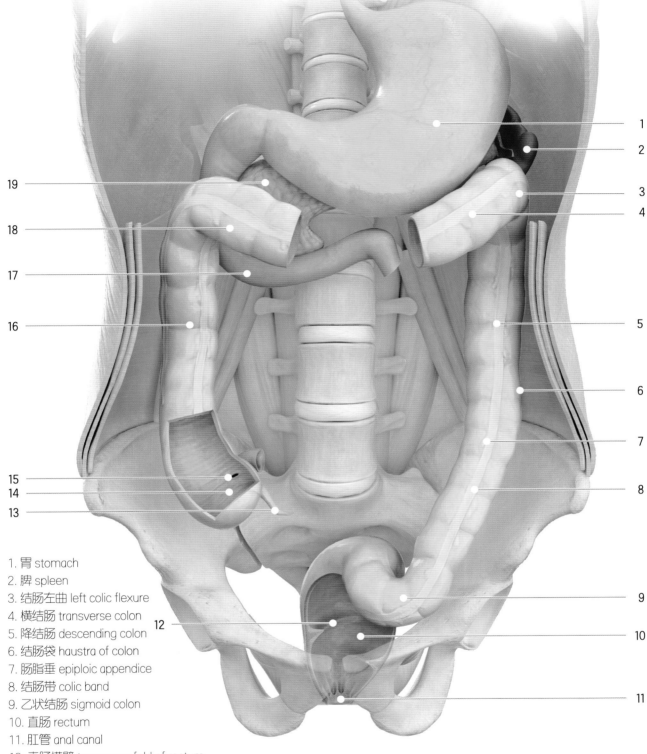

1. 胃 stomach
2. 脾 spleen
3. 结肠左曲 left colic flexure
4. 横结肠 transverse colon
5. 降结肠 descending colon
6. 结肠袋 haustra of colon
7. 肠脂垂 epiploic appendice
8. 结肠带 colic band
9. 乙状结肠 sigmoid colon
10. 直肠 rectum
11. 肛管 anal canal
12. 直肠横襞 transverse fold of rectum
13. 阑尾 vermiform appendix
14. 盲肠 cecum
15. 回盲口 ileocecal orifice
16. 升结肠 ascending colon
17. 十二指肠 duodenum
18. 结肠右曲 right colic flexure
19. 胰 pancreas

外侧面观 Lateral view

图 4-15　大肠
Large intestine

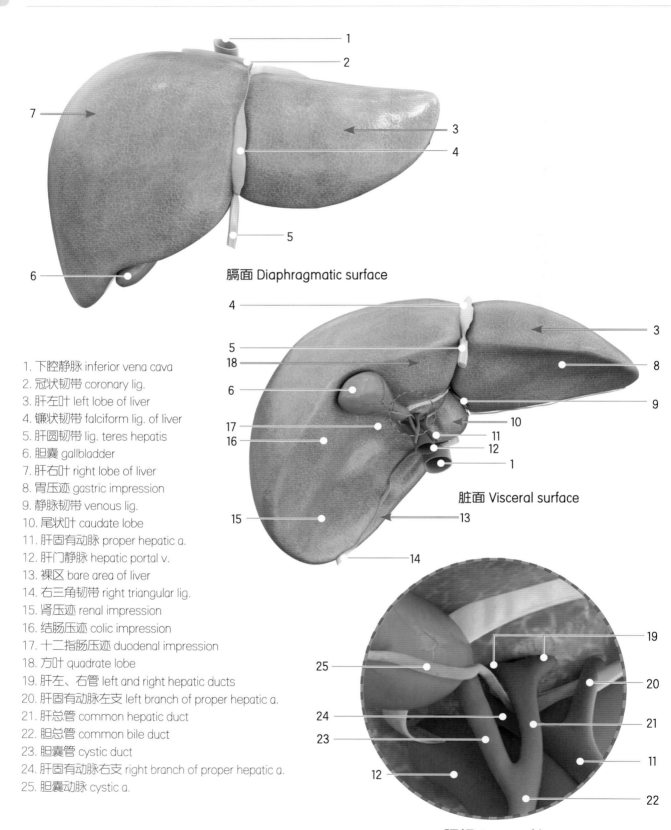

膈面 Diaphragmatic surface

脏面 Visceral surface

肝门 Porta of liver

1. 下腔静脉 inferior vena cava
2. 冠状韧带 coronary lig.
3. 肝左叶 left lobe of liver
4. 镰状韧带 falciform lig. of liver
5. 肝圆韧带 lig. teres hepatis
6. 胆囊 gallbladder
7. 肝右叶 right lobe of liver
8. 胃压迹 gastric impression
9. 静脉韧带 venous lig.
10. 尾状叶 caudate lobe
11. 肝固有动脉 proper hepatic a.
12. 肝门静脉 hepatic portal v.
13. 裸区 bare area of liver
14. 右三角韧带 right triangular lig.
15. 肾压迹 renal impression
16. 结肠压迹 colic impression
17. 十二指肠压迹 duodenal impression
18. 方叶 quadrate lobe
19. 肝左、右管 left and right hepatic ducts
20. 肝固有动脉左支 left branch of proper hepatic a.
21. 肝总管 common hepatic duct
22. 胆总管 common bile duct
23. 胆囊管 cystic duct
24. 肝固有动脉右支 right branch of proper hepatic a.
25. 胆囊动脉 cystic a.

图 4-16　肝
Liver

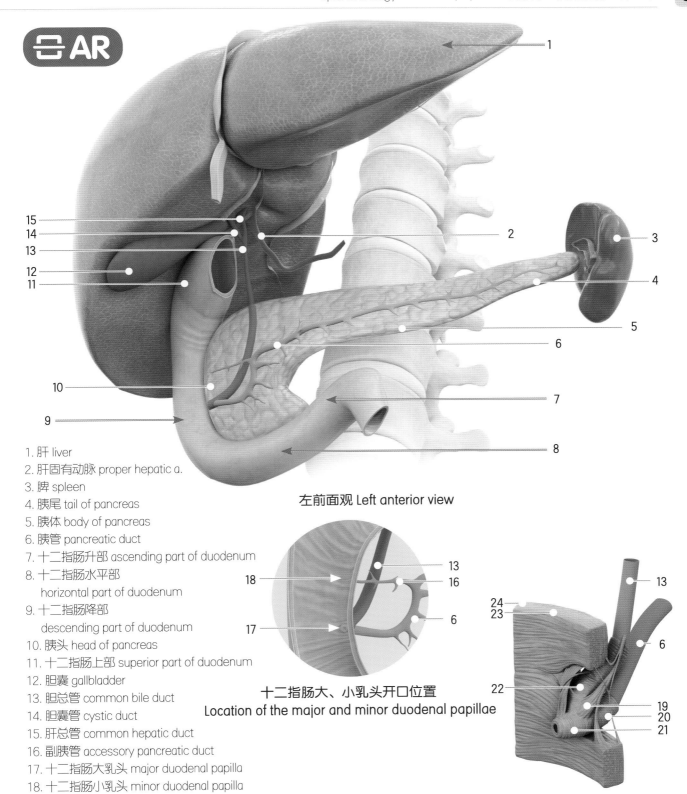

左前面观 Left anterior view

十二指肠大、小乳头开口位置
Location of the major and minor duodenal papillae

胆总管和胰管的括约肌
Sphincter of the common bile and pancreatic ducts

1. 肝 liver
2. 肝固有动脉 proper hepatic a.
3. 脾 spleen
4. 胰尾 tail of pancreas
5. 胰体 body of pancreas
6. 胰管 pancreatic duct
7. 十二指肠升部 ascending part of duodenum
8. 十二指肠水平部 horizontal part of duodenum
9. 十二指肠降部 descending part of duodenum
10. 胰头 head of pancreas
11. 十二指肠上部 superior part of duodenum
12. 胆囊 gallbladder
13. 胆总管 common bile duct
14. 胆囊管 cystic duct
15. 肝总管 common hepatic duct
16. 副胰管 accessory pancreatic duct
17. 十二指肠大乳头 major duodenal papilla
18. 十二指肠小乳头 minor duodenal papilla
19. 纵行肌纤维 longitudinal muscular bundles
20. 胰管括约肌 sphincter of pancreatic duct
21. 肝胰壶腹括约肌 sphincter of hepatopancreatic ampulla
22. 胆总管括约肌 sphincter of common bile duct
23. 十二指肠环形肌 circular muscular fibers of duodenum
24. 十二指肠纵行肌 longitudinal muscular fibers of duodenum

图 4-17 胰、肝外胆道
Pancreas, extrahepatic biliary passages

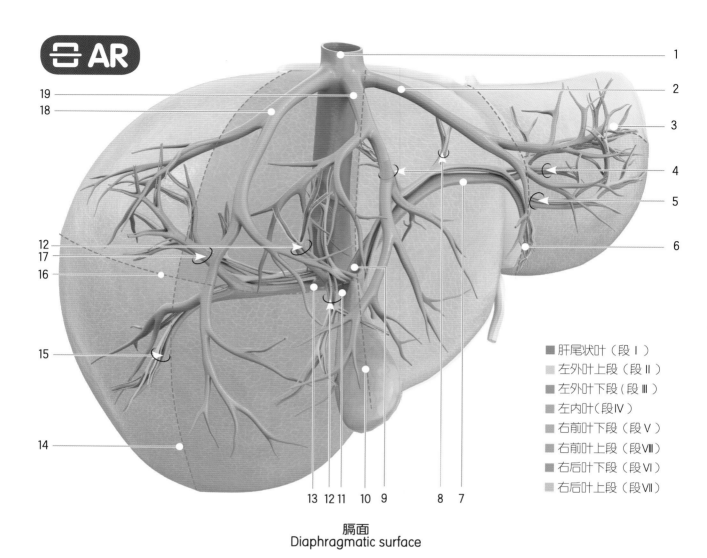

膈面
Diaphragmatic surface

肝尾状叶（段Ⅰ）
左外叶上段（段Ⅱ）
左外叶下段（段Ⅲ）
左内叶（段Ⅳ）
右前叶下段（段Ⅴ）
右前叶上段（段Ⅷ）
右后叶下段（段Ⅵ）
右后叶上段（段Ⅶ）

1. 下腔静脉 inferior vena cava
2. 肝左静脉 left hepatic v.
3. 左段间裂 left intersegmental fissure
4. 左外上支 left laterosuperior branches
5. 左外下支 left lateroinferior branches
6. 左叶间裂 left interlobar fissure
7. 横支 transversal branch
8. 左内支 left medial branches
9. 肝门静脉左支 left branch of hepatic portal v.
10. 正中裂 median fissure

11. 肝门静脉 hepatic portal v.
12. 右前下支 right anteroinferior branches
13. 肝门静脉右支 right branch of hepatic portal v.
14. 右叶间裂 right interlobar fissure
15. 右后下支 right posteroinferior branches
16. 右段间裂 right intersegmental fissure
17. 右后上支 right posterosuperior branches
18. 肝右静脉 right hepatic v.
19. 肝中静脉 intermediate hepatic v.

图 4-18　肝内管道、肝裂和肝段 1
Intrahepatic biliary passage, hepatic fissure and segment of the liver 1

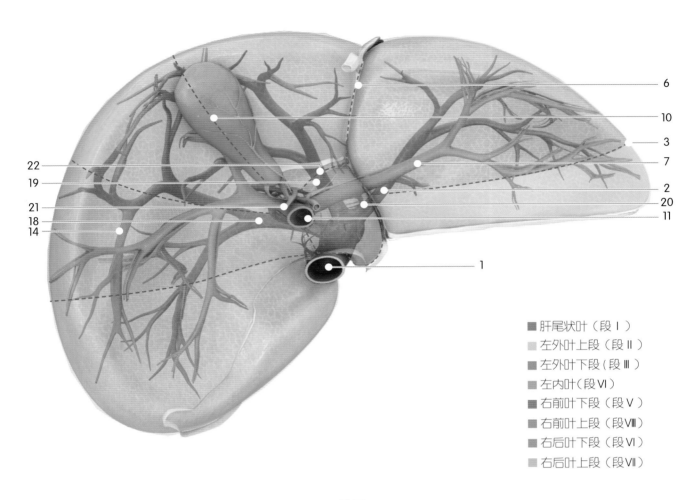

脏面
Visceral surface

■ 肝尾状叶（段Ⅰ）
■ 左外叶上段（段Ⅱ）
■ 左外叶下段（段Ⅲ）
■ 左内叶（段Ⅳ）
■ 右前叶下段（段Ⅴ）
■ 右前叶上段（段Ⅷ）
■ 右后叶下段（段Ⅵ）
■ 右后叶上段（段Ⅶ）

1. 下腔静脉 inferior vena cava
2. 肝左静脉 left hepatic v.
3. 左段间裂 left intersegmental fissure
4. 左外上支 left laterosuperior branches
5. 左外下支 left lateroinferior branches
6. 左叶间裂 left interlobar fissure
7. 横支 transversal branch
8. 左内支 left medial branches
9. 肝门静脉左支 left branch of hepatic portal v.
10. 正中裂 median fissure
11. 肝门静脉 hepatic portal v.

12. 右前下支 right anteroinferior branches
13. 肝门静脉右支 right branch of hepatic portal v.
14. 右叶间裂 right interlobar fissure
15. 右后下支 right posteroinferior branches
16. 右段间裂 right intersegmental fissure
17. 右后上支 right posterosuperior branches
18. 肝右静脉 right hepatic v.
19. 肝中静脉 intermediate hepatic v.
20. 尾状叶支 caudal branches
21. 胆总管 common bile duct
22. 背裂 dorsal fissure

图 4-19　肝内管道、肝裂和肝段 2
Intrahepatic biliary passage, hepatic fissure and segment of the liver 2

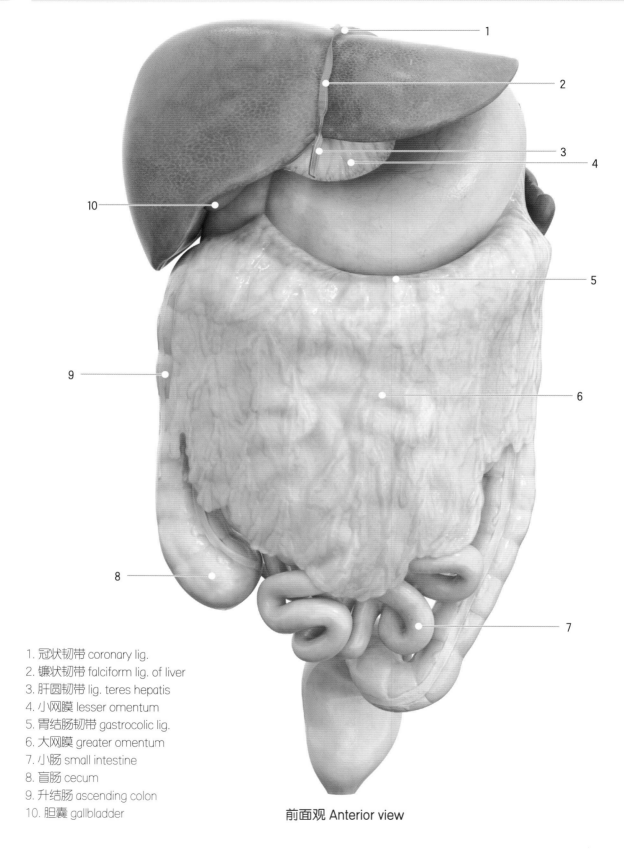

1. 冠状韧带 coronary lig.
2. 镰状韧带 falciform lig. of liver
3. 肝圆韧带 lig. teres hepatis
4. 小网膜 lesser omentum
5. 胃结肠韧带 gastrocolic lig.
6. 大网膜 greater omentum
7. 小肠 small intestine
8. 盲肠 cecum
9. 升结肠 ascending colon
10. 胆囊 gallbladder

前面观 Anterior view

图 4-20　网膜
Omentum

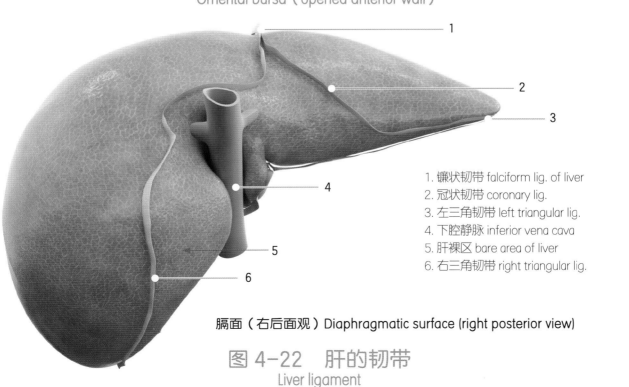

1. 胃左动脉 left gastric a.
2. 左肾上腺 left suprarenal gland
3. 胃脾韧带 gastrosplenic lig.
4. 胃膈韧带 gastrophrenic lig.
5. 胃短动脉 short gastric a.
6. 脾肾韧带 splenorenal lig.
7. 脾动脉 splenic a.
8. 横结肠系膜 transverse mesocolon
9. 大网膜前层 anterior layers of greater omentum
10. 胰十二指肠上前动脉 anterior superior pancreaticoduodenal a.
11. 肝总动脉 common hepatic a.
12. 胃网膜右动脉 right gastroepiploic a.
13. 通过网膜孔内的探针 probe in epiploic (omental) foramen
14. 伸入网膜囊上隐窝的探针 probe in superior recess of omental bursa

图 4-21　网膜囊（打开前壁）
Omental bursa（opened anterior wall）

1. 镰状韧带 falciform lig. of liver
2. 冠状韧带 coronary lig.
3. 左三角韧带 left triangular lig.
4. 下腔静脉 inferior vena cava
5. 肝裸区 bare area of liver
6. 右三角韧带 right triangular lig.

膈面（右后面观）Diaphragmatic surface (right posterior view)

图 4-22　肝的韧带
Liver ligament

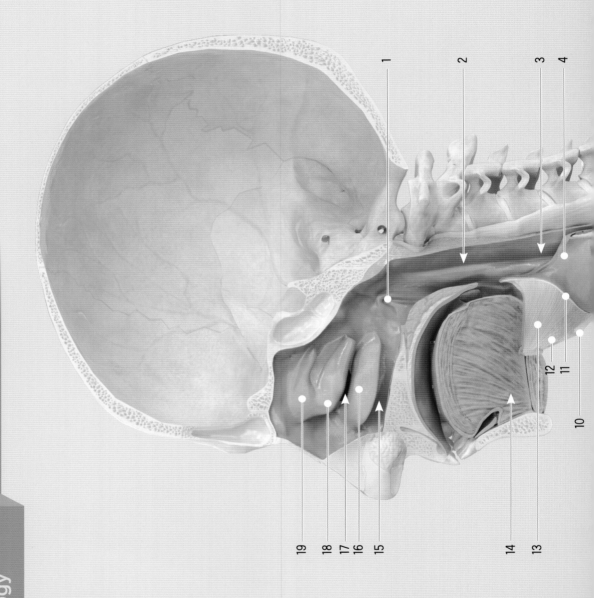

1
2
3
4
12
11
10

19
18
17
16
15

14
13

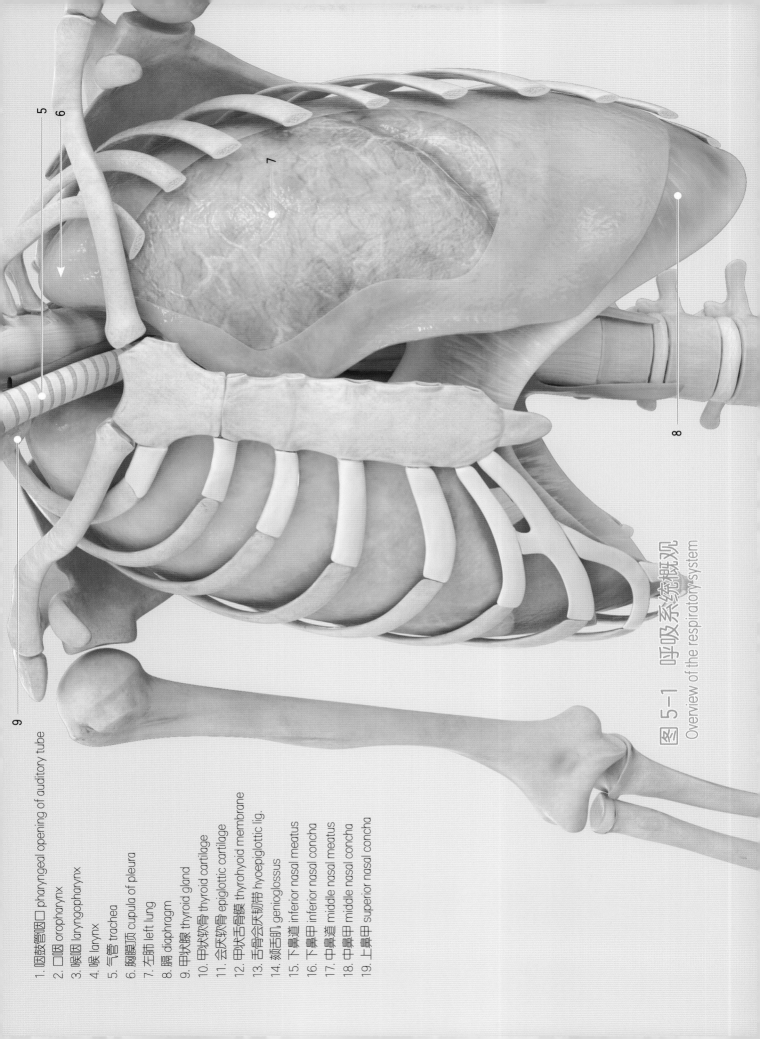

图 5-1 呼吸系统概观 Overview of the respiratory system

1. 咽鼓管咽口 pharyngeal opening of auditory tube
2. 口咽 oropharynx
3. 喉咽 laryngopharynx
4. 喉 larynx
5. 气管 trachea
6. 胸膜顶 cupula of pleura
7. 左肺 left lung
8. 膈 diaphragm
9. 甲状腺 thyroid gland
10. 甲状软骨 thyroid cartilage
11. 会厌软骨 epiglottic cartilage
12. 甲状舌骨膜 thyrohyoid membrane
13. 舌骨会厌韧带 hyoepiglottic lig.
14. 颏舌肌 genioglossus
15. 下鼻道 inferior nasal meatus
16. 下鼻甲 inferior nasal concha
17. 中鼻道 middle nasal meatus
18. 中鼻甲 middle nasal concha
19. 上鼻甲 superior nasal concha

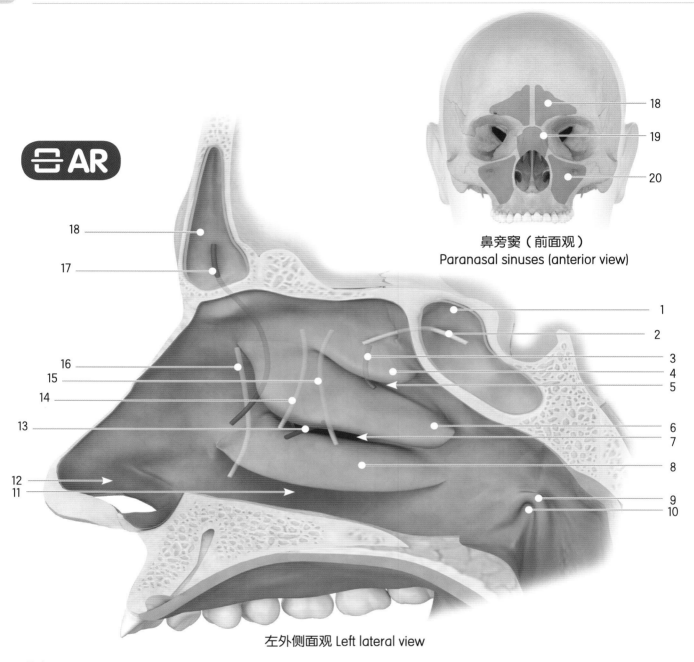

鼻旁窦（前面观）
Paranasal sinuses (anterior view)

左外侧面观 Left lateral view

1. 蝶窦 sphenoidal sinus
2. 通蝶窦的探针 specillum in sphenoidal sinus
3. 通筛窦后组的探针 specillum in posterior group of ethmoidal sinuses
4. 上鼻甲 superior nasal concha
5. 上鼻道 superior nasal meatus
6. 中鼻甲 middle nasal concha
7. 中鼻道 middle nasal meatus
8. 下鼻甲 inferior nasal concha
9. 咽鼓管圆枕 tubal torus
10. 咽鼓管咽口 pharyngeal opening of auditory tube
11. 下鼻道 inferior nasal meatus
12. 鼻阈 nasal limen
13. 通上颌窦的探针 specillum in maxillary sinus
14. 通筛窦前组的探针 specillum in anterior group of sphenoid sinus
15. 通筛窦中组的探针 specillum in middle group of sphenoid sinus
16. 通鼻泪管的探针 specillum in nasolacrimal duct
17. 通额窦的探针 specillum in frontal sinus
18. 额窦 frontal sinus
19. 筛窦 ethmoidal sinus
20. 上颌窦 maxillary sinus

图 5-2　鼻腔外侧壁及鼻旁窦开口
Lateral wall of the nasal cavity and openings of the paranasal sinuses

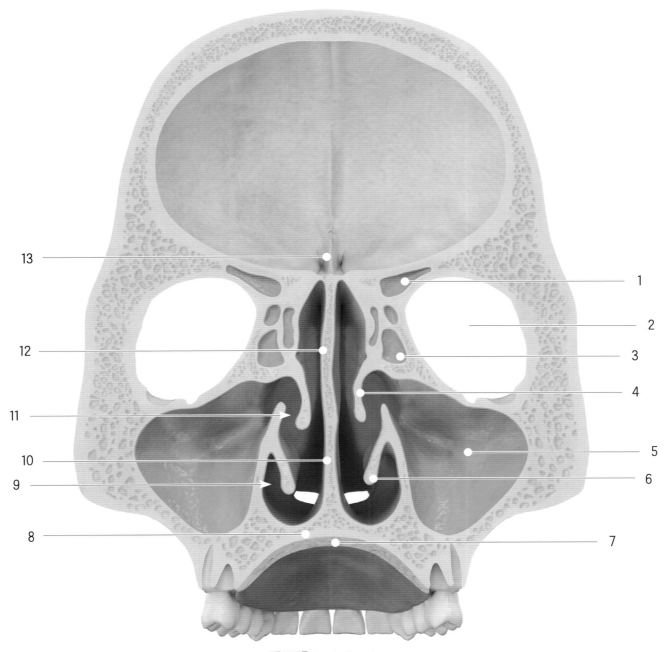

后面观 Posterior view

1. 额窦 frontal sinus
2. 眼眶 orbit
3. 筛骨迷路 ethmoidal labyrinth
4. 中鼻甲 middle nasal concha
5. 上颌窦 maxillary sinus
6. 下鼻甲 inferior nasal concha
7. 口腔黏膜 oral mucosa
8. 硬腭 hard palate
9. 下鼻道 inferior nasal meatus
10. 犁骨 vomer
11. 中鼻道 middle nasal meatus
12. 垂直板 perpendicular plate
13. 鸡冠 crista galli

图 5-3　鼻旁窦冠状断层
Coronal section of the paranasal sinuses

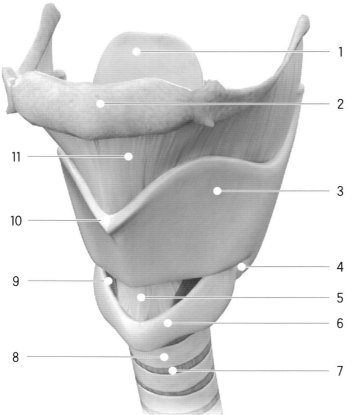

前外侧面观 Anterolateral view

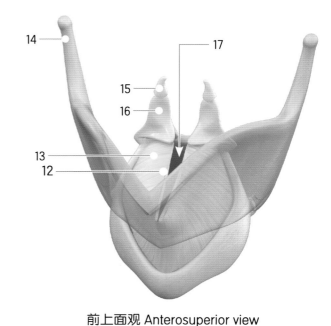

前上面观 Anterosuperior view

1. 会厌软骨 epiglottic cartilage
2. 舌骨体 body of hyoid bone
3. 甲状软骨板 lamina of thyroid cartilage
4. 环甲关节 cricothyroid joint
5. 环甲正中韧带 median cricothyroid lig.
6. 环状软骨弓 arch of cricoid cartilage
7. 环韧带 annular lig.
8. 气管软骨环 tracheal ring
9. 环杓侧肌 lateral cricoarytenoid
10. 喉结 laryngeal prominence
11. 甲状舌骨膜 thyrohyoid membrane
12. 声韧带 vocal lig.
13. 弹性圆锥 conus elasticus
14. 甲状软骨上角 superior cornu of thyroid cartilage
15. 小角软骨 corniculate cartilage
16. 杓状软骨 arytenoid cartilage
17. 声门裂 fissure of glottis
18. 舌骨会厌韧带 hyoepiglottic lig.
19. 方形膜 quadrangular membrane
20. 环杓关节 cricoarytenoid joint
21. 环状软骨板 lamina of cricoid cartilage
22. 膜壁 membranous wall

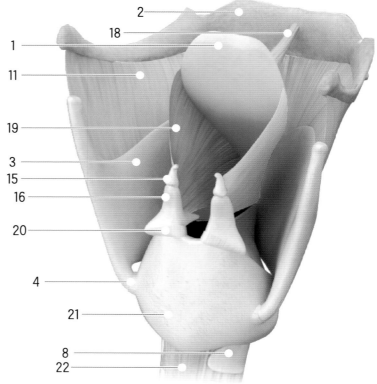

右后外侧面观 Right posterolateral view

图 5-4 喉的软骨及韧带
Cartilages and ligaments of the larynx

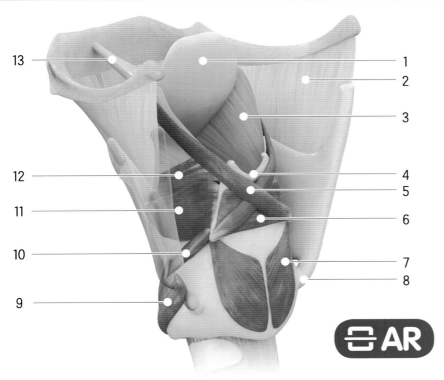

左后外侧面观 Left posterolateral view

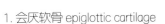

1. 会厌软骨 epiglottic cartilage
2. 甲状舌骨膜 thyrohyoid membrane
3. 方形膜 quadrangular membrane
4. 杓间切迹 interarytenoid notch
5. 杓斜肌 oblique arytenoid
6. 杓横肌 transverse arytenoid
7. 环杓后肌 posterior cricoarytenoid
8. 环甲关节 cricothyroid joint
9. 环甲肌 cricothyroid
10. 环杓侧肌 lateral cricoarytenoid
11. 甲杓肌 thyroarytenoid
12. 甲状会厌肌 thyroepiglottic muscle
13. 舌骨会厌韧带 hyoepiglottic lig.
14. 弹性圆锥 conus elasticus
15. 环甲正中韧带 median cricothyroid lig.

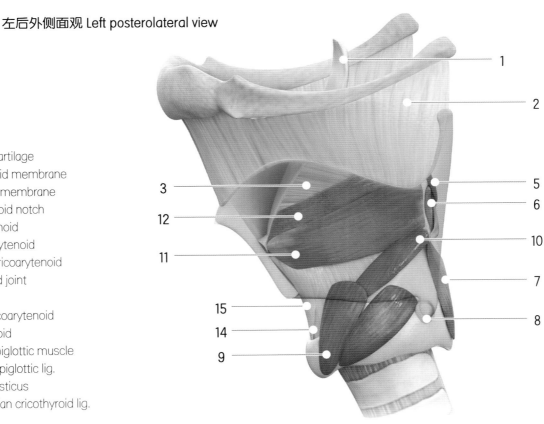

左外侧面观 Left lateral view

图 5-5　喉肌
Laryngeal muscles

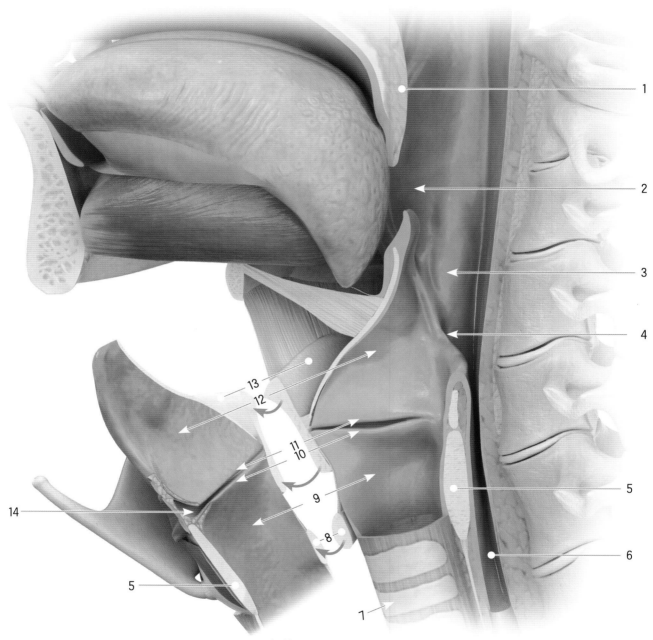

矢状面 Sagittal section

1. 软腭 soft palate
2. 口咽 oropharynx
3. 喉咽 laryngopharynx
4. 喉口 aperture of larynx
5. 环状软骨板 lamina of cricoid cartilage
6. 食管 esophagus
7. 气管 trachea

8. 环状软骨弓 arch of cricoid cartilage
9. 声门下腔 infraglottic cavity
10. 声襞 vocal fold
11. 前庭襞 vestibular fold
12. 喉前庭 laryngeal vestibule
13. 甲状软骨 thyroid cartilage
14. 喉室 ventricle of larynx

图 5-6　喉矢状切面
Sagittal section of the larynx

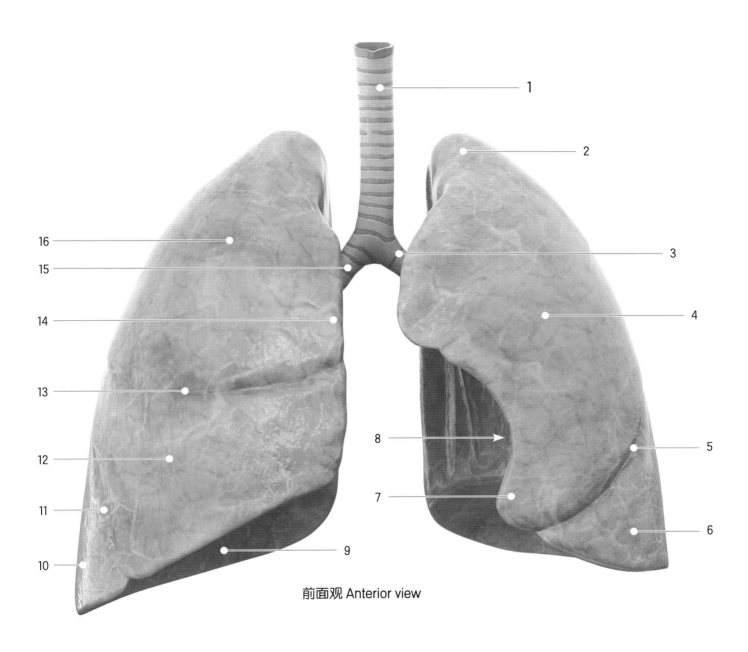

前面观 Anterior view

1. 气管 trachea	9. 肺底 base of lung
2. 肺尖 apex of lung	10. 右肺下叶 inferior lobe of right lung
3. 左主支气管 left principal bronchus	11. 右肺斜裂 oblique fissure of right lung
4. 左肺上叶 superior lobe of left lung	12. 右肺中叶 middle lobe of right lung
5. 左肺斜裂 oblique fissure of left lung	13. 右肺水平裂 horizontal fissure of right lung
6. 左肺下叶 inferior lobe of left lung	14. 右肺前缘 anterior border of right lung
7. 左肺小舌 lingula of left lung	15. 右主支气管 right principal bronchus
8. 心切迹 cardiac notch	16. 右肺上叶 superior lobe of right lung

图 5-7　气管、支气管和肺
Trachea, bronchi and lungs

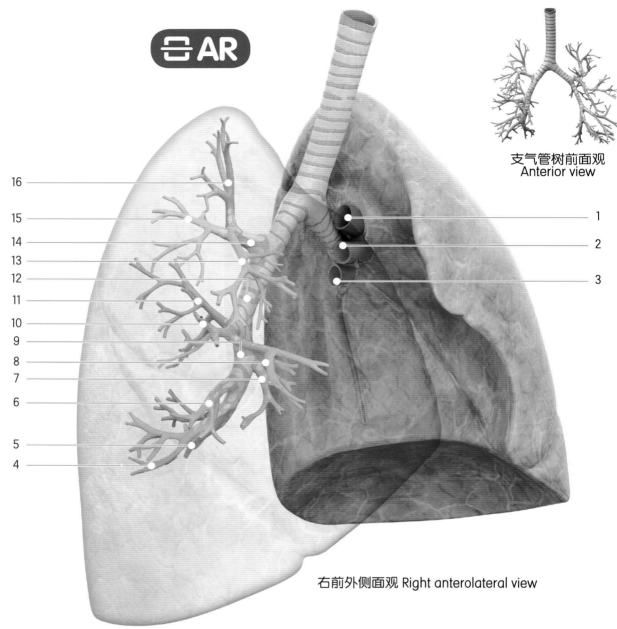

支气管树前面观
Anterior view

右前外侧面观 Right anterolateral view

1. 左肺动脉 left pulmonary a.
2. 左肺上静脉 left superior pulmonary v.
3. 左肺下静脉 left inferior pulmonary v.
4. 右肺下叶外侧底段支气管 right lateral basal segmental bronchus in inferior lobe
5. 右肺下叶后底段支气管 right posterior basal segmental bronchus in inferior lobe
6. 右肺下叶前底段支气管 right anterior basal segmental bronchus in inferior lobe
7. 右肺下叶内侧底段支气管 right medial basal segmental bronchus in inferior lobe
8. 右肺中叶内侧段支气管 right medial segmental bronchus in middle lobe
9. 右肺下叶支气管 right inferior lobar bronchus
10. 右肺中叶外侧段支气管 right lateral segmental bronchus in middle lobe
11. 右肺下叶上段支气管 right superior segmental bronchus in inferior lobe
12. 右肺中间支气管 right intermediate bronchus
13. 右肺上叶前段支气管 right anterior segmental bronchus in superior lobe
14. 右肺上叶支气管 right superior lobar bronchus
15. 右肺上叶后段支气管 right posterior segmental bronchus in superior lobe
16. 右肺上叶尖段支气管 right apical segmental bronchus in superior lobe

图 5-8　支气管树、右肺段支气管及左肺门
Bronchial tree, right segmental bronchi and left hilum of lung

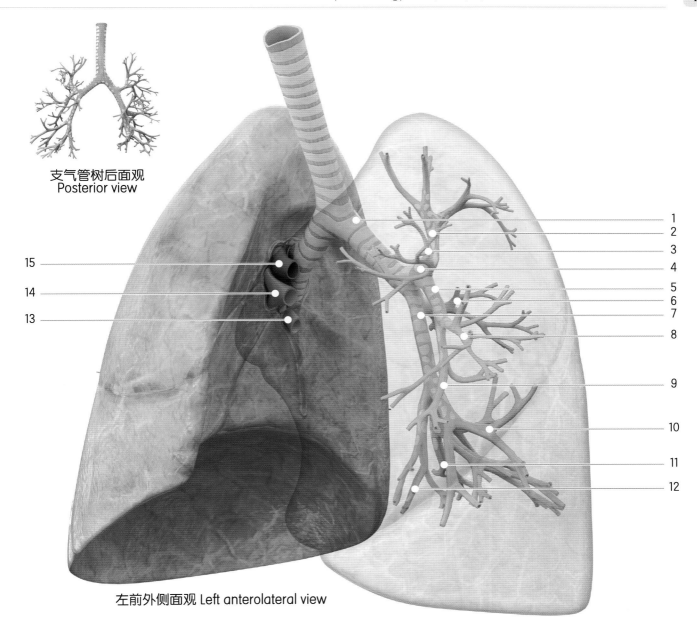

支气管树后面观
Posterior view

左前外侧面观 Left anterolateral view

1. 左主支气管 left principal bronchus
2. 左肺尖后段支气管 left apicoposterior segmental bronchus
3. 左肺上叶前段支气管 left anterior segmental bronchus in superior lobe
4. 左肺上叶支气管 left superior lobar bronchus
5. 支气管舌干 lingular bronchial trunk
6. 左肺下叶上段支气管 left superior segmental bronchus in inferior lobe
7. 左肺下叶支气管 left inferior lobar bronchus
8. 左肺上叶上舌段支气管 left superior lingular segmental bronchus in superior lobe

9. 左肺上叶下舌段支气管 left inferior lingular segmental bronchus in superior lobe
10. 左肺下叶内前底段支气管 left medioanterior basal segmental bronchus in inferior lobe
11. 左肺外侧底段支气管 left lateral basal segmental bronchus
12. 左肺下叶后底段支气管 left posterior basal segmental bronchus in inferior lobe
13. 右肺下静脉 right inferior pulmonary v.
14. 右肺上静脉 right superior pulmonary v.
15. 右肺动脉 right pulmonary a.

图 5-9　支气管树、左肺段支气管及右肺门
Bronchial tree, left segmental bronchi and right hilum of lung

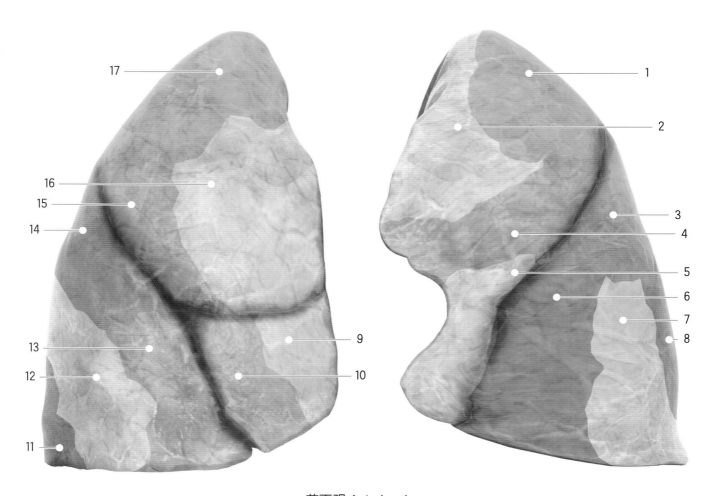

前面观 Anterior view

1. 左肺上叶尖后段 apicoposterior segment in superior lobe of left lung
2. 左肺上叶前段 anterior segment in superior lobe of left lung
3. 左肺下叶上段 superior segment in inferior lobe of left lung
4. 左肺上叶上舌段 superior lingular segment in superior lobe of left lung
5. 左肺上叶下舌段 inferior lingular segment in superior lobe of left lung
6. 左肺下叶内前底段 medioanterior basal segment in inferior lobe of left lung
7. 左肺下叶外侧底段 lateral basal segment in inferior lobe of left lung
8. 左肺下叶后底段 posterior basal segment in inferior lobe of left lung

9. 右肺中叶内侧段 medial segment in middle lobe of right lung
10. 右肺中叶外侧段 lateral segment in middle lobe of right lung
11. 右肺下叶后底段 posterior basal segment in superior lobe of right lung
12. 右肺下叶外侧底段 lateral basal segment in inferior lobe of right lung
13. 右肺下叶内侧底段 medial basal segment in inferior lobe of right lung
14. 右肺下叶上段 upper segment in inferior lobe of right lung
15. 右肺上叶后段 posterior segment in superior lobe of right lung
16. 右肺上叶前段 anterior segment in superior lobe of right lung
17. 右肺上叶尖段 apical segment in superior lobe of right lung

图 5-10　肺段 1
Pulmonary segments 1

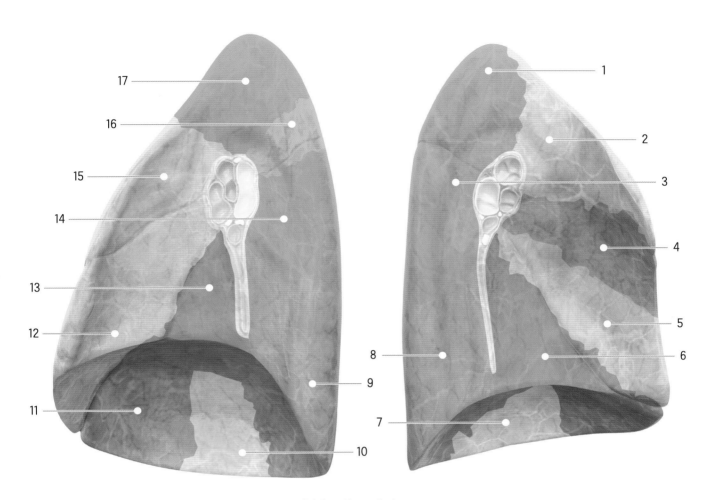

内侧面观 Medial view

1. 左肺上叶尖后段 apicoposterior segment in superior lobe of left lung
2. 左肺上叶前段 anterior segment in superior lobe of left lung
3. 左肺下叶上段 superior segment in inferior lobe of left lung
4. 左肺上叶上舌段 superior lingular segment in superior lobe of left lung
5. 左肺上叶下舌段 inferior lingular segment in superior lobe of left lung
6. 左肺下叶内前底段 medioanterior basal segment in inferior lobe of left lung
7. 左肺下叶外侧底段 lateral basal segment in inferior lobe of left lung
8. 左肺下叶后底段 posterior basal segment in inferior lobe of left lung
9. 右肺下叶后底段 posterior basal segment in inferior lobe of right lung
10. 右肺下叶外侧底段 lateral basal segment in inferior lobe of right lung
11. 右肺下叶前底段 anterior basal segment in inferior lobe of right lung
12. 右肺中叶内侧段 medial segment in middle lobe of right lung
13. 右肺下叶内侧底段 anterior basal segment in inferior lobe of right lung
14. 右肺下叶上段 upper segment in inferior lobe of right lung
15. 右肺上叶前段 anterior segment in superior lobe of right lung
16. 右肺上叶后段 posterior segment in superior lobe of right lung
17. 右肺上叶尖段 apical segment in superior lobe of right lung

图 5-11 肺段 2
Pulmonary segments 2

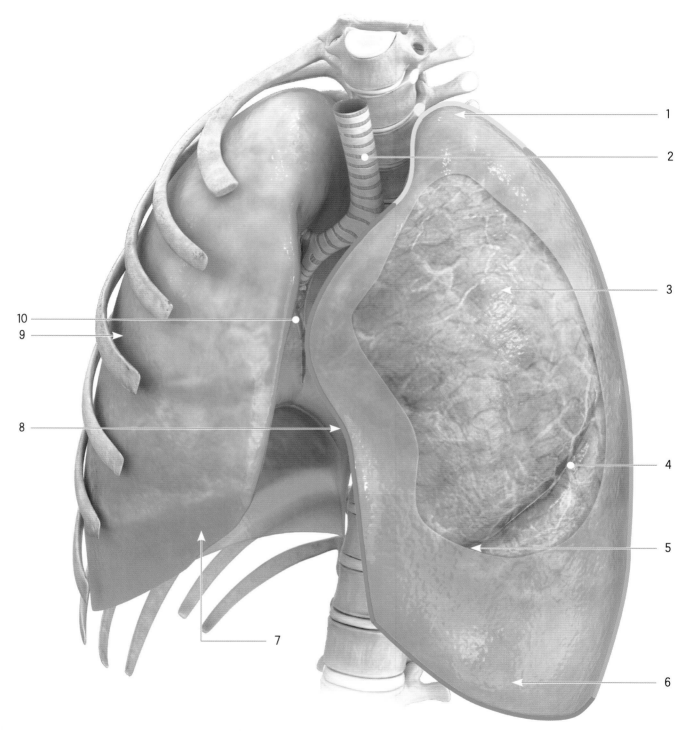

1. 胸膜顶 cupula of pleura
2. 气管 trachea
3. 左肺脏胸膜 visceral pleura of left lung
4. 左肺斜裂 oblique fissure of left lung
5. 左肺胸膜腔 pleural cavity of left lung
6. 肋膈隐窝 costodiaphragmatic recess
7. 膈胸膜 diaphragmatic pleura
8. 胸膜前线 anterior pleural line
9. 肋胸膜 costal pleura
10. 肺韧带 pulmonary ligament

图 5-12 胸膜
Pleura

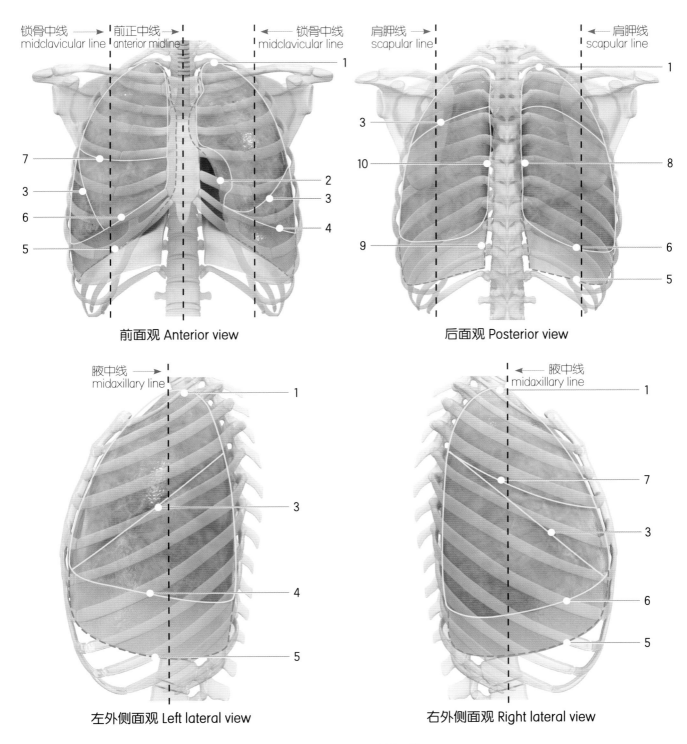

锁骨中线 midclavicular line → ← 前正中线 anterior midline → ← 锁骨中线 midclavicular line

7
3
6
5
1
2
3
4

前面观 Anterior view

肩胛线 scapular line → ← 肩胛线 scapular line

3
10
9
1
8
6
5

后面观 Posterior view

腋中线 midaxillary line →

1
3
4
5

左外侧面观 Left lateral view

← 腋中线 midaxillary line

1
7
3
6
5

右外侧面观 Right lateral view

1. 胸膜顶 cupula of pleura
2. 胸膜前线 anterior pleural line
3. 斜裂 oblique fissure
4. 左肺下缘 inferior border of left lung
5. 胸膜下线 subpleural line
6. 右肺下缘 inferior border of right lung
7. 右肺水平裂 horizontal fissure of right lung
8. 右肺后缘 posterior border of right lung
9. 胸膜后线 posterior pleural line
10. 左肺后缘 posterior border of left lung

图 5-13　肺及胸膜的体表投影
Surface projection of the lungs and pleura

第6章 内脏学
Splanchnology

泌尿生殖系统
Urogenital System

1. 左肾上腺　left suprarenal gland
2. 左肾　left kidney
3. 输尿管　ureter
4. 膀胱　urinary bladder
5. 前列腺　prostate
6. 附睾　epididymis
7. 睾丸　testis
8. 阴茎　penis
9. 输精管　deferent duct
10. 肾盂　renal pelvis
11. 右肾上腺　right suprarenal gland
12. 输卵管　uterine tube
13. 卵巢　ovary
14. 子宫　uterus
15. 前庭球　bulb of vestibule
16. 前庭大腺　greater vestibular gland

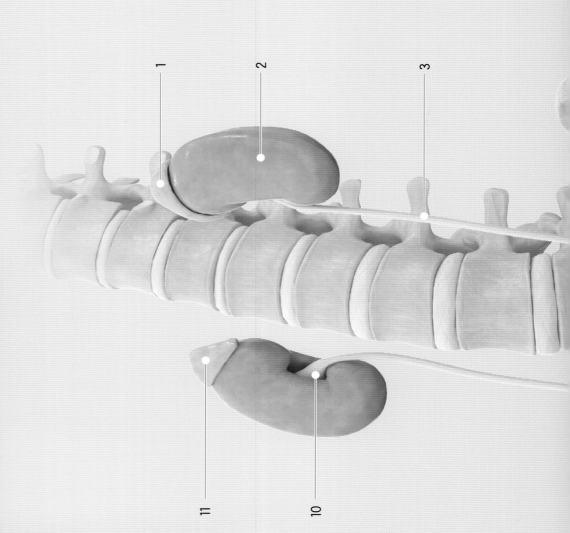

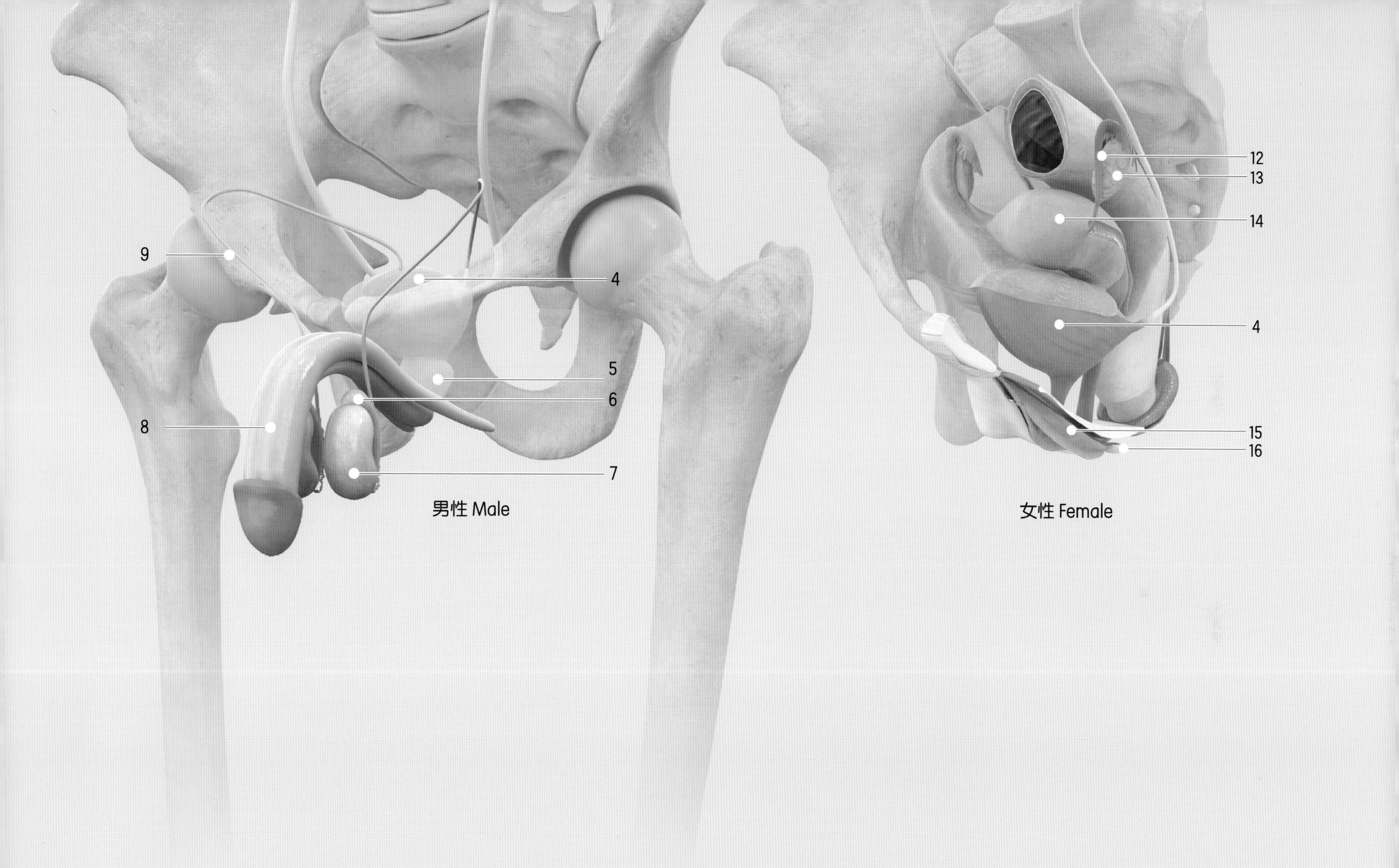

12
13
14

4

15
16

女性 Female

4

5
6

7

男性 Male

9

8

图 6-1 泌尿生殖系统概观
Overview of the urogenital system

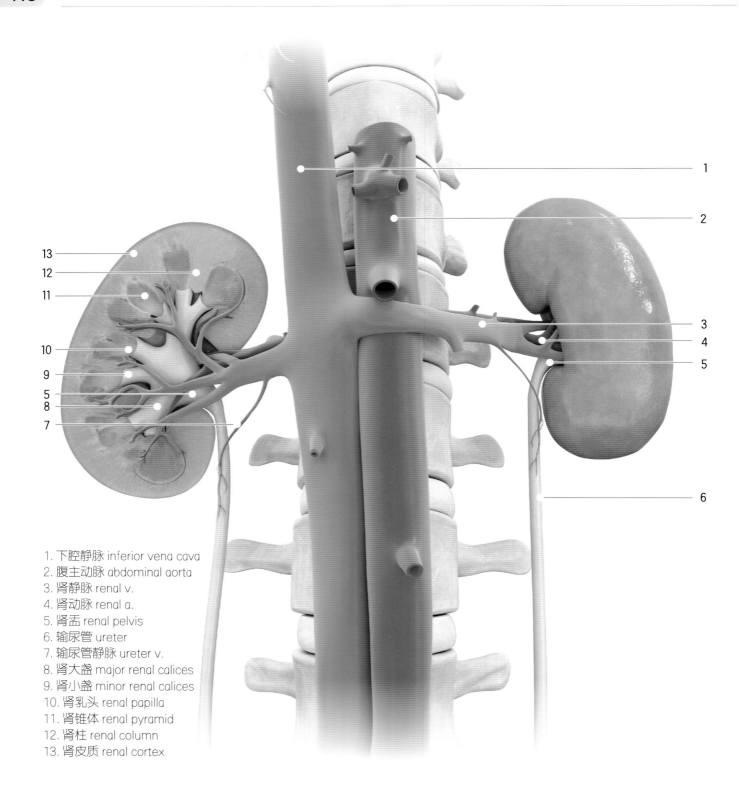

1. 下腔静脉 inferior vena cava
2. 腹主动脉 abdominal aorta
3. 肾静脉 renal v.
4. 肾动脉 renal a.
5. 肾盂 renal pelvis
6. 输尿管 ureter
7. 输尿管静脉 ureter v.
8. 肾大盏 major renal calices
9. 肾小盏 minor renal calices
10. 肾乳头 renal papilla
11. 肾锥体 renal pyramid
12. 肾柱 renal column
13. 肾皮质 renal cortex

图 6-2　肾、输尿管及血管
Kidneys, ureters and blood vessels

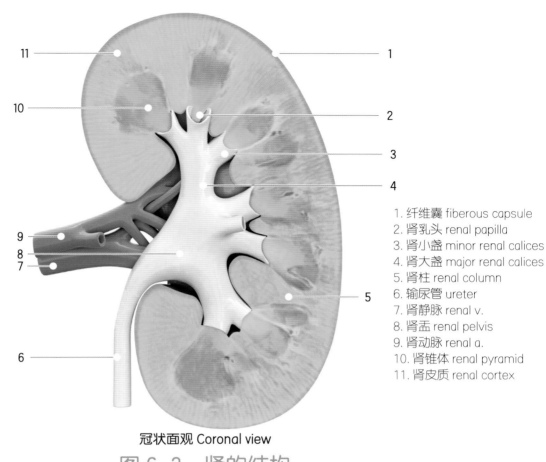

1. 纤维囊 fiberous capsule
2. 肾乳头 renal papilla
3. 肾小盏 minor renal calices
4. 肾大盏 major renal calices
5. 肾柱 renal column
6. 输尿管 ureter
7. 肾静脉 renal v.
8. 肾盂 renal pelvis
9. 肾动脉 renal a.
10. 肾锥体 renal pyramid
11. 肾皮质 renal cortex

冠状面观 Coronal view

图 6-3 肾的结构
Structures of the kidney

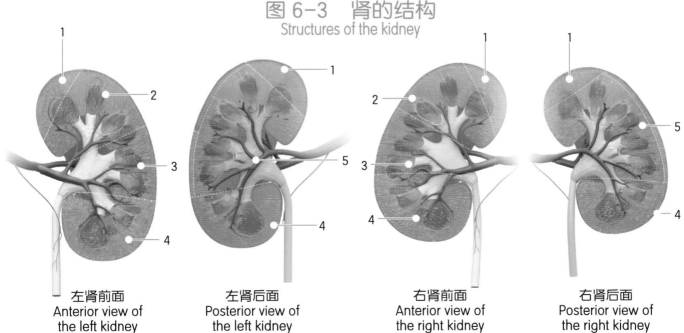

左肾前面
Anterior view of
the left kidney

左肾后面
Posterior view of
the left kidney

右肾前面
Anterior view of
the right kidney

右肾后面
Posterior view of
the right kidney

1. 上段 superior segment（apical）
2. 上前段 superior anterior segment（upper）
3. 下前段 inferior anterior segment（middle）

4. 下段 inferior segment（lower）
5. 后段 posterior segment

图 6-4 肾段动脉模式图
Diagram of the renal segmental arteries

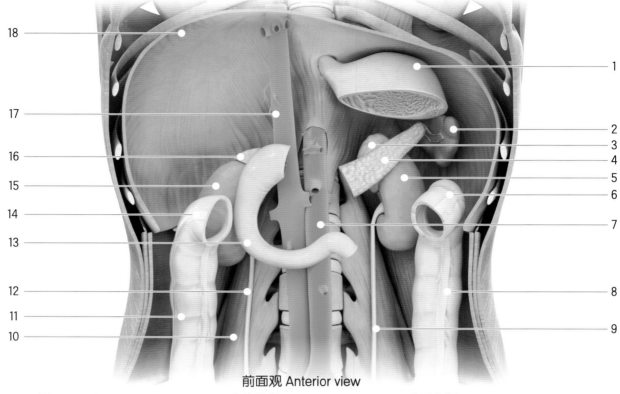

前面观 Anterior view

1. 胃 stomach
2. 脾 spleen
3. 左肾上腺 left suprarenal gland
4. 胰 pancreas
5. 左肾 left kidney
6. 结肠左曲 left colic flexure
7. 腹主动脉 abdominal aorta
8. 降结肠 descending colon
9. 左输尿管 left ureter
10. 腰大肌 psoas major
11. 升结肠 ascending colon
12. 右输尿管 right ureter
13. 十二指肠 duodenum
14. 结肠右曲 right colic flexure
15. 右肾 right kidney
16. 右肾上腺 right suprarenal gland
17. 下腔静脉 inferior vena cava
18. 膈 diaphragm

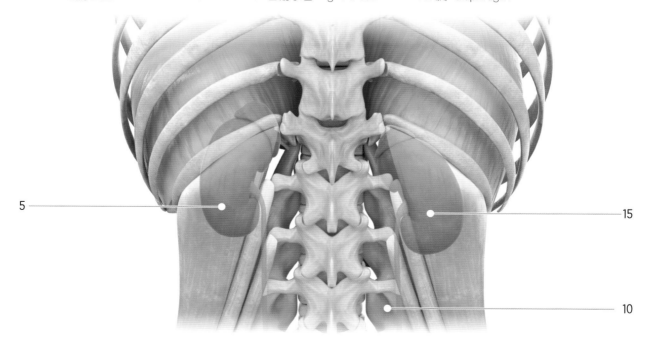

后面观 Posterior view

图 6-5 肾的位置和毗邻
Position and relations of the kidneys

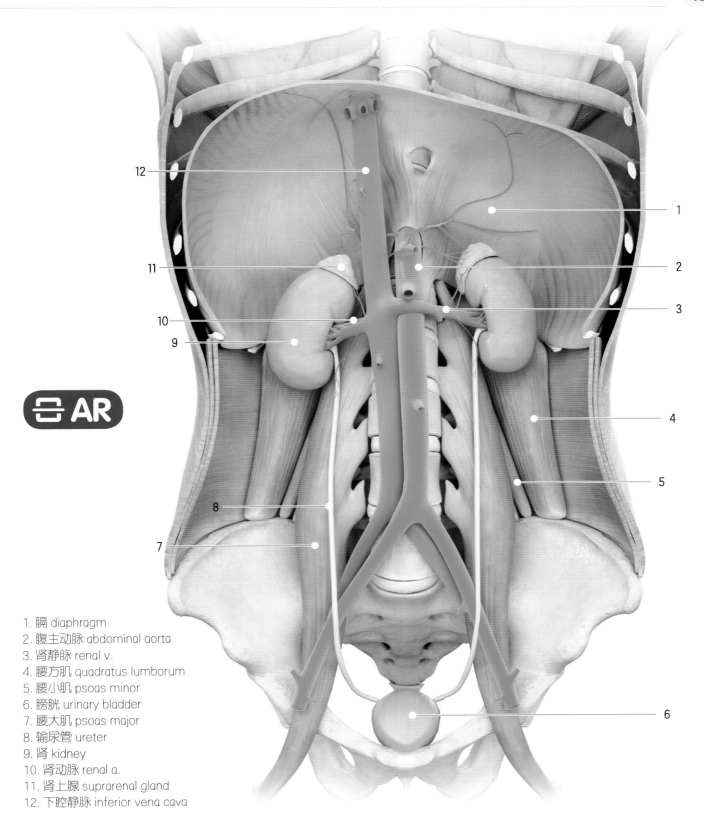

1. 膈 diaphragm
2. 腹主动脉 abdominal aorta
3. 肾静脉 renal v.
4. 腰方肌 quadratus lumborum
5. 腰小肌 psoas minor
6. 膀胱 urinary bladder
7. 腰大肌 psoas major
8. 输尿管 ureter
9. 肾 kidney
10. 肾动脉 renal a.
11. 肾上腺 suprarenal gland
12. 下腔静脉 inferior vena cava

图 6-6　腹后壁（肾及输尿管的位置）
Posterior abdominal wall (with the kidneys and ureters in situ)

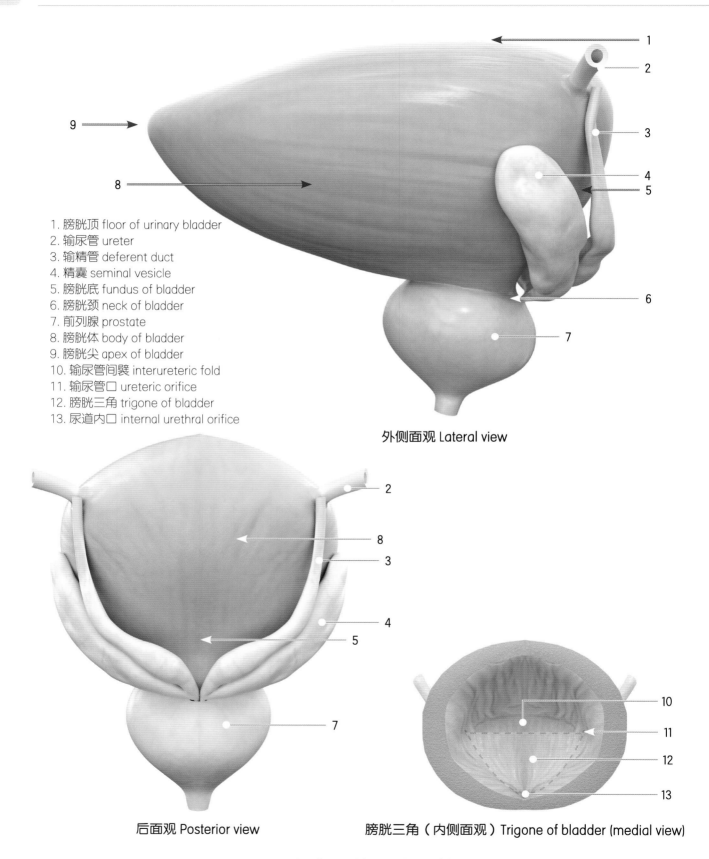

1. 膀胱顶 floor of urinary bladder
2. 输尿管 ureter
3. 输精管 deferent duct
4. 精囊 seminal vesicle
5. 膀胱底 fundus of bladder
6. 膀胱颈 neck of bladder
7. 前列腺 prostate
8. 膀胱体 body of bladder
9. 膀胱尖 apex of bladder
10. 输尿管间襞 interureteric fold
11. 输尿管口 ureteric orifice
12. 膀胱三角 trigone of bladder
13. 尿道内口 internal urethral orifice

外侧面观 Lateral view

后面观 Posterior view

膀胱三角（内侧面观）Trigone of bladder (medial view)

图 6-7 膀胱、前列腺及精囊腺
Urinary bladder, prostate and seminal vesicle

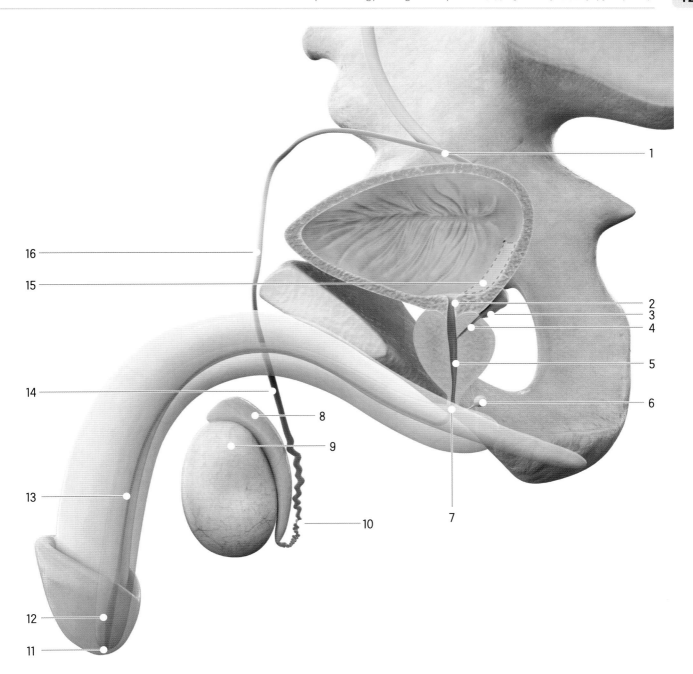

1. 输精管盆部 pelvic part of deferent duct
2. 尿道内口 internal urethral orifice
3. 输精管壶腹 ampulla of deferent duct
4. 射精管 ejaculatory duct
5. 尿道前列腺部 prostatic part of urethra
6. 尿道球 bulb of urethra
7. 尿道膜部 membranous part of urethra
8. 附睾 epididymis
9. 睾丸 testis
10. 输精管睾丸部 testicular part of deferent duct
11. 尿道外口 external orifice of urethra
12. 尿道舟状窝 navicular fossa of urethra
13. 尿道海绵体部 cavernous part of urethra
14. 输精管精索部 spermatic cord part of deferent duct
15. 膀胱三角 trigone of bladder
16. 输精管腹股沟管部 inguinal canal part of deferent duct

图 6-8　男性生殖系统正中矢状面
Median sagittal section of the male urogenital system

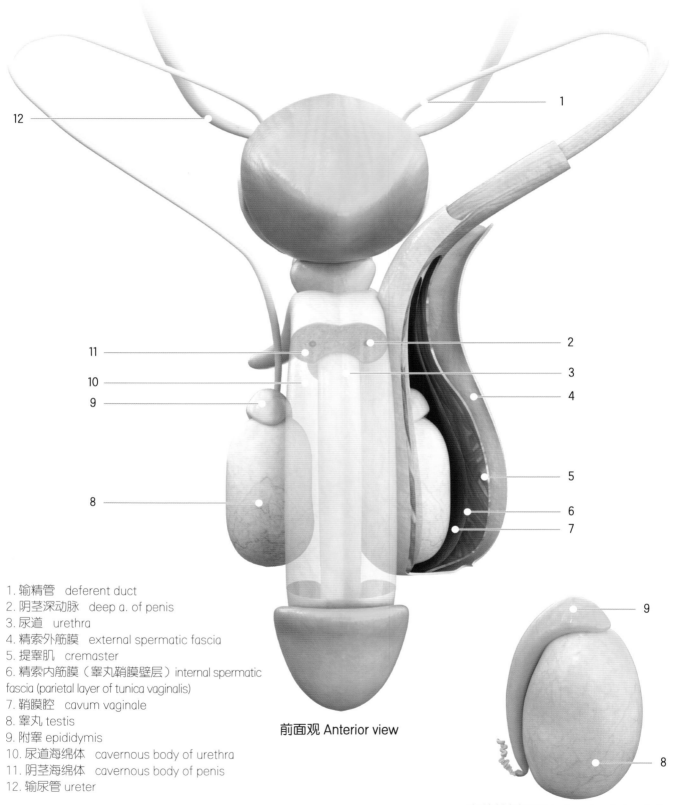

1. 输精管　deferent duct
2. 阴茎深动脉　deep a. of penis
3. 尿道　urethra
4. 精索外筋膜　external spermatic fascia
5. 提睾肌　cremaster
6. 精索内筋膜（睾丸鞘膜壁层）internal spermatic fascia (parietal layer of tunica vaginalis)
7. 鞘膜腔　cavum vaginale
8. 睾丸　testis
9. 附睾　epididymis
10. 尿道海绵体　cavernous body of urethra
11. 阴茎海绵体　cavernous body of penis
12. 输尿管　ureter

前面观 Anterior view

左前外侧面观 Left anterolateral view

图 6-9　阴茎、睾丸和附睾 1
Penis, testis and epididymis 1

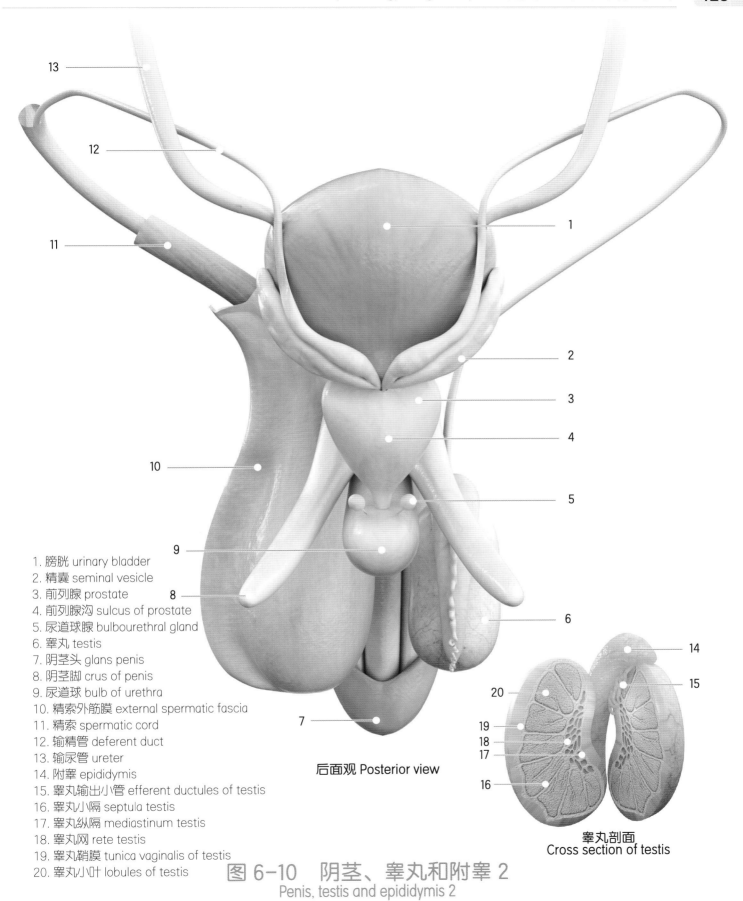

1. 膀胱 urinary bladder
2. 精囊 seminal vesicle
3. 前列腺 prostate
4. 前列腺沟 sulcus of prostate
5. 尿道球腺 bulbourethral gland
6. 睾丸 testis
7. 阴茎头 glans penis
8. 阴茎脚 crus of penis
9. 尿道球 bulb of urethra
10. 精索外筋膜 external spermatic fascia
11. 精索 spermatic cord
12. 输精管 deferent duct
13. 输尿管 ureter
14. 附睾 epididymis
15. 睾丸输出小管 efferent ductules of testis
16. 睾丸小隔 septula testis
17. 睾丸纵隔 mediastinum testis
18. 睾丸网 rete testis
19. 睾丸鞘膜 tunica vaginalis of testis
20. 睾丸小叶 lobules of testis

后面观 Posterior view

睾丸剖面
Cross section of testis

图 6-10　阴茎、睾丸和附睾 2
Penis, testis and epididymis 2

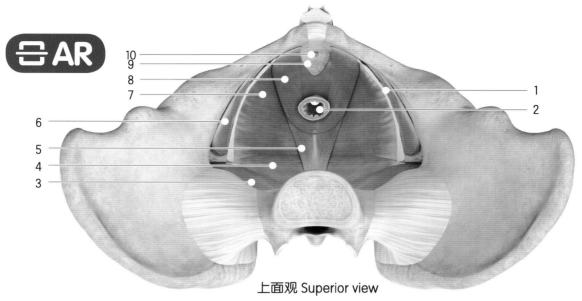

上面观 Superior view

1. 肛提肌腱弓 tendinous arch of levator ani
2. 直肠 rectum
3. 梨状肌 piriformis
4. 尾骨肌 coccygeus
5. 耻尾肌 pubococcygeus
6. 闭孔内肌 obturator internus
7. 髂尾肌 iliococcygeus
8. 耻骨直肠肌 puborectalis
9. 尿生殖膈 urogenital diaphragm
10. 尿道 urethra

图 6-11   男性盆肌
Male pelvic muscles

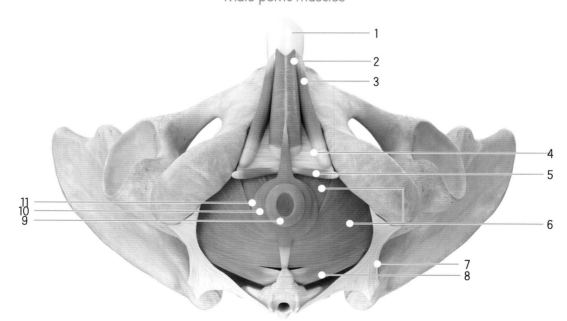

下面观 Inferior view

1. 阴茎深筋膜 deep fascia of penis
2. 球海绵体肌 bulbocavernosus
3. 坐骨海绵体肌 ischiocavernosus
4. 尿生殖膈下筋膜 inferior fascia of urogenital diaphragm
5. 会阴浅横肌 superficial transverse muscle of perineum
6. 肛提肌 levator ani
7. 骶结节韧带 sacrotuberous lig.
8. 尾骨肌 coccygeus
9. 肛门外括约肌（皮下）external anal sphincter (subcutaneous part)
10. 肛门外括约肌（浅部）external anal sphincter (superficial part)
11. 肛门外括约肌（深部）external anal sphincter (deep part)

图 6-12   男会阴肌
Male perineum muscles

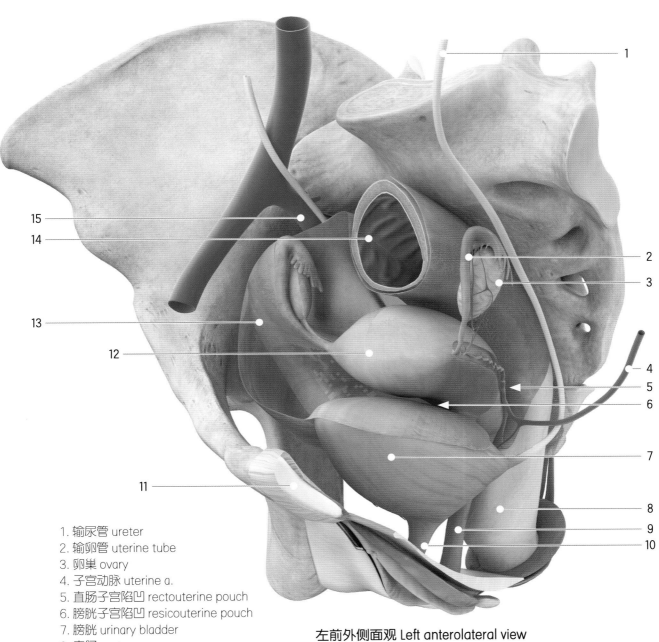

1. 输尿管 ureter
2. 输卵管 uterine tube
3. 卵巢 ovary
4. 子宫动脉 uterine a.
5. 直肠子宫陷凹 rectouterine pouch
6. 膀胱子宫陷凹 resicouterine pouch
7. 膀胱 urinary bladder
8. 直肠 rectum
9. 阴道 vagina
10. 尿道 urethra
11. 耻骨联合 pubic symphysis
12. 子宫 uterus
13. 子宫阔韧带 broad lig. of uterus
14. 直肠 rectum
15. 髂内动脉 internal iliac a.

左前外侧面观 Left anterolateral view

图 6-13　女性盆腔器官
Female pelvic organs

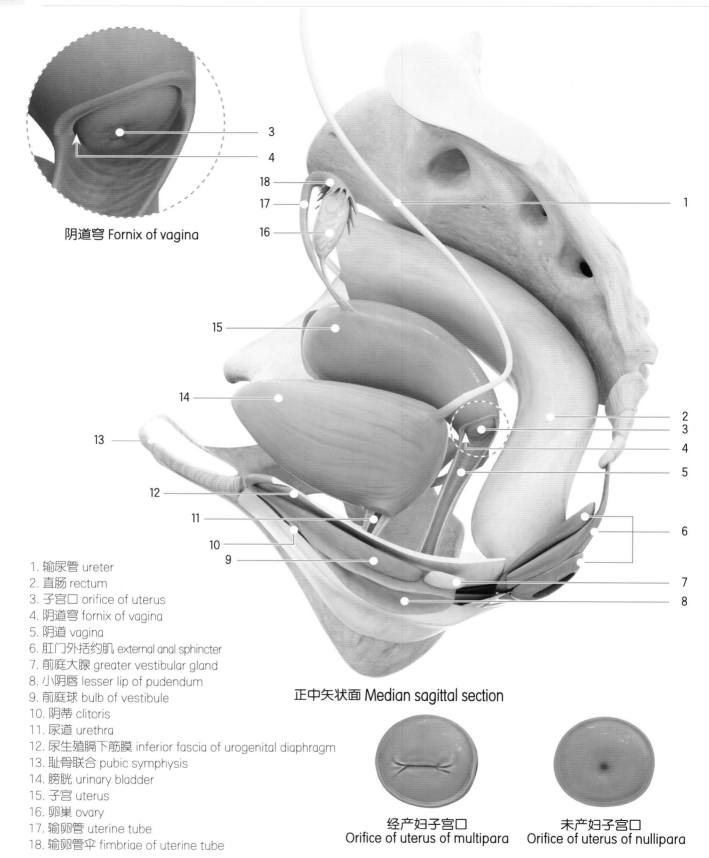

阴道穹 Fornix of vagina

1. 输尿管 ureter
2. 直肠 rectum
3. 子宫口 orifice of uterus
4. 阴道穹 fornix of vagina
5. 阴道 vagina
6. 肛门外括约肌 external anal sphincter
7. 前庭大腺 greater vestibular gland
8. 小阴唇 lesser lip of pudendum
9. 前庭球 bulb of vestibule
10. 阴蒂 clitoris
11. 尿道 urethra
12. 尿生殖膈下筋膜 inferior fascia of urogenital diaphragm
13. 耻骨联合 pubic symphysis
14. 膀胱 urinary bladder
15. 子宫 uterus
16. 卵巢 ovary
17. 输卵管 uterine tube
18. 输卵管伞 fimbriae of uterine tube

正中矢状面 Median sagittal section

经产妇子宫口
Orifice of uterus of multipara

未产妇子宫口
Orifice of uterus of nullipara

图 6-14　女性生殖系统
Female urogenital system

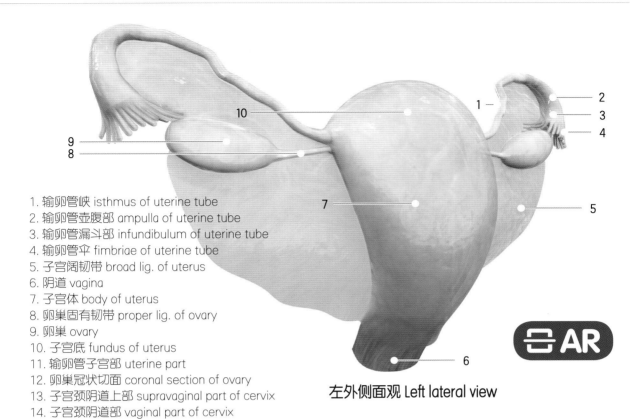

1. 输卵管峡 isthmus of uterine tube
2. 输卵管壶腹部 ampulla of uterine tube
3. 输卵管漏斗部 infundibulum of uterine tube
4. 输卵管伞 fimbriae of uterine tube
5. 子宫阔韧带 broad lig. of uterus
6. 阴道 vagina
7. 子宫体 body of uterus
8. 卵巢固有韧带 proper lig. of ovary
9. 卵巢 ovary
10. 子宫底 fundus of uterus
11. 输卵管子宫部 uterine part
12. 卵巢冠状切面 coronal section of ovary
13. 子宫颈阴道上部 supravaginal part of cervix
14. 子宫颈阴道部 vaginal part of cervix
15. 子宫口 orifice of uterus
16. 子宫颈管 canal of cervix of uterus
17. 子宫峡 isthmus of uterus
18. 子宫腔 cavity of uterus

左外侧面观 Left lateral view

冠状面 Coronal section

图 6-15　女性内生殖器（冠状面）
Female internal genital organs (coronal plane)

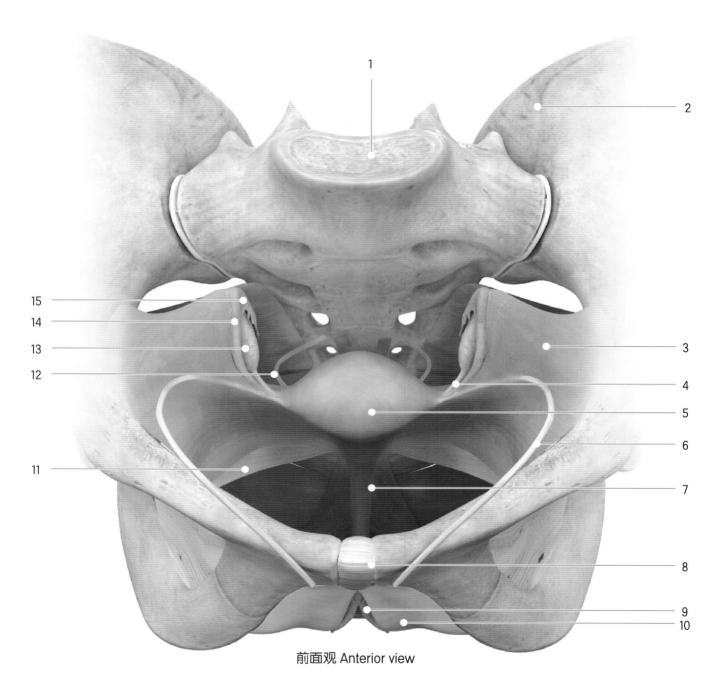

前面观 Anterior view

1. 骶骨 sacrum
2. 髋骨 hip bone
3. 子宫阔韧带 broad lig. of uterus
4. 卵巢固有韧带 proper lig. of ovary
5. 子宫 uterus
6. 子宫圆韧带 round lig. of uterus
7. 阴道 vagina
8. 耻骨联合 pubic symphysis
9. 小阴唇 lesser lip of pudendum
10. 会阴浅筋膜 superficial fascia of perineum
11. 子宫主韧带 cardinal lig. of uterus
12. 子宫骶韧带 uterosacral lig.
13. 卵巢 ovary
14. 输卵管 uterine tube
15. 输卵管伞 fimbriae of uterine tube

图 6-16 子宫固定装置模式图
Diagram of the fixed installation of uterus

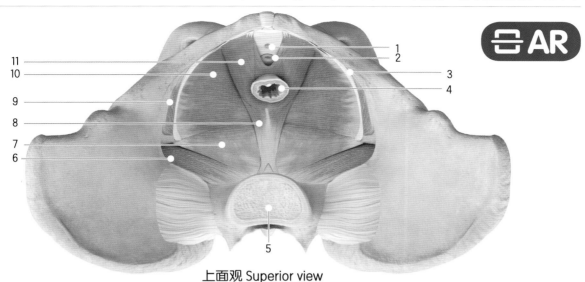

上面观 Superior view

1. 尿道 urethra
2. 阴道口 vaginal orifice
3. 肛提肌腱弓 tendinous arch of levator ani
4. 直肠 rectum
5. 骶骨 sacrum
6. 梨状肌 piriformis
7. 尾骨肌 coccygeus
8. 耻尾肌 pubococcygeus
9. 闭孔内肌 obturator internus
10. 髂尾肌 iliococcygeus
11. 耻骨直肠肌 puborectalis

图 6-17　女性盆肌
Female pelvic muscles

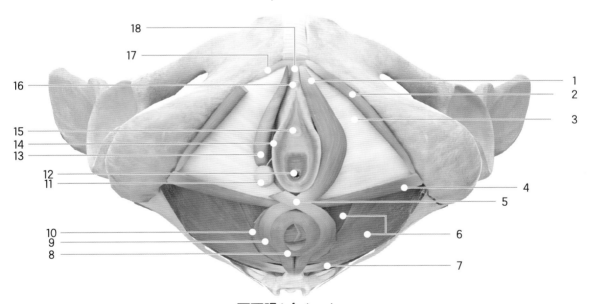

下面观 Inferior view

1. 球海绵体肌 bulbocavernosus
2. 坐骨海绵体肌 ischiocavernosus
3. 尿生殖膈下筋膜 inferior fascia of urogenital diaphragm
4. 会阴浅横肌 superficial transverse muscle of perineum
5. 会阴中心腱 perineal central tendon
6. 肛提肌 levator ani
7. 尾骨肌 coccygeus
8. 肛门外括约肌（皮下）external anal sphincter (subcutaneous part)
9. 肛门外括约肌（浅部）external anal sphincter (superficial part)
10. 肛门外括约肌（深部）external anal sphincter (deep part)
11. 前庭大腺 greater vestibular gland
12. 阴道口 vaginal orifice
13. 前庭球 bulb of vestibule
14. 小阴唇 lesser lip of pudendum
15. 尿道外口 external orifice of urethra
16. 阴蒂 clitoris
17. 阴蒂脚 crus of clitoris
18. 阴蒂体 body of clitoris

图 6-18　女会阴肌
Female perineum muscles

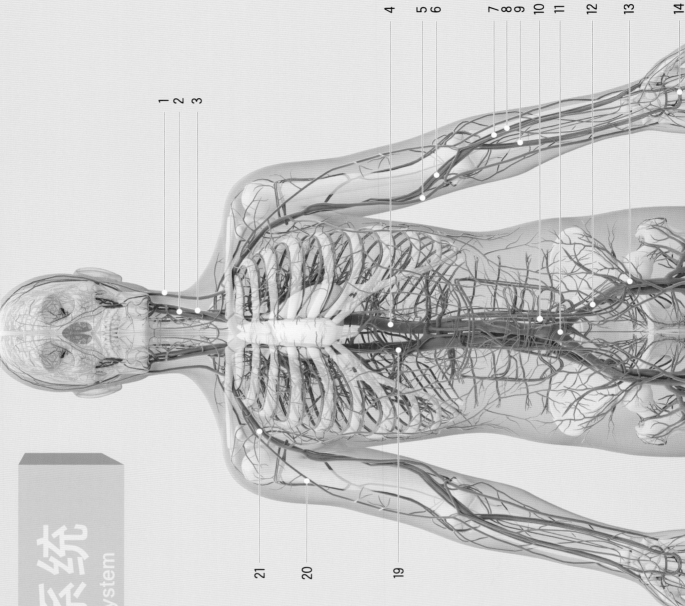

第7章 心血管系统
Cardiovascular System

1. 颈外静脉 external jugular v.
2. 颈总动脉 common carotid a.
3. 颈内静脉 internal jugular v.
4. 胸主动脉 thoracic aorta
5. 贵要静脉 basilic v.
6. 肱动脉 brachial a.
7. 前臂正中静脉 median antebrachial v.
8. 桡动脉 radial a.
9. 尺动脉 ulnar a.
10. 肠系膜下动脉 inferior mesenteric a.
11. 腹主动脉 abdominal aorta
12. 髂总动脉 common iliac a.
13. 髂外动脉 external iliac a.
14. 掌浅弓 superficial palmar arch
15. 胫前动脉 anterior tibial a.
16. 大隐静脉 great saphenous v.
17. 股动脉 femoral a.
18. 股深动脉 deep femoral a.
19. 下腔静脉 inferior vena cava
20. 头静脉 cephalic v.
21. 腋静脉 axillary v.

15
16

18
17

图 7-1 心血管系统概观
Overview of the cardiovascular system

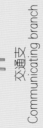

侧支循环　Collateral circulation

侧支吻合　Collateral anastomoses

动、静脉吻合　Arteriovenous anastomosis

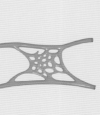

动脉网　Arterial rete

动脉弓　Arterial arcades

交通支　Communicating branch

血管吻合和侧支循环示意图
Vascular anastomosis and collateral circulation

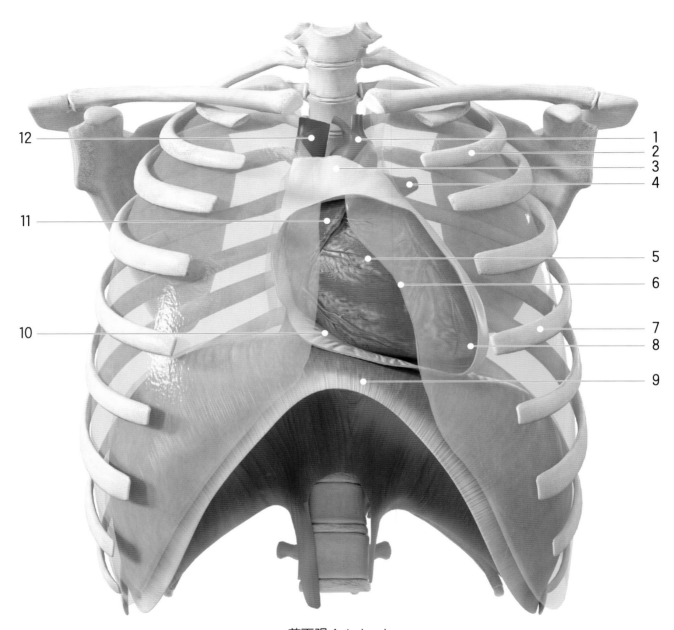

前面观 Anterior view

1. 主动脉弓 aortic arch
2. 第 2 肋 2nd rib
3. 心包 pericardium
4. 左肺动脉 left pulmonary a.
5. 右心室 right ventricle
6. 胸膜前线 anterior pleural line

7. 第 5 肋 5th rib
8. 心尖 cardiac apex
9. 膈 diaphragm
10. 心包腔 pericardial cavity
11. 右心耳 right auricle
12. 上腔静脉 superior vena cava

图 7-2　心的位置
Location of the heart

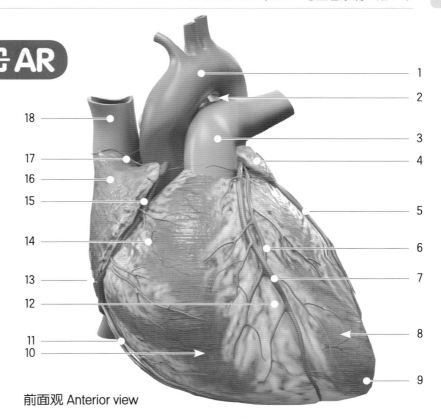

1. 主动脉弓 aortic arch
2. 动脉韧带 arterial lig.
3. 肺动脉干 pulmonary trunk
4. 左心耳 left auricle
5. 左缘支 left marginal branch
6. 心大静脉 great cardiac v.
7. 前室间支 anterior interventricular branch
8. 左心室 left ventricle
9. 心尖 cardiac apex
10. 右心室 right ventricle
11. 右缘支 right marginal branch
12. 前室间沟 anterior interventricular groove
13. 右房支 right atrial branch
14. 右室前支 anterior right ventricular branch
15. 右冠状动脉 right coronary a.
16. 右心耳 right auricle
17. 窦房结支 branch of sinuatrial node
18. 上腔静脉 superior vena cava
19. 右肺动脉 right pulmonary a.
20. 右肺静脉 right pulmonary v.
21. 冠状窦 coronary sinus
22. 下腔静脉 inferior vena cava
23. 心中静脉 middle cardiac v.
24. 后室间支 posterior interventricular branch
25. 右室后支 posterior branch of right ventricle
26. 后室间沟 posterior interventricular groove
27. 左肺静脉 left pulmonary v.
28. 左肺动脉 left pulmonary a.

前面观 Anterior view

后下面观 Posteroinferior view

图 7-3　心的外形
External features of the heart

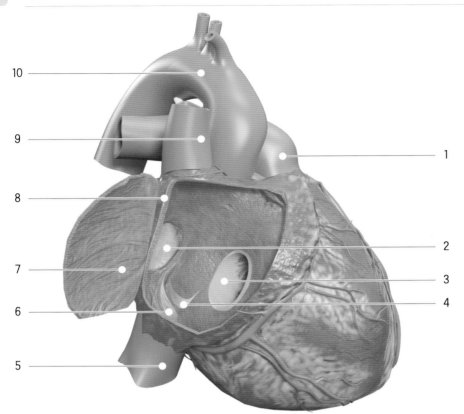

内侧面观 Medial view

图 7-4　右心房
Right atrium

1. 肺动脉干 pulmonary trunk
2. 卵圆窝 fossa ovalis
3. 右房室口 right atrioventricular orifice
4. 冠状窦瓣 valve of coronary sinus
5. 下腔静脉 inferior vena cava
6. 下腔静脉瓣 valve of inferior vena cava
7. 梳状肌 pectinate muscle
8. 界嵴 crista terminalis
9. 上腔静脉 superior vena cava
10. 主动脉弓 aortic arch

1. 主动脉弓 aortic arch
2. 肺动脉瓣 pulmonary valve
3. 动脉圆锥 conus arteriosus
4. 隔侧乳头肌 septal papillary muscle
5. 隔缘肉柱 septomarginal trabecula
6. 前乳头肌 anterior papillary muscle
7. 腱索 chordae tendineae
8. 隔侧尖 septal cusp
9. 前尖 anterior cusp
10. 室上嵴 supraventricular crest
11. 右心耳 right auricle

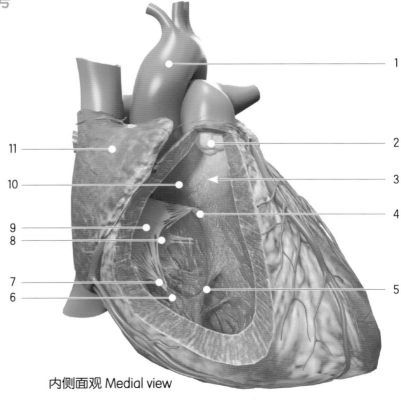

内侧面观 Medial view

图 7-5　右心室
Right ventricle

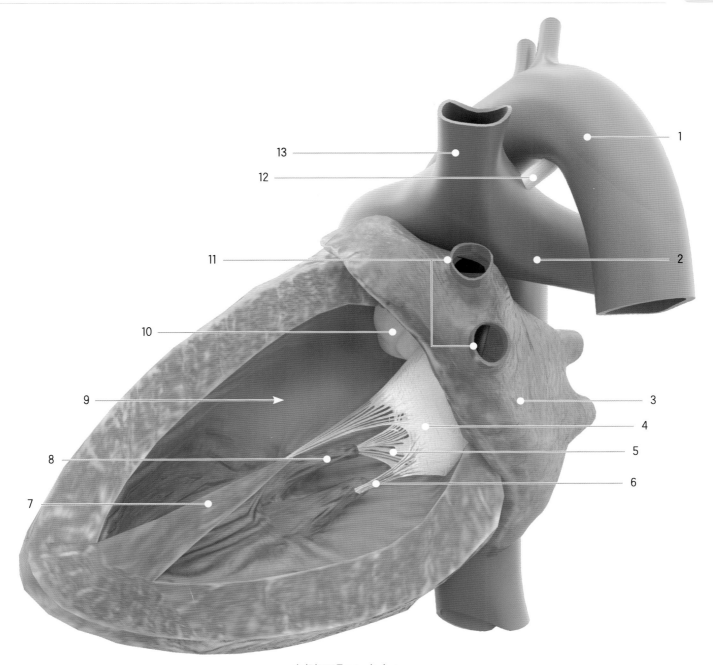

内侧面观 Medial view

1. 主动脉 aorta
2. 右肺动脉 right pulmonary a.
3. 左心房 left atrium
4. 二尖瓣前尖 anterior cusp of mitral valve
5. 二尖瓣后尖 posterior cusp of mitral valve
6. 腱索 chordae tendineae
7. 前乳头肌 anterior papillary muscle
8. 后乳头肌 posterior papillary muscle
9. 左心室 left ventricle
10. 主动脉瓣 aortic valve
11. 左肺静脉 left pulmonary v.
12. 动脉韧带 arterial lig.
13. 左肺动脉 left pulmonary a.

图 7-6 左心室
Left ventricle

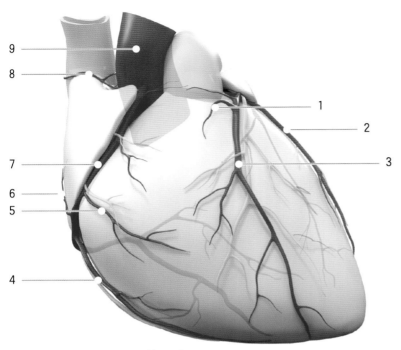

前面观 Anterior view

1. 动脉圆锥支 branch of arterial conus
2. 左缘支 left marginal branch
3. 前室间支 anterior interventricular branch
4. 右缘支 right marginal branch
5. 右室前支 anterior right ventricular branch
6. 右房支 right atrial branch
7. 右冠状动脉 right coronary a.
8. 窦房结支 branch of sinuatrial node
9. 升主动脉 ascending aorta
10. 冠状窦 coronary sinus
11. 后室间支 posterior interventricular branch
12. 右室后支 posterior branch of right ventricle
13. 左室后支 posterior branch of left ventricle
14. 旋支 circumflex branch
15. 左冠状动脉 left coronary a.

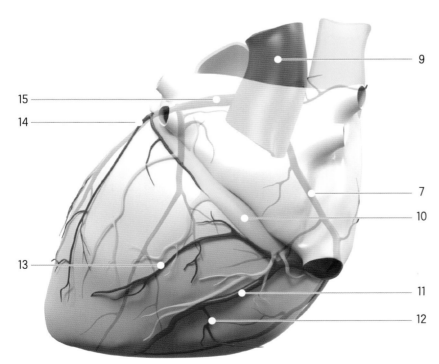

后面观 Posterior view

图 7-7　冠状动脉
Coronary arteries

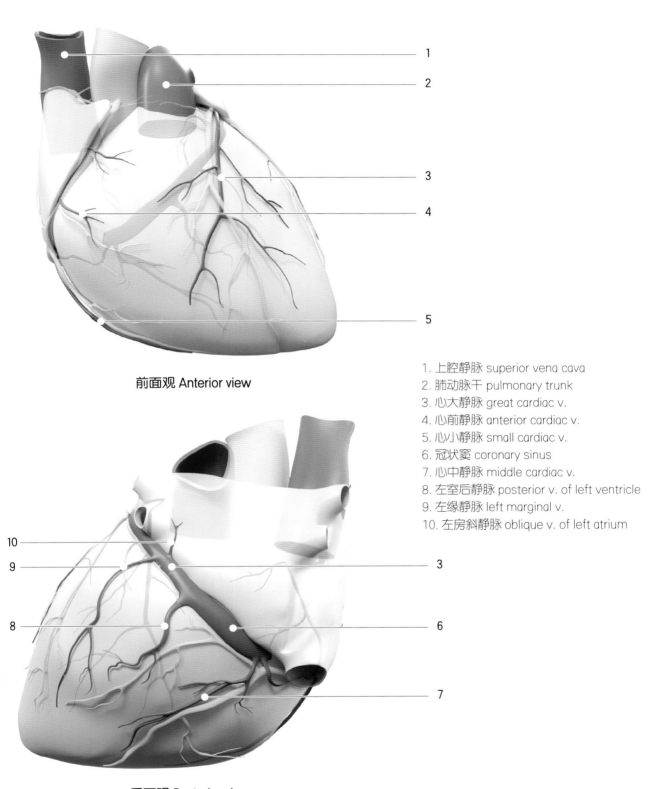

前面观 Anterior view

后面观 Posterior view

1. 上腔静脉 superior vena cava
2. 肺动脉干 pulmonary trunk
3. 心大静脉 great cardiac v.
4. 心前静脉 anterior cardiac v.
5. 心小静脉 small cardiac v.
6. 冠状窦 coronary sinus
7. 心中静脉 middle cardiac v.
8. 左室后静脉 posterior v. of left ventricle
9. 左缘静脉 left marginal v.
10. 左房斜静脉 oblique v. of left atrium

图 7-8 心的静脉
Cardiac veins

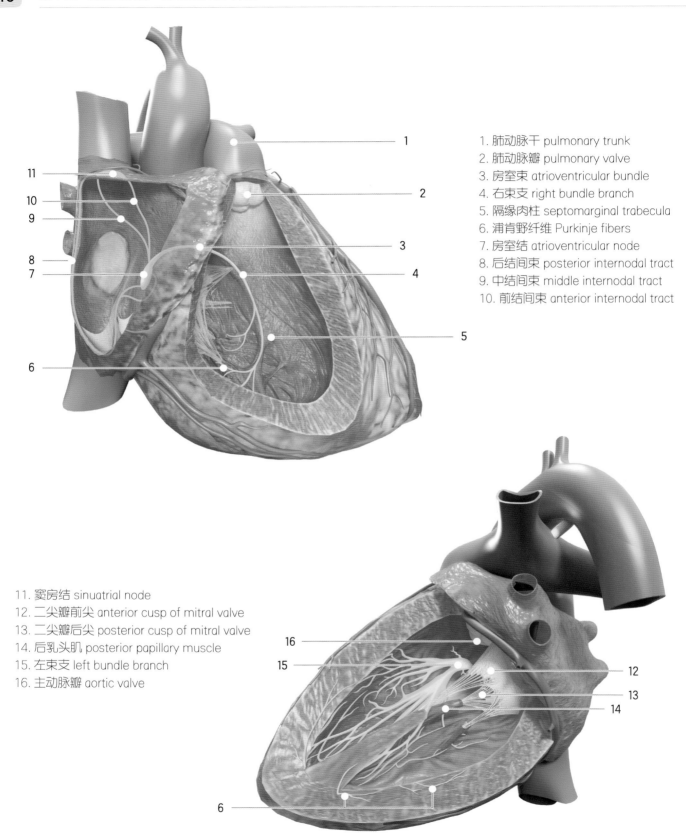

1. 肺动脉干 pulmonary trunk
2. 肺动脉瓣 pulmonary valve
3. 房室束 atrioventricular bundle
4. 右束支 right bundle branch
5. 隔缘肉柱 septomarginal trabecula
6. 浦肯野纤维 Purkinje fibers
7. 房室结 atrioventricular node
8. 后结间束 posterior internodal tract
9. 中结间束 middle internodal tract
10. 前结间束 anterior internodal tract

11. 窦房结 sinuatrial node
12. 二尖瓣前尖 anterior cusp of mitral valve
13. 二尖瓣后尖 posterior cusp of mitral valve
14. 后乳头肌 posterior papillary muscle
15. 左束支 left bundle branch
16. 主动脉瓣 aortic valve

图 7-9　心的传导系统
Conduction system of the heart

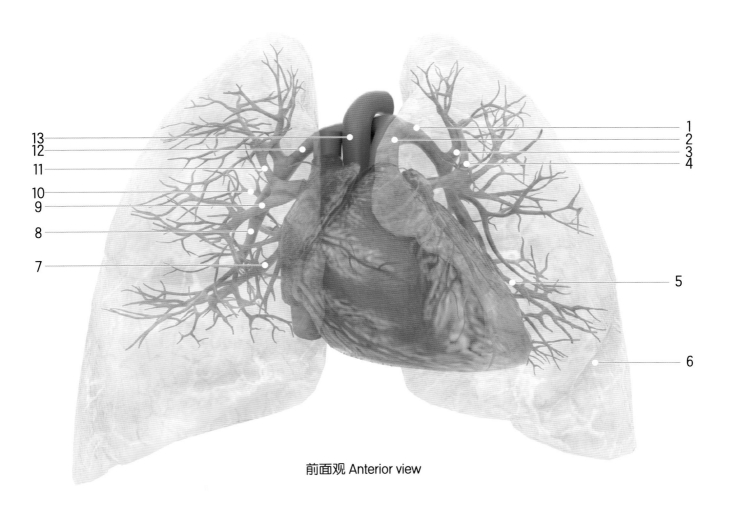

前面观 Anterior view

1. 左肺动脉 left pulmonary a.
2. 肺动脉干 pulmonary trunk
3. 左肺上叶动脉 a. of superior lobe of left lung
4. 左肺上叶静脉 v. of superior lobe of left lung
5. 左肺下叶静脉 v. of inferior lobe of left lung
6. 左肺斜裂 oblique fissure of left lung
7. 右肺下叶静脉 v. of inferior lobe of right lung

8. 右肺下叶动脉 a. of inferior lobe of right lung
9. 右肺中叶静脉 v. of middle lobe of right lung
10. 右肺叶间动脉 interbobar a. of right lung
11. 右肺上叶静脉 v. of superior lobe of right lung
12. 右肺动脉 right pulmonary a.
13. 升主动脉 ascending aorta

图 7-10　肺循环
Pulmonary circulation

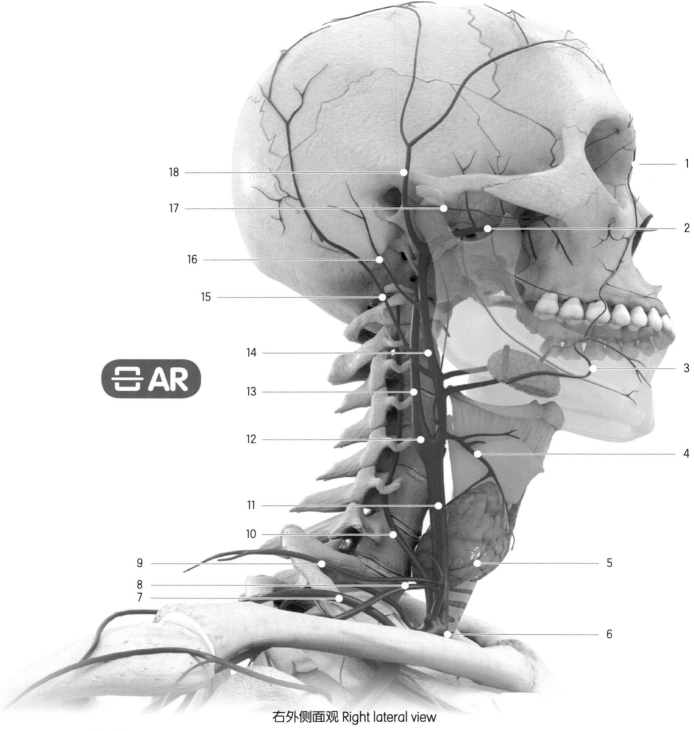

右外侧面观 Right lateral view

1. 内眦动脉 angular a.
2. 上颌动脉 maxillary a.
3. 面动脉 facial a.
4. 甲状腺上动脉 superior thyroid a.
5. 甲状腺下动脉 inferior thyroid a.
6. 锁骨下动脉 subclavian a.

7. 肩胛背动脉 dorsal scapular a.
8. 肩胛上动脉 suprascapular a.
9. 颈横动脉 transverse cervical a.
10. 椎动脉 vertebral a.
11. 颈总动脉 common carotid a.
12. 颈动脉窦 carotid sinus

13. 颈内动脉 internal carotid a.
14. 颈外动脉 external carotid a.
15. 枕动脉 occipital a.
16. 耳后动脉 posterior auricular a.
17. 面横动脉 transverse facial a.
18. 颞浅动脉 superficial temporal a.

图 7-11　头颈部动脉 1
Arteries of the head and neck 1

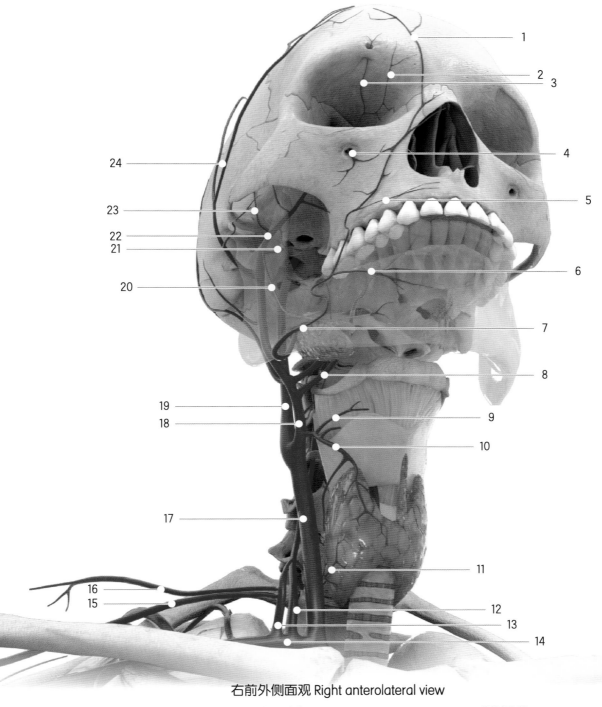

右前外侧面观 Right anterolateral view

1. 内眦动脉 angular a.
2. 滑车上动脉 supratrochlear a.
3. 眶上动脉 supraorbital a.
4. 眶下动脉 infraorbital a.
5. 上唇动脉 superior labial a.
6. 下唇动脉 inferior labial a.
7. 面动脉 facial a.
8. 舌动脉 lingual a.
9. 喉上动脉 superior laryngeal a.
10. 甲状腺上动脉 superior thyroid a.
11. 甲状腺下动脉 inferior thyroid a.
12. 椎动脉 vertebral a.
13. 甲状颈干 thyrocervical trunk
14. 锁骨下动脉 subclavian a.
15. 肩胛上动脉 suprascapular a.
16. 颈横动脉 transverse cervical a.
17. 颈总动脉 common carotid a.
18. 颈外动脉 external carotid a.
19. 颈内动脉 internal carotid a.
20. 下牙槽动脉 inferior alveolar a.
21. 脑膜中动脉 middle meningeal a.
22. 上颌动脉 maxillary a.
23. 颞深动脉 deep temporal a.
24. 颞浅动脉 superficial temporal a.

图 7-12　头颈部动脉 2
Arteries of the head and neck 2

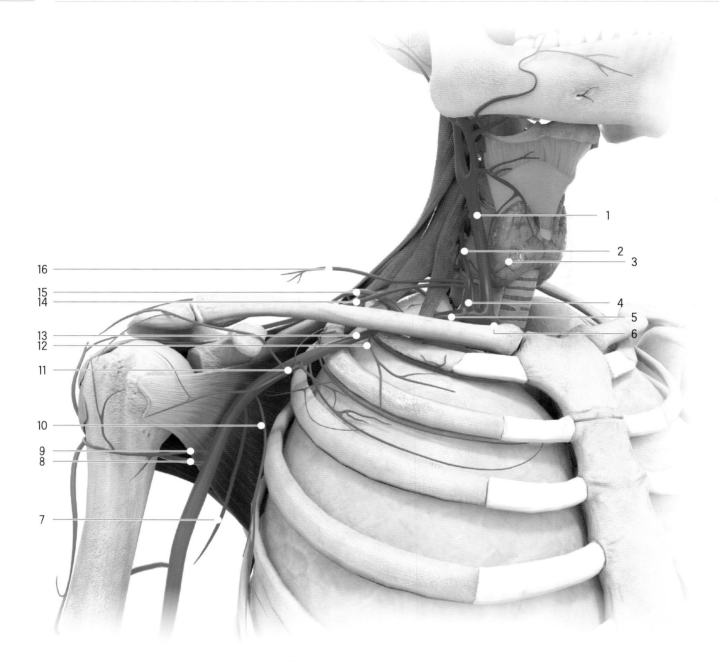

右前外侧面观 Right anterolateral view

1. 右颈总动脉 right common carotid a.
2. 椎动脉 vertebral a.
3. 甲状腺下动脉 inferior thyroid a.
4. 甲状颈干 thyrocervical trunk
5. 右锁骨下动脉 right subclavian a.
6. 头臂干 brachiocephalic trunk
7. 肩胛下动脉 subscapular a.
8. 旋肱后动脉 posterior humeral circumflex a.

9. 旋肱前动脉 anterior humeral circumflex a.
10. 胸外侧动脉 lateral thoracic a.
11. 胸肩峰动脉 thoracoacromial a.
12. 胸上动脉 superior thoracic a.
13. 腋动脉 axillary a.
14. 肩胛上动脉 suprascapular a.
15. 肩胛背动脉 dorsal scapular a.
16. 颈横动脉 transverse cervical a.

图 7-13　锁骨下动脉和腋动脉 1
Subclavian artery and axillary artery 1

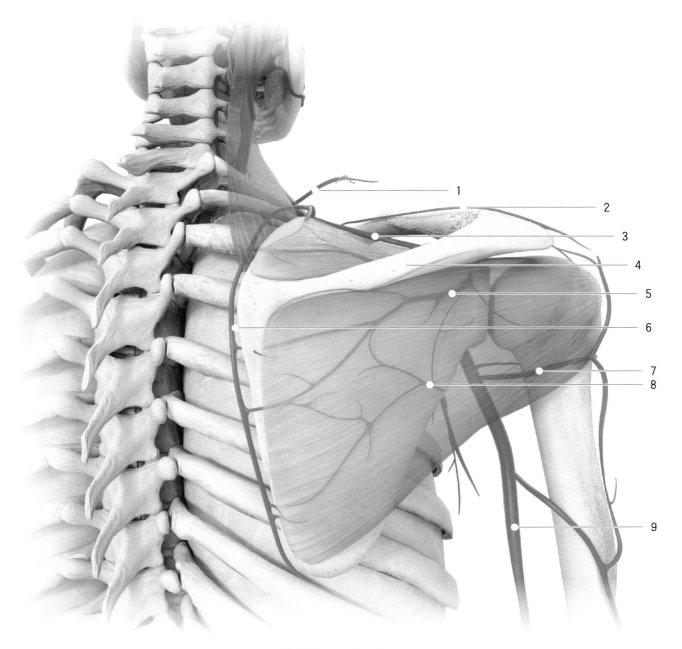

后面观 Posterior view

1. 颈横动脉 transverse cervical a.
2. 肩胛上动脉 suprascapular a.
3. 胸肩峰动脉的肩峰支 acromial branch of thoracoacromial a.
4. 肩胛冈 spine of scapula
5. 肩胛上动脉的冈下支 acromial branch of suprascapular a.
6. 肩胛背动脉 dorsal scapular a.
7. 旋肱后动脉 posterior humeral circumflex a.
8. 旋肩胛动脉 circumflex scapular a.
9. 肱动脉 brachial a.

图 7-14　锁骨下动脉和腋动脉 2
Subclavian artery and axillary artery 2

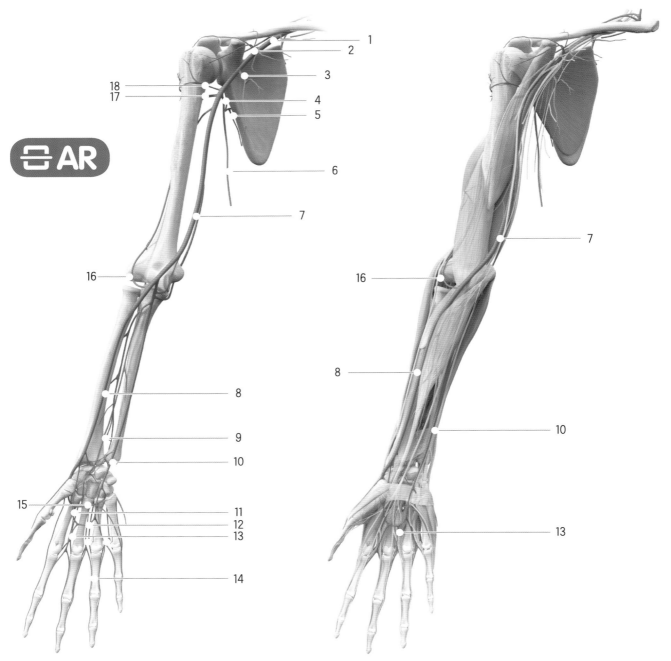

前面观 Anterior view

1. 腋动脉 axillary a.
2. 胸肩峰动脉 thoracoacromial a.
3. 胸外侧动脉 lateral thoracic a.
4. 肩胛下动脉 subscapular a.
5. 旋肩胛动脉 circumflex scapular a.
6. 胸背动脉 thoracodorsal a.

7. 肱动脉 brachial a.
8. 桡动脉 radial a.
9. 骨间前动脉 anterior interosseous a.
10. 尺动脉 ulnar a.
11. 掌浅支 superficial palmar branch
12. 掌浅弓 superficial palmar arch

13. 指掌侧总动脉 common palmar digital a.
14. 指掌侧固有动脉 proper palmar digital a.
15. 掌深弓 deep palmar arch
16. 桡侧返动脉 radial recurrent a.
17. 旋肱后动脉 posterior humeral circumflex a.
18. 旋肱前动脉 anterior humeral circumflex a.

图 7-15　上肢的动脉 1
Arteries of the upper limb 1

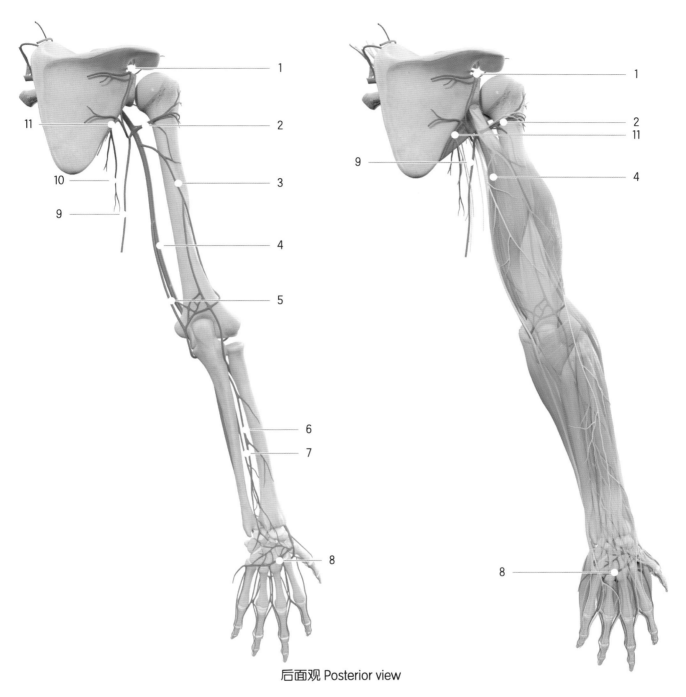

后面观 Posterior view

1. 肩胛背动脉 dorsal scapular a.
2. 旋肱后动脉 posterior humeral circumflex a.
3. 肱深动脉 deep brachial a.
4. 肱动脉 brachial a.
5. 尺侧上副动脉 superior ulnar collateral a.
6. 骨间后动脉 posterior interosseous a.

7. 骨间前动脉 anterior interosseous a.
8. 腕背侧弓 dorsal carpal arch
9. 胸外侧动脉 lateral thoracic a.
10. 胸背动脉 thoracodorsal a.
11. 旋肩胛动脉 circumflex scapular a.

图 7-16 上肢的动脉 2
Arteries of the upper limb 2

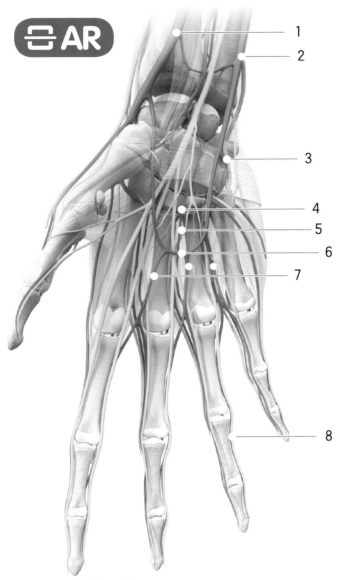

前面观 Anterior view

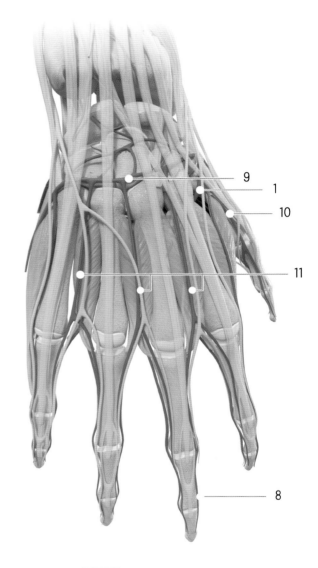

后面观 Posterior view

1. 桡动脉 radial a.
2. 尺动脉 ulnar a.
3. 掌深支 deep palmar branch
4. 掌深弓 deep palmar arch
5. 掌心动脉 palmar metacarpal a.
6. 掌浅弓 superficial palmar arch

7. 指掌侧总动脉 common palmar digital a.
8. 指掌侧固有动脉 proper palmar digital a.
9. 腕背侧弓 dorsal carpal arch
10. 拇主要动脉 principal a. of thumb
11. 指背动脉 dorsal digital a.

图 7-17　手的动脉
Arteries of the hand

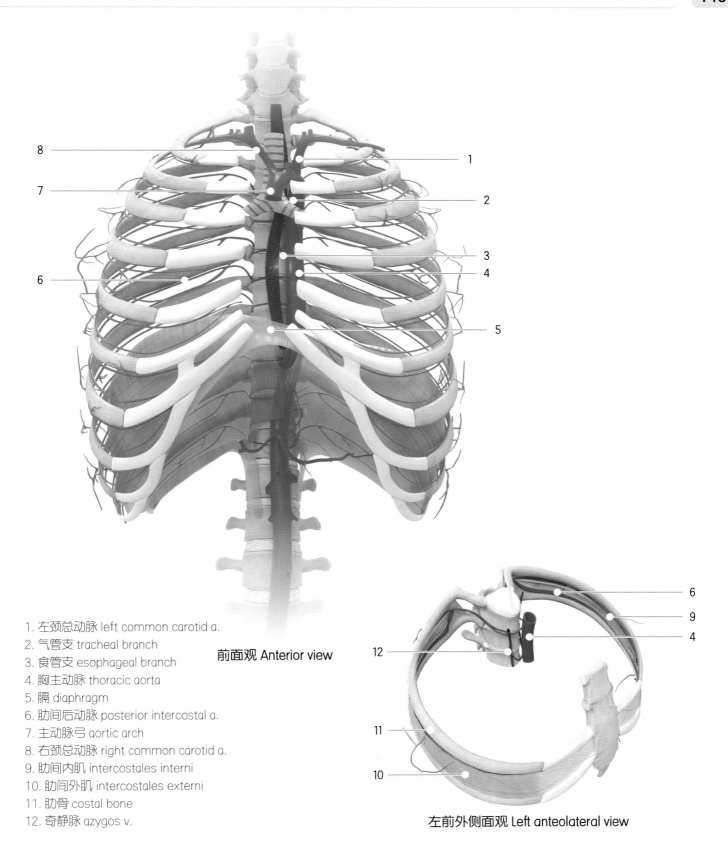

1. 左颈总动脉 left common carotid a.
2. 气管支 tracheal branch
3. 食管支 esophageal branch
4. 胸主动脉 thoracic aorta
5. 膈 diaphragm
6. 肋间后动脉 posterior intercostal a.
7. 主动脉弓 aortic arch
8. 右颈总动脉 right common carotid a.
9. 肋间内肌 intercostales interni
10. 肋间外肌 intercostales externi
11. 肋骨 costal bone
12. 奇静脉 azygos v.

前面观 Anterior view

左前外侧面观 Left anteolateral view

图 7-18 胸部动脉
Arteries of the thorax

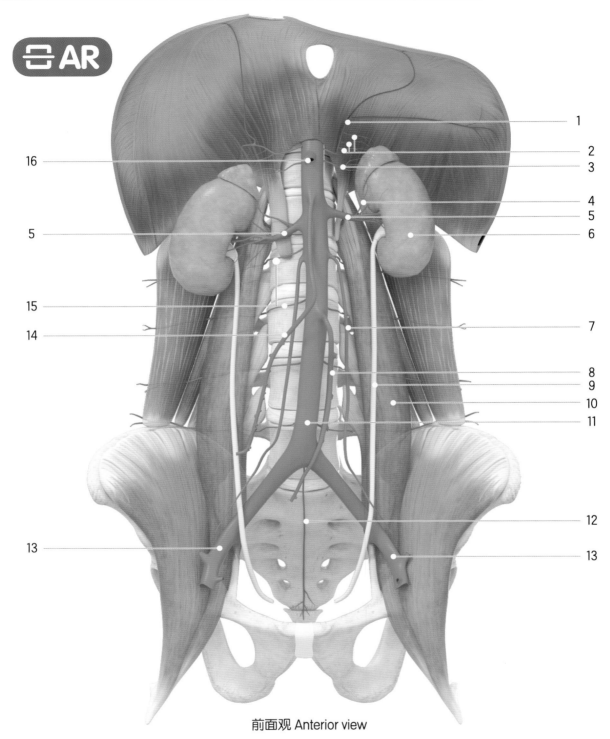

前面观 Anterior view

1. 膈下动脉 inferior phrenic a.
2. 肾上腺上动脉 superior suprarenal a.
3. 肾上腺中动脉 middle suprarenal a.
4. 肾上腺下动脉 inferior suprarenal a.
5. 肾动脉 renal a.
6. 左肾 left kidney
7. 性腺动脉 gonadal a.
8. 肠系膜下动脉 inferior mesenteric a.
9. 输尿管 ureter
10. 腰大肌 psoas major
11. 腹主动脉 abdominal aorta
12. 骶正中动脉 median sacral a.
13. 髂总动脉 common iliac a.
14. 肠系膜上动脉 superior mesenteric a.
15. 腰动脉 lumbar a.
16. 腹腔干 celiac trunk

图 7-19　腹部动脉
Arteries of the abdomen

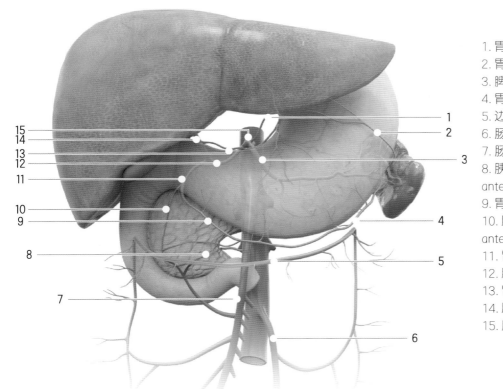

1. 胃左动脉 left gastric a.
2. 胃后动脉 posterior gastric a.
3. 脾动脉 splenic a.
4. 胃网膜左动脉 left gastroepiploic a.
5. 边缘动脉 marginal a.
6. 肠系膜下动脉 inferior mesenteric a.
7. 肠系膜上动脉 superior mesenteric a.
8. 胰十二指肠前下动脉 anteroinferior pancreaticoduodenal a.
9. 胃网膜右动脉 right gastroepiploic a.
10. 胰十二指肠前上动脉 anterosuperior pancreaticoduodenal a.
11. 胃十二指肠动脉 gastroduodenal a.
12. 肝总动脉 common hepatic a.
13. 胃右动脉 right gastric a.
14. 肝固有动脉 proper hepatic a.
15. 腹腔干 celiac trunk

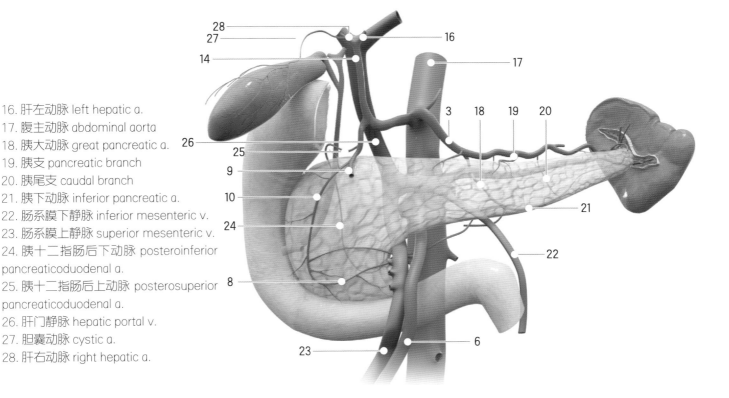

16. 肝左动脉 left hepatic a.
17. 腹主动脉 abdominal aorta
18. 胰大动脉 great pancreatic a.
19. 胰支 pancreatic branch
20. 胰尾支 caudal branch
21. 胰下动脉 inferior pancreatic a.
22. 肠系膜下静脉 inferior mesenteric v.
23. 肠系膜上静脉 superior mesenteric v.
24. 胰十二指肠后下动脉 posteroinferior pancreaticoduodenal a.
25. 胰十二指肠后上动脉 posterosuperior pancreaticoduodenal a.
26. 肝门静脉 hepatic portal v.
27. 胆囊动脉 cystic a.
28. 肝右动脉 right hepatic a.

图 7-20 腹主动脉不成对脏支
Unpaired visceral branches of the abdominal aorta

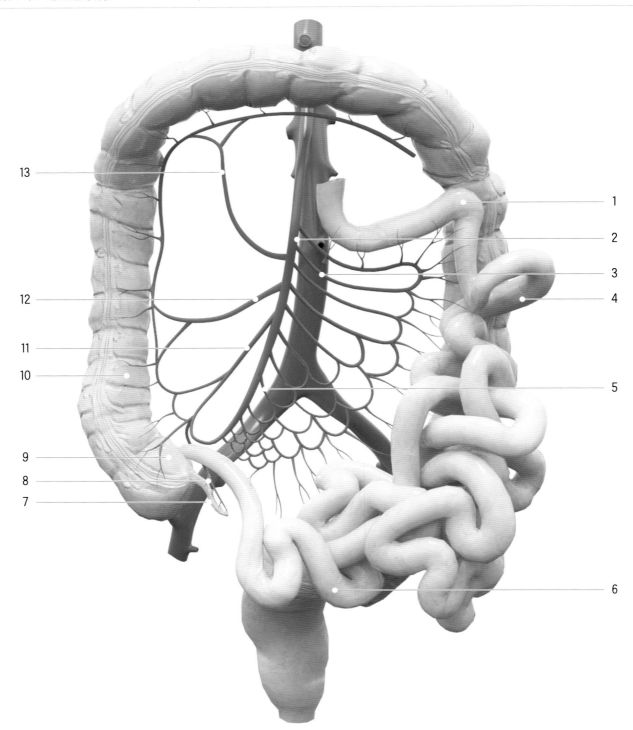

13

1

2

3

4

12

11

10

5

9

8

7

6

前面观 Anterior view

1. 十二指肠空肠曲 duodenojejunal flexure
2. 肠系膜上动脉 superior mesenteric a.
3. 空肠动脉 jejunal a.
4. 空肠 jejunum
5. 回肠动脉 ileal a.
6. 回肠 ileum
7. 阑尾 vermiform appendix
8. 阑尾动脉 appendicular a.
9. 盲肠 cecum
10. 升结肠 ascending colon
11. 回结肠动脉 ileocolic a.
12. 右结肠动脉 right colic a.
13. 中结肠动脉 middle colic a.

图 7-21 肠系膜上动脉及其分支
Superior mesenteric artery and its branches

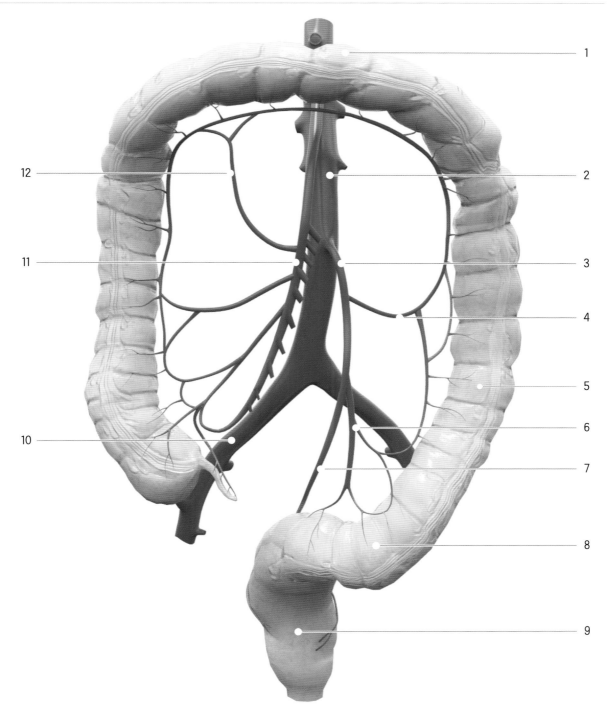

前面观 Anterior view

1. 横结肠 transverse colon
2. 腹主动脉 abdominal aorta
3. 肠系膜下动脉 inferior mesenteric a.
4. 左结肠动脉 left colic a.
5. 降结肠 descending colon
6. 乙状结肠动脉 sigmoid colic a.
7. 直肠上动脉 superior rectal a.
8. 乙状结肠 sigmoid colon
9. 直肠 rectum
10. 髂总动脉 common iliac a.
11. 肠系膜上动脉 superior mesenteric a.
12. 中结肠动脉 middle colic a.

图 7-22　肠系膜下动脉及其分支
Inferior mesenteric artery and its branches

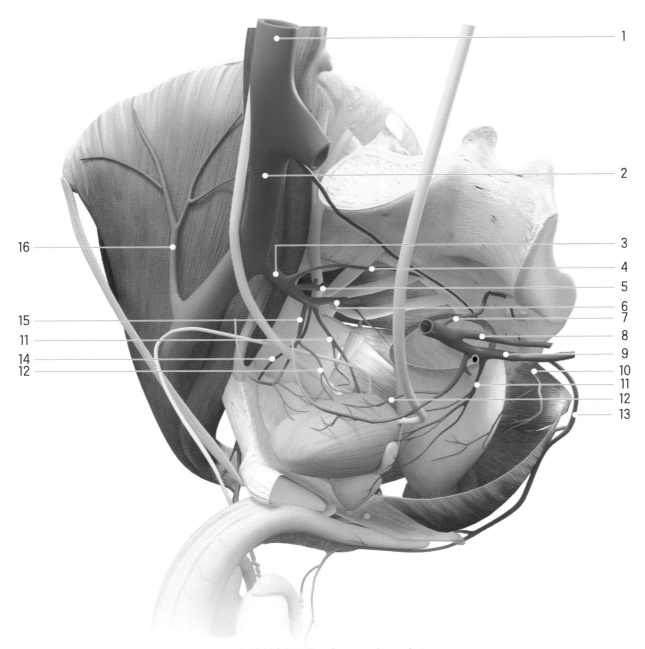

左前外侧面观 Left anterolateral view

1. 腹主动脉 abdominal aorta
2. 髂总动脉 common iliac a.
3. 髂内动脉 internal iliac a.
4. 骶外侧动脉 lateral sacral a.
5. 臀上动脉 superior gluteal a.
6. 臀下动脉 inferior gluteal a.
7. 髂腰动脉 iliolumbar a.
8. 髂内动脉后干 posterior trunk of internal iliac a.
9. 髂内动脉前干 anterior trunk of internal iliac a.
10. 直肠下动脉 inferior rectal a.
11. 膀胱下动脉 inferior vesical a.
12. 膀胱上动脉 superior vesical a.
13. 阴部内动脉 internal pudendal a.
14. 闭孔动脉 obturator a.
15. 脐动脉 umbilical a.
16. 腹壁下动脉 inferior epigastric a.

图 7-23　男性盆腔动脉
Arteries of the male pelvic

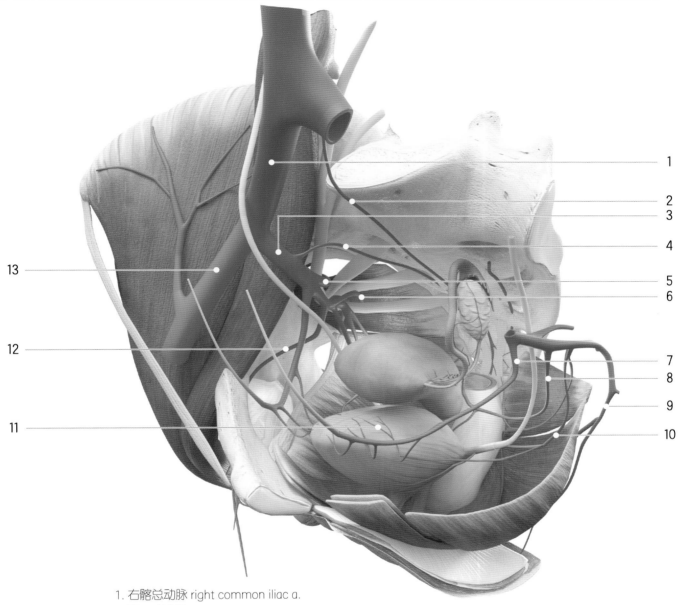

1
2
3
4
5
6
7
8
9
10
11
12
13

左前外侧面观 Left anterolateral view

1. 右髂总动脉 right common iliac a.
2. 骶正中动脉 median sacral a.
3. 髂内动脉 internal iliac a.
4. 骶外侧动脉 lateral sacral a.
5. 臀上动脉 superior gluteal a.
6. 臀下动脉 inferior gluteal a.
7. 脐动脉 umbilical a.
8. 子宫动脉 uterine a.
9. 阴部内动脉 internal pudendal a.
10. 膀胱下动脉 inferior vesical a.
11. 膀胱上动脉 superior vesical a.
12. 闭孔动脉 obturator a.
13. 髂外动脉 external iliac a.

图 7-24　女性盆腔动脉
Arteries of the female pelvic

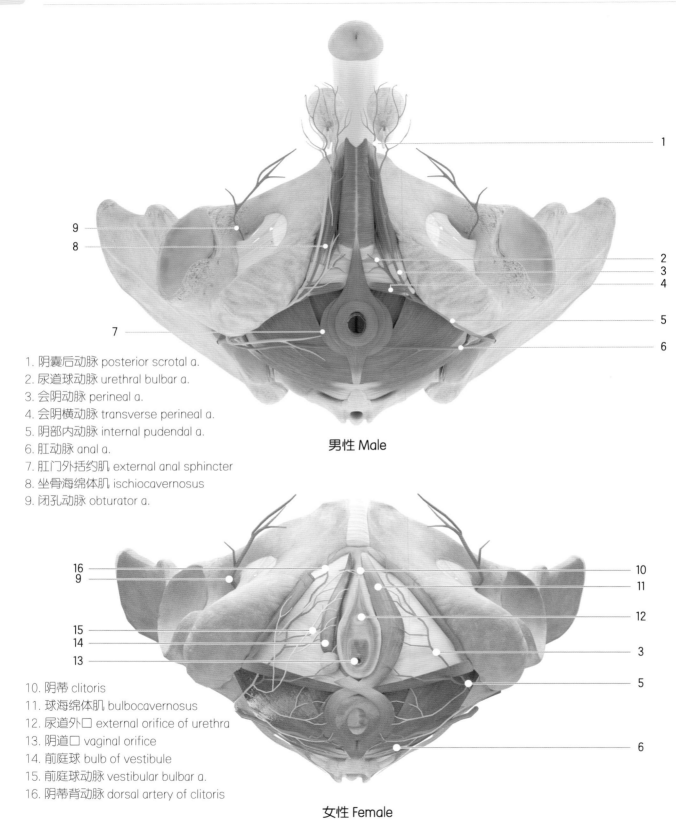

1. 阴囊后动脉 posterior scrotal a.
2. 尿道球动脉 urethral bulbar a.
3. 会阴动脉 perineal a.
4. 会阴横动脉 transverse perineal a.
5. 阴部内动脉 internal pudendal a.
6. 肛动脉 anal a.
7. 肛门外括约肌 external anal sphincter
8. 坐骨海绵体肌 ischiocavernosus
9. 闭孔动脉 obturator a.

男性 Male

10. 阴蒂 clitoris
11. 球海绵体肌 bulbocavernosus
12. 尿道外口 external orifice of urethra
13. 阴道口 vaginal orifice
14. 前庭球 bulb of vestibule
15. 前庭球动脉 vestibular bulbar a.
16. 阴蒂背动脉 dorsal artery of clitoris

女性 Female

图 7-25　会阴部动脉
Arteries of the perineum

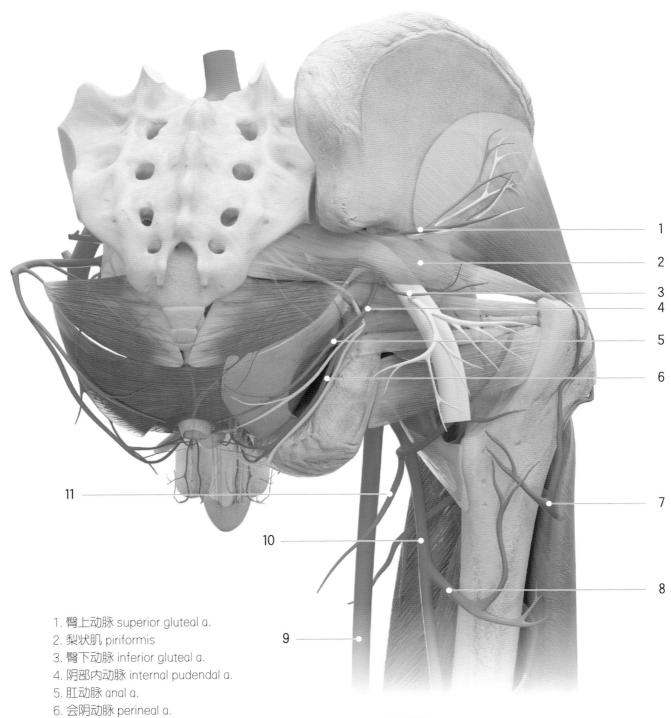

1. 臀上动脉 superior gluteal a.
2. 梨状肌 piriformis
3. 臀下动脉 inferior gluteal a.
4. 阴部内动脉 internal pudendal a.
5. 肛动脉 anal a.
6. 会阴动脉 perineal a.
7. 旋股外侧动脉 lateral femoral circumflex a.
8. 穿动脉 perforating a.
9. 股动脉 femoral a.
10. 股深动脉 deep femoral a.
11. 旋股内侧动脉 medial femoral circumflex a.

后面观 Posterior view

图 7-26　臀部和股后部动脉
Arteries of the gluteal region and posterior aspect of the thigh

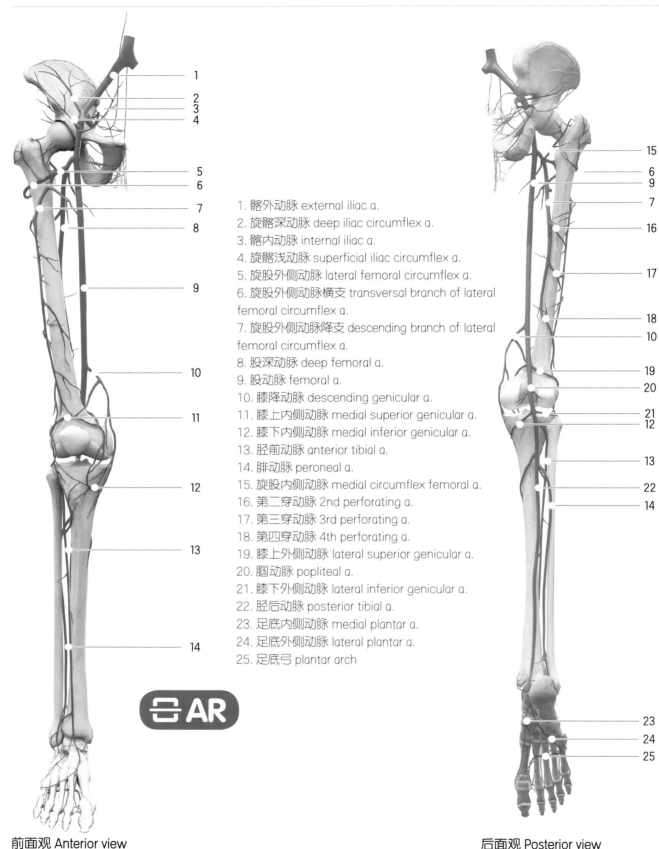

1. 髂外动脉 external iliac a.
2. 旋髂深动脉 deep iliac circumflex a.
3. 髂内动脉 internal iliac a.
4. 旋髂浅动脉 superficial iliac circumflex a.
5. 旋股外侧动脉 lateral femoral circumflex a.
6. 旋股外侧动脉横支 transversal branch of lateral femoral circumflex a.
7. 旋股外侧动脉降支 descending branch of lateral femoral circumflex a.
8. 股深动脉 deep femoral a.
9. 股动脉 femoral a.
10. 膝降动脉 descending genicular a.
11. 膝上内侧动脉 medial superior genicular a.
12. 膝下内侧动脉 medial inferior genicular a.
13. 胫前动脉 anterior tibial a.
14. 腓动脉 peroneal a.
15. 旋股内侧动脉 medial circumflex femoral a.
16. 第二穿动脉 2nd perforating a.
17. 第三穿动脉 3rd perforating a.
18. 第四穿动脉 4th perforating a.
19. 膝上外侧动脉 lateral superior genicular a.
20. 腘动脉 popliteal a.
21. 膝下外侧动脉 lateral inferior genicular a.
22. 胫后动脉 posterior tibial a.
23. 足底内侧动脉 medial plantar a.
24. 足底外侧动脉 lateral plantar a.
25. 足底弓 plantar arch

前面观 Anterior view

后面观 Posterior view

图 7-27 下肢的动脉
Arteries of the lower limb

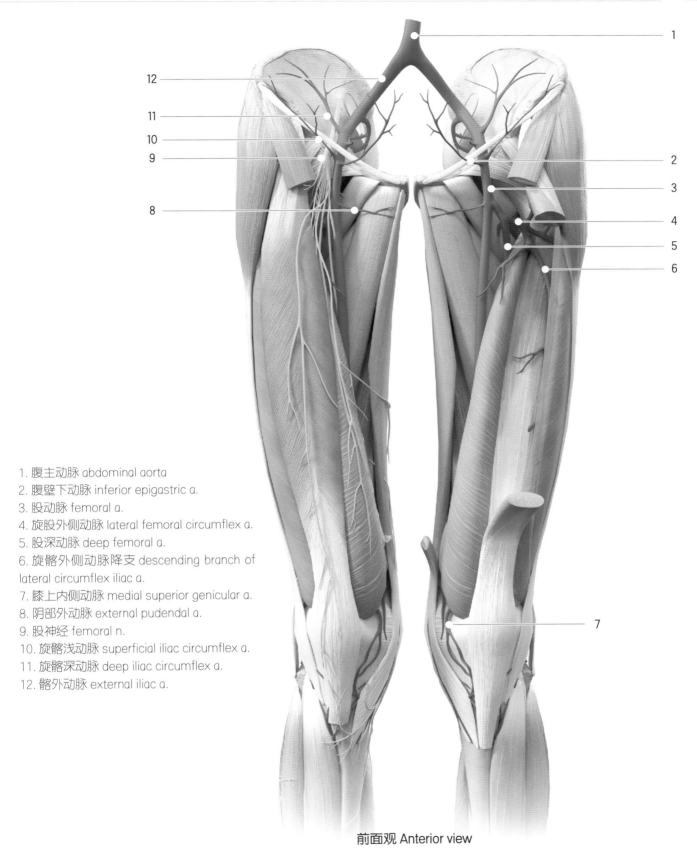

1. 腹主动脉 abdominal aorta
2. 腹壁下动脉 inferior epigastric a.
3. 股动脉 femoral a.
4. 旋股外侧动脉 lateral femoral circumflex a.
5. 股深动脉 deep femoral a.
6. 旋髂外侧动脉降支 descending branch of lateral circumflex iliac a.
7. 膝上内侧动脉 medial superior genicular a.
8. 阴部外动脉 external pudendal a.
9. 股神经 femoral n.
10. 旋髂浅动脉 superficial iliac circumflex a.
11. 旋髂深动脉 deep iliac circumflex a.
12. 髂外动脉 external iliac a.

前面观 Anterior view

图 7-28　股动脉及其分支
Femoral artery and its branches

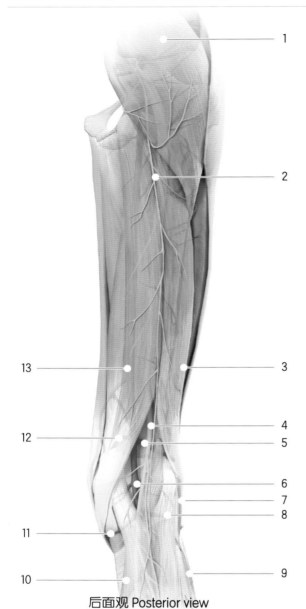

后面观 Posterior view

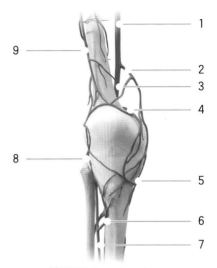

前面观 Anterior view

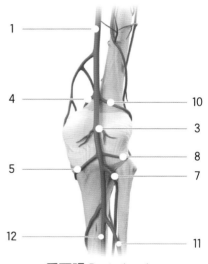

后面观 Posterior view

1. 臀大肌 gluteus maximus
2. 股后皮神经 posterior femoral cutaneous n.
3. 股二头肌 biceps femoris
4. 胫神经 tibial n.
5. 膝上外侧动脉 lateral superior genicular a.
6. 腘动脉 popliteal a.
7. 腓总神经 common peroneal n.
8. 膝下外侧动脉 lateral inferior genicular a.
9. 腓肠肌外侧头 lateral head of gastrocnemius
10. 腓肠肌内侧头 medial head of gastrocnemius
11. 膝下内侧动脉 medial inferior genicular a.
12. 膝上内侧动脉 medial superior genicular a.
13. 股动脉 femoral a.

1. 股动脉 femoral a.
2. 膝降动脉 descending genicular a.
3. 腘动脉 popliteal a.
4. 膝上内侧动脉 superior medial genicular a.
5. 膝下内侧动脉 medial inferior genicular a.
6. 胫前返动脉 anterior tibial recurrent a.
7. 胫前动脉 anterior tibial a.
8. 膝下外侧动脉 lateral inferior genicular a.
9. 降支 descending branch
10. 膝上外侧动脉 lateral superior genicular a.
11. 腓动脉 peroneal a.
12. 胫后动脉 posterior tibial a.

图 7-29　股后部动脉
Arteries of the posterior region of thigh

图 7-30　膝关节周围动脉
Peripheral arteries of the knee joint

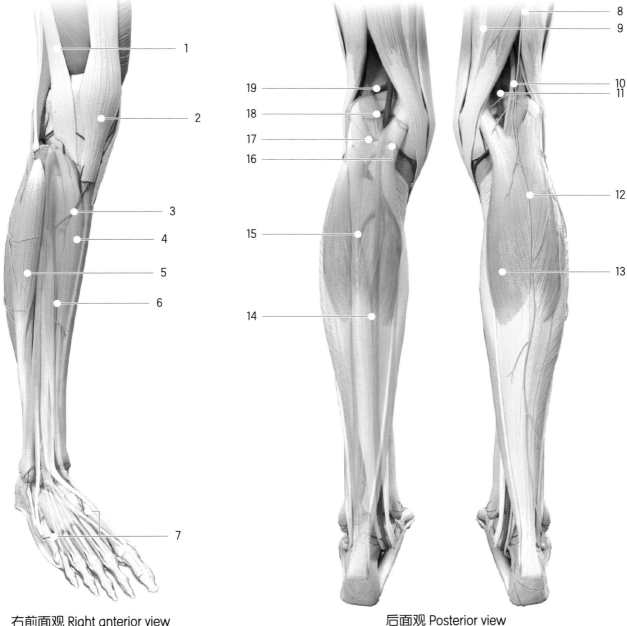

右前面观 Right anterior view

后面观 Posterior view

1. 髂胫束 iliotibial tract
2. 髌韧带 patellar lig.
3. 胫前返动脉 anterior tibial recurrent a.
4. 胫骨前肌 tibialis anterior
5. 腓骨长肌 peroneus longus
6. 胫前动脉 anterior tibial a.
7. 足背动脉 dorsal a. of foot
8. 股后皮神经 posterior femoral cutaneous n.
9. 半膜肌 semimembranosus
10. 胫神经 tibial n.

11. 腘动脉 popliteal a.
12. 腓肠内侧皮神经 medial sural cutaneous n.
13. 腓肠肌 gastrocnemius
14. 胫后动脉 posterior tibial a.
15. 腓动脉 peroneal a.
16. 膝下内侧动脉 medial inferior genicular a.
17. 膝下外侧动脉 lateral inferior genicular a.
18. 膝中动脉 middle genicular a.
19. 膝上外侧动脉 lateral superior genicular a.

图 7-31 小腿的动脉
Arteries of the leg

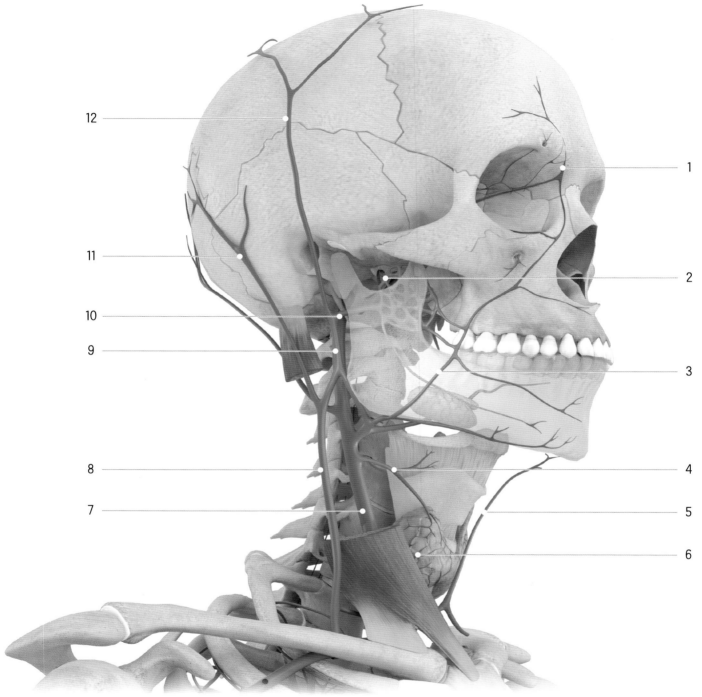

右前外侧面观 Right anterolateral view

1. 内眦静脉 angular v.
2. 翼静脉丛 pterygoid venous plexus
3. 面静脉 facial v.
4. 甲状腺上静脉 superior thyroid v.
5. 颈前静脉 anterior jugular v.
6. 甲状腺中静脉 middle thyroid v.
7. 颈内静脉 internal jugular v.
8. 颈外静脉 external jugular v.
9. 下颌后静脉 retromandibular v.
10. 上颌静脉 maxillary v.
11. 枕静脉 occipital v.
12. 颞浅静脉 superficial temporal v.

图 7-32 头颈部静脉
Veins of the head and neck

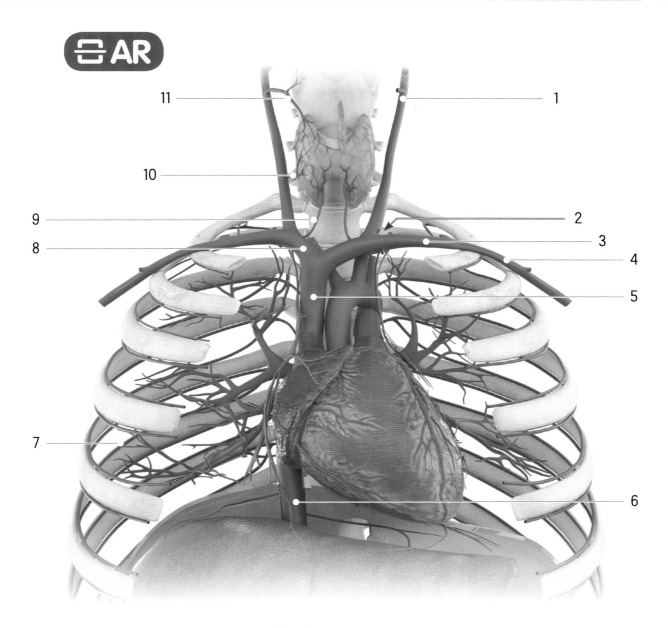

前面观 Anterior view

1. 左颈内静脉 left internal jugular v.
2. 静脉角 venous angle
3. 左锁骨下静脉 left subclavian v.
4. 腋静脉 axillary v.
5. 上腔静脉 superior vena cava
6. 下腔静脉 inferior vena cava
7. 肋间后静脉 posterior intercostal v.
8. 右头臂静脉 right brachiocephalic v.
9. 甲状腺下静脉 inferior thyroid v.
10. 甲状腺中静脉 middle thyroid v.
11. 甲状腺上静脉 superior thyroid v.

图 7-33　上腔静脉及其属支
Superior vena cava and its tributaries

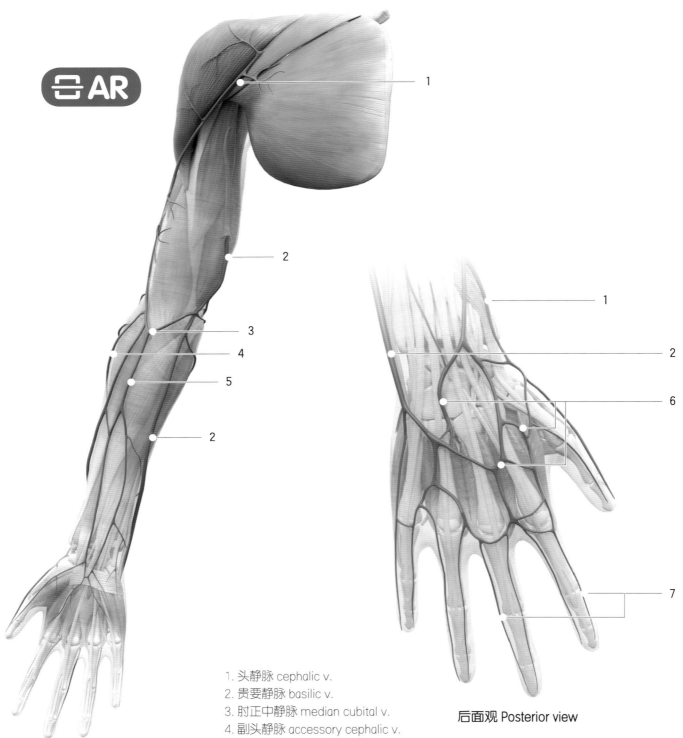

前面观 Anterior view

后面观 Posterior view

1. 头静脉 cephalic v.
2. 贵要静脉 basilic v.
3. 肘正中静脉 median cubital v.
4. 副头静脉 accessory cephalic v.
5. 前臂正中静脉 median antebrachial v.
6. 手背静脉网 dorsal venous rete of hand
7. 指掌侧固有静脉 proper palmar digital v.

图 7-34　上肢浅静脉
Superficial veins of the upper limb

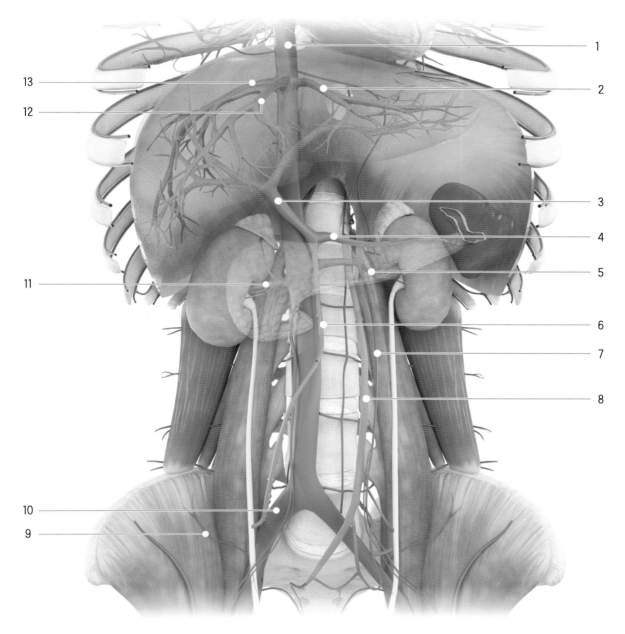

前面观 Anterior view

1. 下腔静脉 inferior vena cava
2. 肝左静脉 left hepatic v.
3. 肝门静脉 hepatic portal v.
4. 脾静脉 splenic v.
5. 左肾静脉 left renal v.
6. 肠系膜上静脉 superior mesenteric v.
7. 睾丸静脉 testicular v.
8. 肠系膜下静脉 inferior mesenteric v.
9. 腹壁静脉 epigastric v.
10. 右髂总静脉 right common iliac v.
11. 右肾静脉 right renal v.
12. 肝中静脉 intermediate hepatic v.
13. 肝右静脉 right hepatic v.

图 7-35 下腔静脉、肝门静脉及其属支
Inferior vena cava,hepatic portal vein and their tributaries

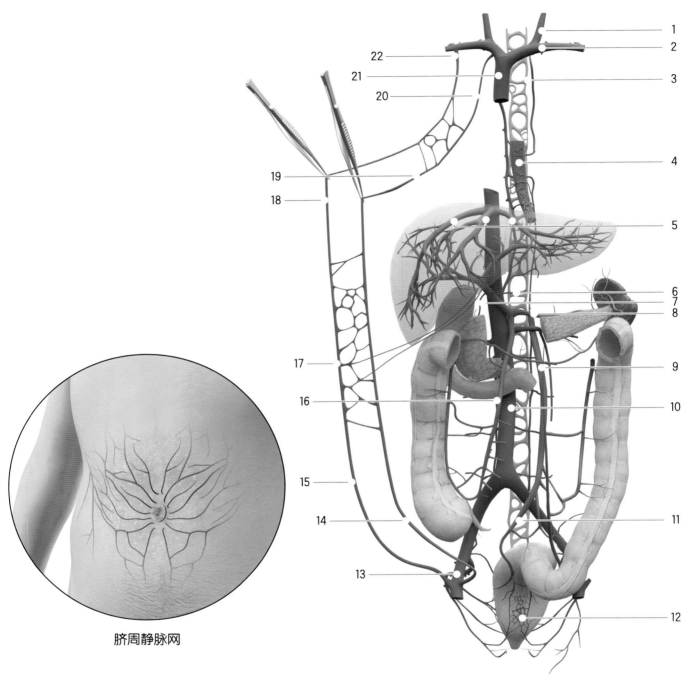

脐周静脉网

1. 左颈内静脉 left internal jugular v.
2. 左锁骨下静脉 left subclavian v.
3. 脊柱静脉丛 vertebral venous plexus
4. 食管静脉 esophageal v.
5. 肝静脉 hepatic v.
6. 胃左静脉 left gastric v.
7. 胃右静脉 right gastric v.
8. 脾静脉 splenic v.

9. 肠系膜下静脉 inferior mesenteric v.
10. 下腔静脉 inferior vena cava
11. 直肠上静脉 superior rectal v.
12. 直肠静脉丛 rectal venous plexus
13. 髂外静脉 external iliac v.
14. 腹壁下静脉 inferior epigastric v.
15. 腹壁浅静脉 superficial epigastric v.
16. 肠系膜上静脉 superior mesenteric v.

17. 附脐静脉 paraumbilical v.
18. 胸腹壁静脉 thoracoepigastric v.
19. 腹壁上静脉 superior epigastric v.
20. 胸廓内静脉 internal thoracic v.
21. 上腔静脉 superior vena cava
22. 胸外侧静脉 lateral thoracic v.

图 7-36　肝门静脉与上、下腔静脉吻合模式图
Diagram of the anastomosis of hepatic portal vein, superior vena cava and inferior vena cava

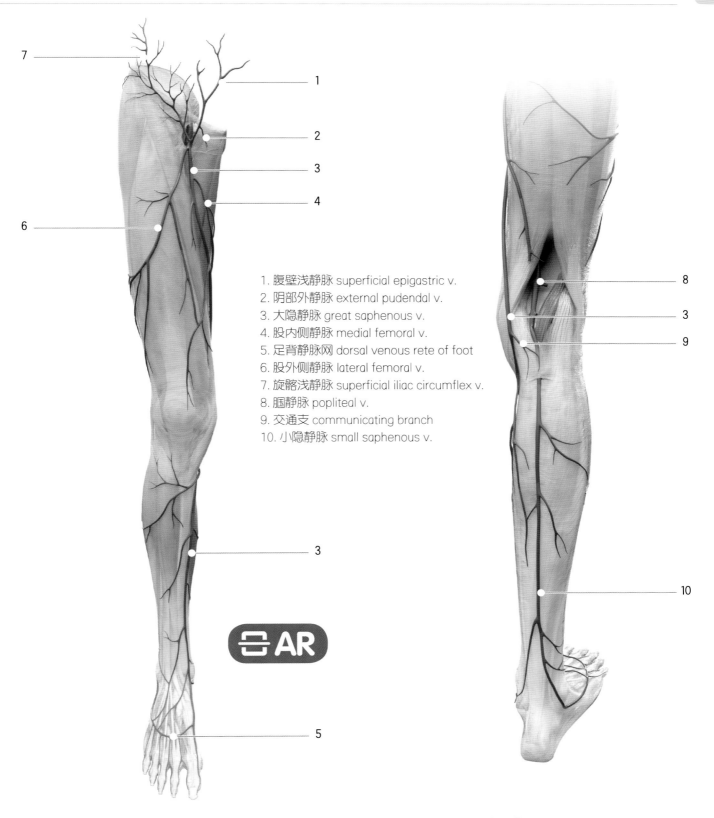

1. 腹壁浅静脉 superficial epigastric v.
2. 阴部外静脉 external pudendal v.
3. 大隐静脉 great saphenous v.
4. 股内侧静脉 medial femoral v.
5. 足背静脉网 dorsal venous rete of foot
6. 股外侧静脉 lateral femoral v.
7. 旋髂浅静脉 superficial iliac circumflex v.
8. 腘静脉 popliteal v.
9. 交通支 communicating branch
10. 小隐静脉 small saphenous v.

前面观 Anterior view

后面观 Posterior view

图 7-37　下肢浅静脉
Superficial veins of the lower limb

1

2

3

4

5

6

7

10

11

12

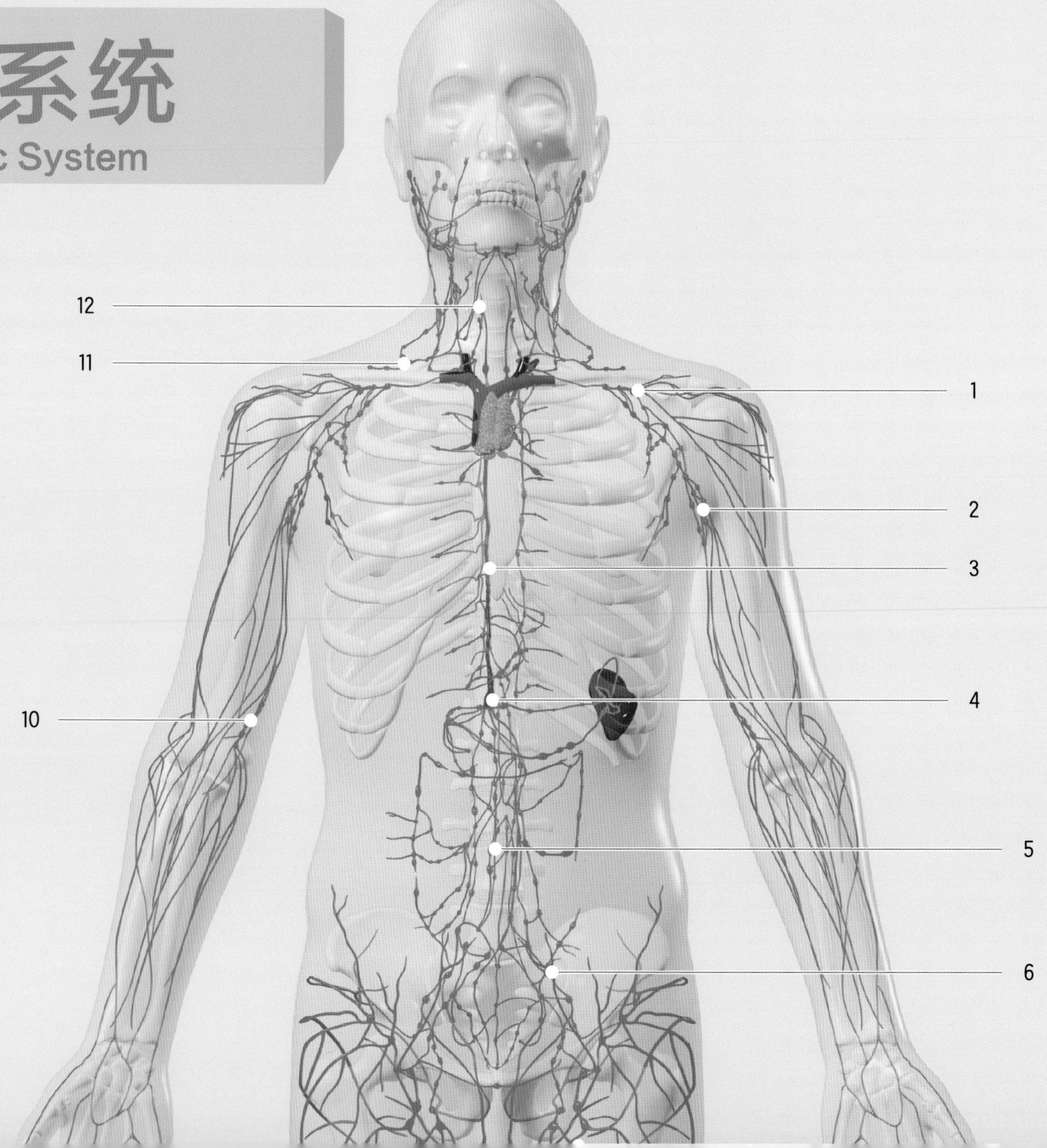

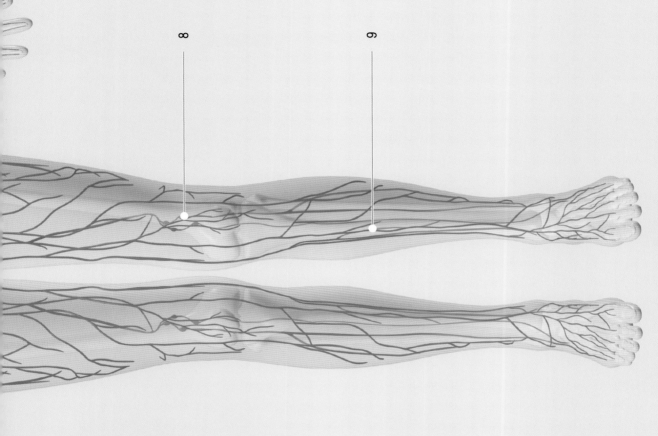

8

9

图 8-1　淋巴系统概观
Overview of the lymphatic system

1. 锁骨下淋巴结 subclavicular lymph nodes
2. 中央淋巴结 central lymph nodes
3. 胸导管 thoracic duct
4. 乳糜池 cisterna chyli
5. 腰淋巴结 lumbar lymph nodes
6. 髂淋巴结 iliac lymph nodes
7. 腹股沟浅淋巴结 superficial inguinal lymph nodes
8. 腘淋巴结 popliteal lymph nodes
9. 浅淋巴管 superficial lymphatic vessels
10. 肘淋巴结 cubital lymph nodes
11. 锁骨上淋巴结 supraclavicular lymph nodes
12. 甲状腺淋巴结 thyroid lymph nodes

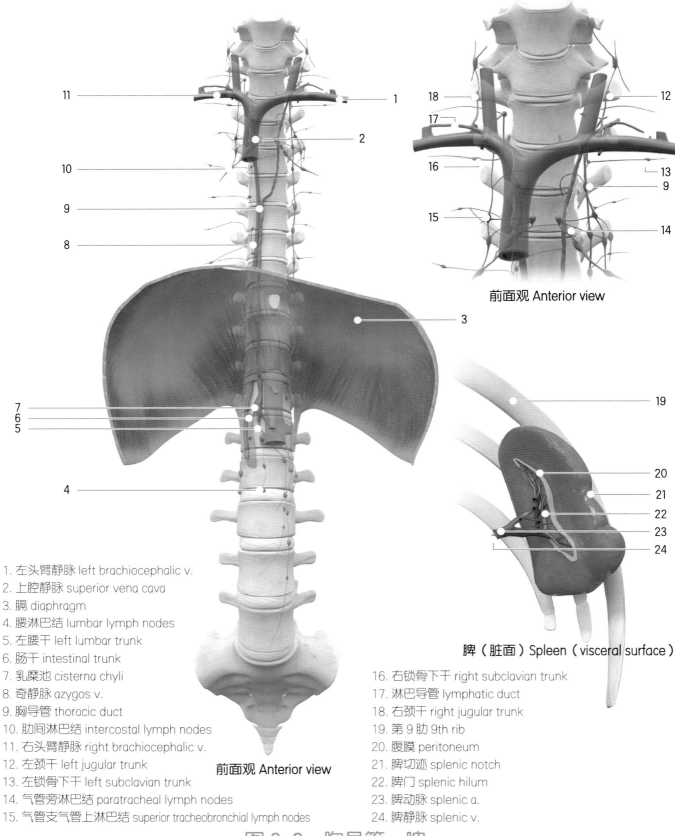

前面观 Anterior view

前面观 Anterior view

脾（脏面）Spleen（visceral surface）

1. 左头臂静脉 left brachiocephalic v.
2. 上腔静脉 superior vena cava
3. 膈 diaphragm
4. 腰淋巴结 lumbar lymph nodes
5. 左腰干 left lumbar trunk
6. 肠干 intestinal trunk
7. 乳糜池 cisterna chyli
8. 奇静脉 azygos v.
9. 胸导管 thoracic duct
10. 肋间淋巴结 intercostal lymph nodes
11. 右头臂静脉 right brachiocephalic v.
12. 左颈干 left jugular trunk
13. 左锁骨下干 left subclavian trunk
14. 气管旁淋巴结 paratracheal lymph nodes
15. 气管支气管上淋巴结 superior tracheobronchial lymph nodes

16. 右锁骨下干 right subclavian trunk
17. 淋巴导管 lymphatic duct
18. 右颈干 right jugular trunk
19. 第 9 肋 9th rib
20. 腹膜 peritoneum
21. 脾切迹 splenic notch
22. 脾门 splenic hilum
23. 脾动脉 splenic a.
24. 脾静脉 splenic v.

图 8-2　胸导管、脾
Thoracic duct, spleen

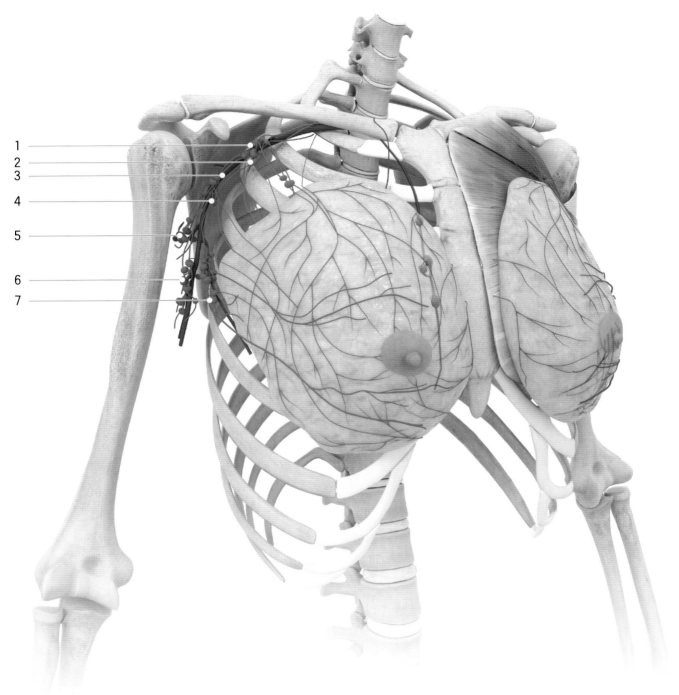

右前外侧面观 Right anterolateral view

1. 尖淋巴结 apical lymph nodes
2. 中央淋巴结 central lymph nodes
3. 锁骨下静脉 subclavian v.
4. 外侧淋巴结 lateral lymph nodes
5. 肱外侧淋巴结 humeral lateral lymph nodes
6. 肩胛下淋巴结 subscapular lymph nodes
7. 胸肌淋巴结 pectoral lymph nodes

图 8-3　腋淋巴结和乳房淋巴管
Axillary lymph nodes and breast lymphatic vessels

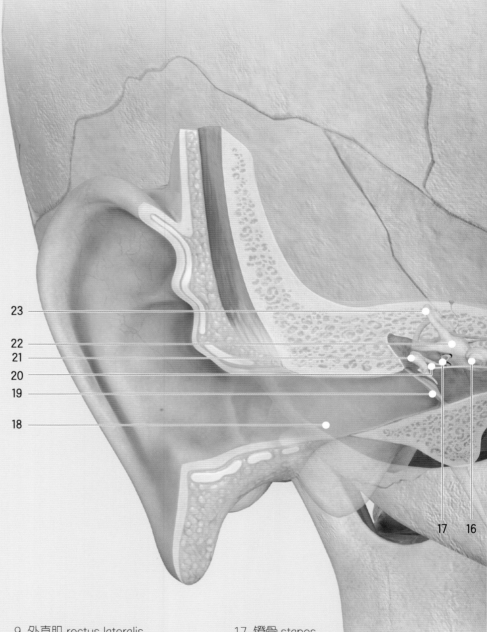

1. 蜗神经 cochlear n.
2. 前庭神经 vestibular n.
3. 面神经 facial n.
4. 泪腺 lacrimal gland
5. 上睑提肌 levator palpebrae superioris
6. 上斜肌 obliquus superior
7. 上直肌 rectus superior
8. 瞳孔 pupil

9. 外直肌 rectus lateralis
10. 巩膜 sclera
11. 下直肌 rectus inferior
12. 下斜肌 obliquus inferior
13. 鼓膜张肌 tensor tympani
14. 咽鼓管 pharyngotympanic tube
15. 腭帆张肌 tensor veli palatini
16. 耳蜗 cochlea

17. 镫骨 stapes
18. 外耳道 external acoustic meatus
19. 鼓膜 tympanic membrane
20. 砧骨 incus
21. 锤骨 malleus
22. 前庭 vestibule
23. 半规管 semicircular canal

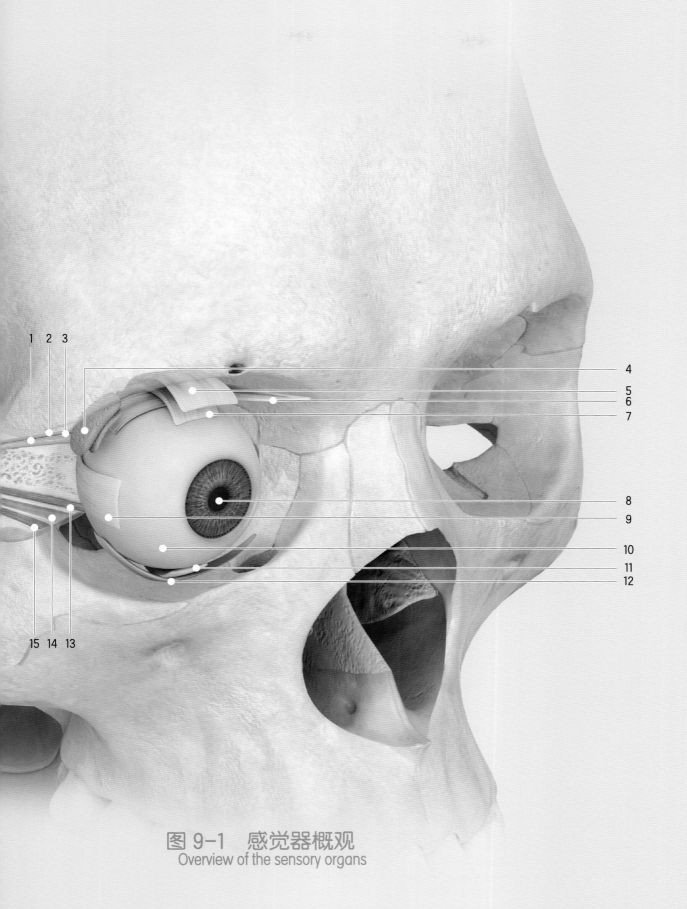

图 9-1　感觉器概观
Overview of the sensory organs

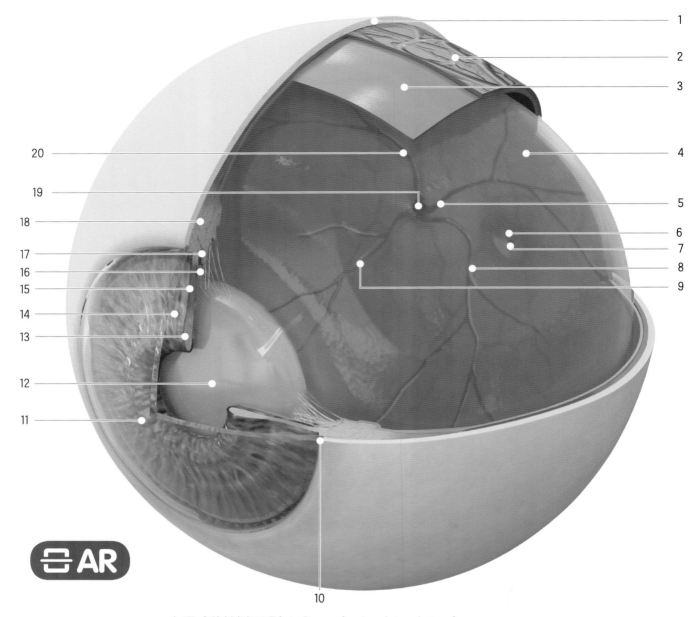

左眼（前外侧面观）Left eye（anterolateral view）

1. 巩膜 sclera
2. 脉络膜 choroid
3. 视网膜 retina
4. 玻璃体 vitreous body
5. 视网膜颞侧上小动脉 superior temporal arteriole of retina
6. 黄斑 macula lutea
7. 中央凹 fovea centralis
8. 视网膜颞侧下小动脉 inferior temporal arteriole of retina
9. 视网膜鼻侧下小动脉 inferior nasal arteriole of retina
10. 巩膜静脉窦 sinus venosus sclerae

11. 角膜 cornea
12. 晶状体 lens
13. 瞳孔括约肌 sphincter pupillae
14. 虹膜 iris
15. 瞳孔开大肌 dilator pupillae
16. 睫状小带 ciliary zonule
17. 睫状突 ciliary processes
18. 睫状肌 ciliary muscle
19. 视神经盘 optic disc
20. 视网膜鼻侧上小动脉 superior nasal arteriole of retina

图 9-2　眼球的结构
Structure of the eyeball

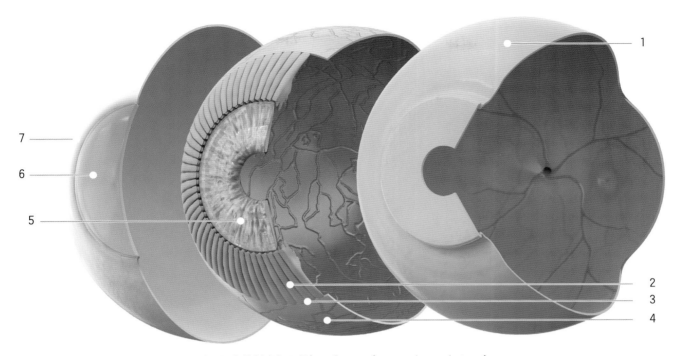

左眼（前外侧面观）Left eye（anterolateral view）

1. 视网膜 retina
2. 睫状体 ciliary body
3. 锯状缘 ora serrata
4. 脉络膜 choroid
5. 虹膜 iris
6. 角膜 cornea
7. 角膜缘 limbus corneae

图 9-3　眼球壁
Wall of the eyeball

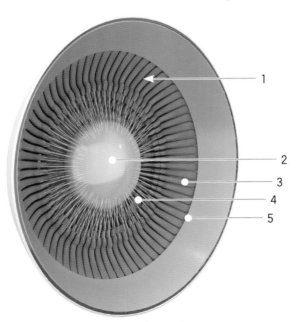

后外侧面观 Posterolateral view

1. 睫状环 ciliary ring
2. 晶状体 lens
3. 睫状突 ciliary processes
4. 睫状小带 ciliary zonule
5. 锯状缘 ora serrata

图 9-4　虹膜、睫状体及晶状体
Iris, ciliary body and lens

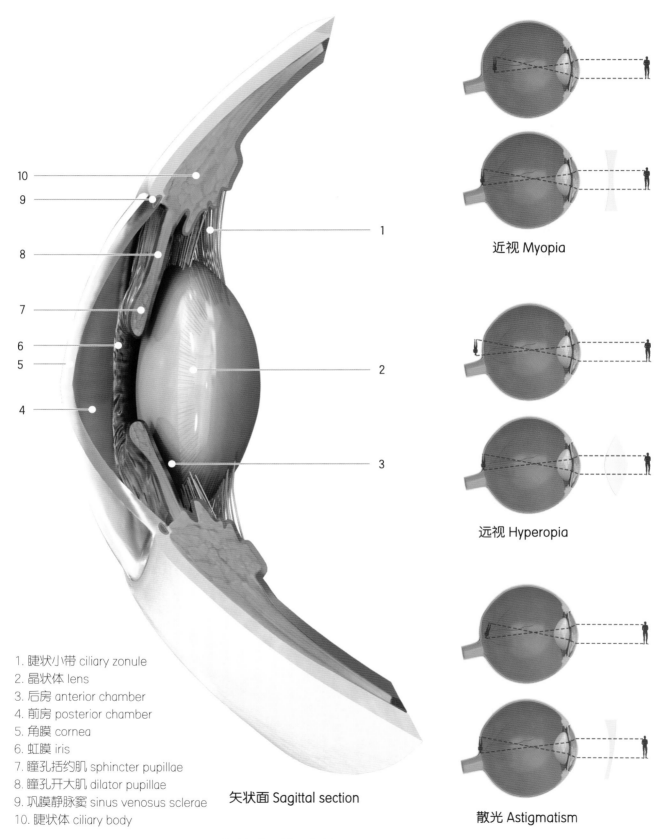

1. 睫状小带 ciliary zonule
2. 晶状体 lens
3. 后房 anterior chamber
4. 前房 posterior chamber
5. 角膜 cornea
6. 虹膜 iris
7. 瞳孔括约肌 sphincter pupillae
8. 瞳孔开大肌 dilator pupillae
9. 巩膜静脉窦 sinus venosus sclerae
10. 睫状体 ciliary body

矢状面 Sagittal section

近视 Myopia

远视 Hyperopia

散光 Astigmatism

图 9-5　眼球前部的结构
Structure of the anterior part of the eyeball

图 9-6　晶状体调节异常及校正
Dysregulation and correction of the crystalline lens

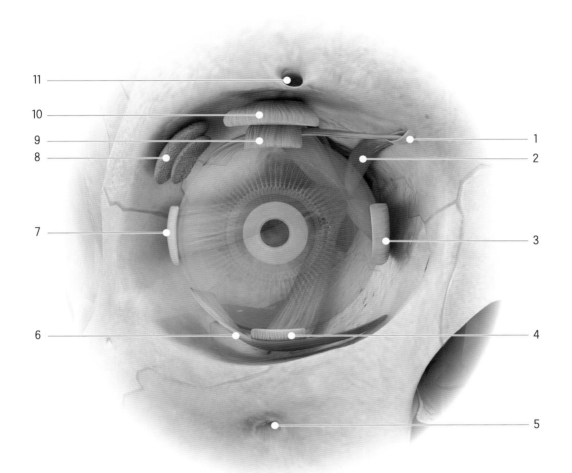

前面观 Anterior view

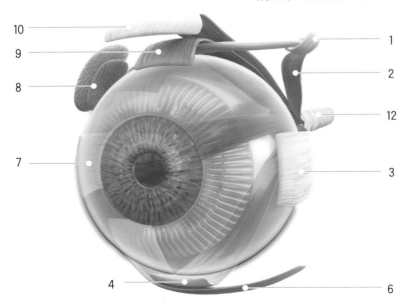

前内侧面观 Anteromedial view

1. 滑车 trochlea
2. 上斜肌 obliquus superior
3. 内直肌 rectus medialis
4. 下直肌 rectus inferior
5. 眶下孔 infraorbital foramen
6. 下斜肌 obliquus inferior
7. 外直肌 rectus lateralis
8. 泪腺 lacrimal gland
9. 上直肌 rectus superior
10. 上睑提肌 levator palpebrae superioris
11. 眶上孔 supraorbital foramen
12. 总腱环 common tendinous ring

图 9-7 眼球外肌
Ocular muscles

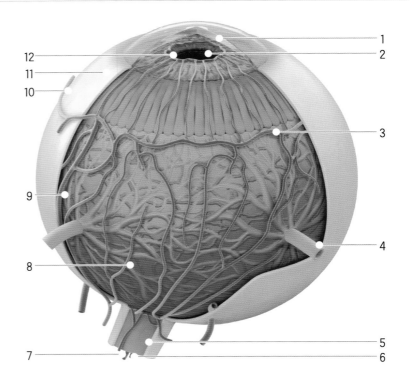

1. 角膜 cornea
2. 瞳孔 pupil
3. 虹膜动脉大环 greater arterial circle of iris
4. 涡静脉 vorticose v.
5. 视神经 optic n.
6. 视网膜中央动脉 central artery of retina
7. 视网膜中央静脉 central vein of retina
8. 睫后短动脉 short posterior ciliary a.
9. 睫后长动脉 long posterior ciliary a.
10. 睫前动脉 anterior ciliary a.
11. 巩膜 sclera
12. 虹膜动脉小环 lesser arterial circle of iris

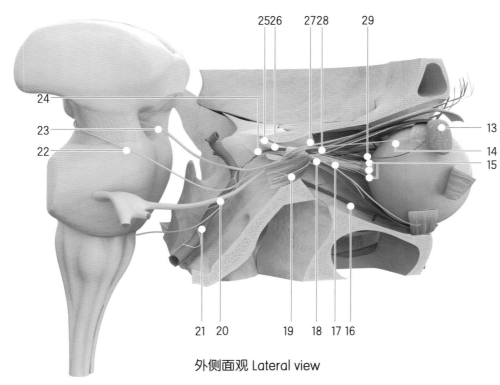

13. 泪腺 lacrimal gland
14. 泪腺神经 lacrimal n.
15. 睫状短神经 short ciliary n.
16. 眼下静脉 inferior ophthalmic v.
17. 睫状神经节 ciliary ganglion
18. 动眼神经下支
   inferior branch of oculomotor n.
19. 展神经 abducent n.
20. 眼神经 ophthalmic n.
21. 颈内动脉 internal carotid a.
22. 滑车神经 trochlear n.
23. 动眼神经 oculomotor n.
24. 眼动脉 ophthalmic a.
25. 视神经 optic n.
26. 眼静脉 ophthalmic v.
27. 额神经 frontal n.
28. 动眼神经上支
   superior branch of oculomotor n.
29. 鼻睫神经 nasociliary n.

外侧面观 Lateral view

图 9-8 眼球血管及神经
Blood vessels and nerves of the eyeball

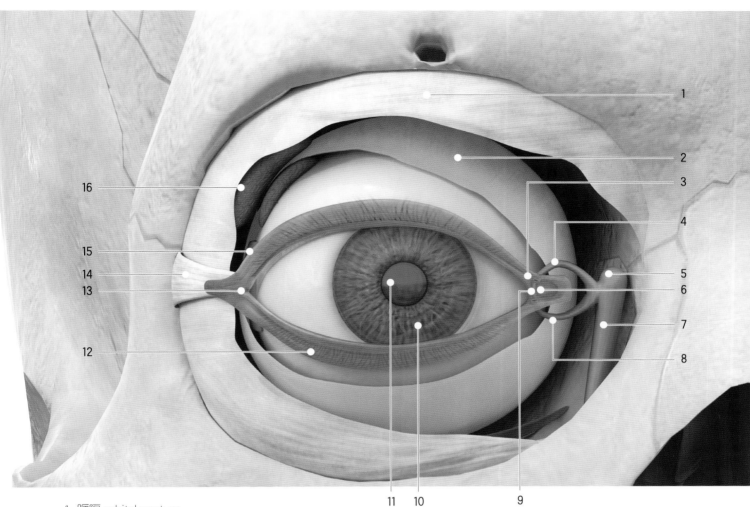

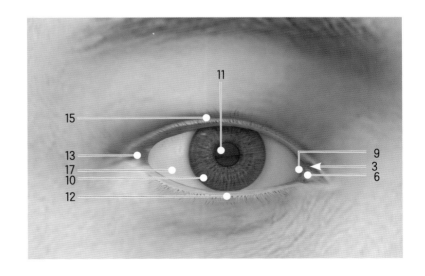

1. 眶隔 orbital septum
2. 眼球筋膜鞘 sheath of eyeball
3. 泪点 lacrimal punctum
4. 上泪小管 superior lacrimal ductule
5. 泪囊 lacrimal sac
6. 泪阜 lacrimal caruncle
7. 鼻泪管 nasolacrimal duct
8. 下泪小管 inferior lacrimal ductule
9. 半月襞 semilunar fold
10. 虹膜 iris
11. 瞳孔 pupil
12. 下睑 inferior palpebrae
13. 外眦 lateral angle of eye
14. 睑外侧韧带 lateral palpebral ligament
15. 上睑 superior palpebrae
16. 泪腺 lacrimal gland
17. 球结膜 bulbar conjunctiva

图 9-9 泪器
Lacrimal apparatus

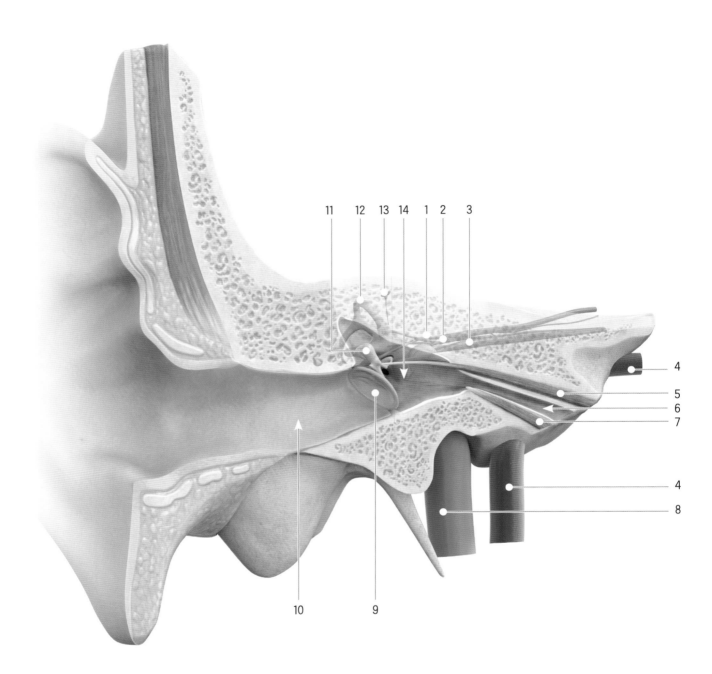

1. 面神经　facial n.
2. 前庭神经 vestibular n.
3. 蜗神经 cochlear n.
4. 颈内动脉 internal carotid a.
5. 鼓膜张肌 tensor tympani
6. 咽鼓管 pharyngotympanic tube
7. 腭帆张肌 tensor veli palatini
8. 颈内静脉 internal jugular v.
9. 鼓膜 tympanic membrane
10. 外耳道 external acoustic meatus
11. 锤骨 malleus
12. 骨半规管 bony semicircular canals
13. 内淋巴囊 endolymphatic sac
14. 鼓室 tympanic cavity

图 9-10　前庭蜗器模式图
Diagram of the vestibulocochlear organ

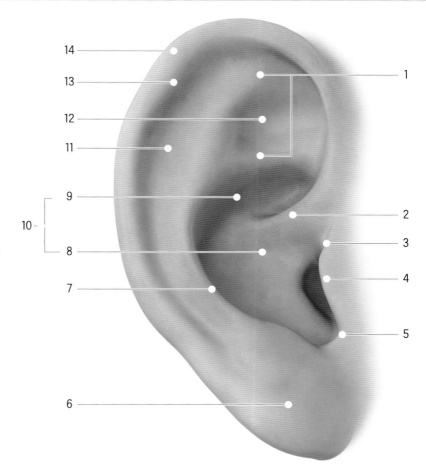

1. 对耳轮脚 crura of antihelix
2. 耳轮脚 crus of helix
3. 耳前切迹 anterior notch of ear
4. 耳屏 tragus
5. 耳屏间切迹 intertragic notch
6. 耳垂 auricular lobule
7. 对耳轮 antihelix
8. 耳甲腔 cavity of auricular concha
9. 耳甲艇 cymba of auricular concha
10. 耳甲 auricular concha
11. 耳舟 scapha
12. 三角窝 triangular fossa
13. 耳郭结节 auricular tubercle
14. 耳轮 helix

图 9-11 耳郭
Auricle

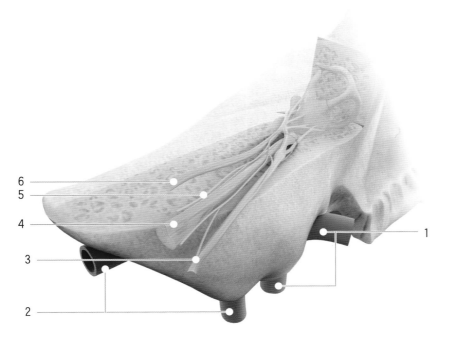

1. 颈内静脉 internal jugular v.
2. 颈内动脉 internal carotid a.
3. 前庭神经 vestibular n.
4. 蜗神经 cochlear n.
5. 中间神经 intermediate n.
6. 面神经 facial n.

图 9-12 前庭蜗神经、面神经和内耳门
Vestibulocochlear nerve, facial nerve and internal acoustic pore

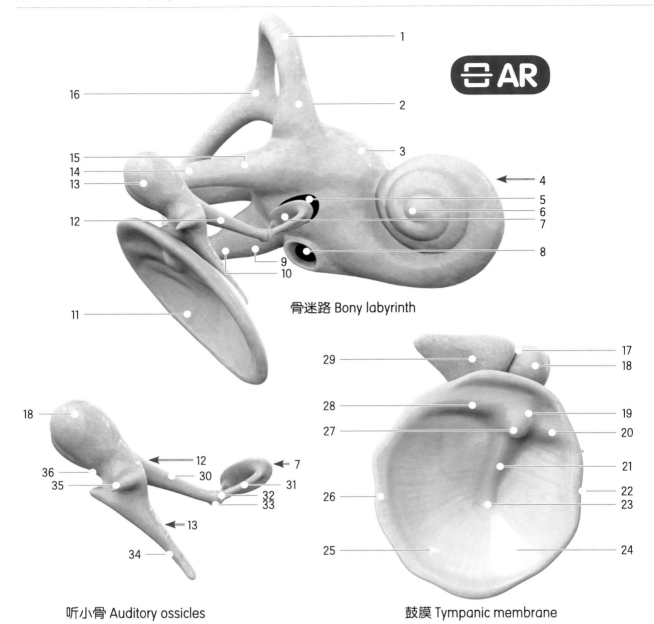

骨迷路 Bony labyrinth

听小骨 Auditory ossicles

鼓膜 Tympanic membrane

1. 前半规管 anterior semicircular canal
2. 前骨壶腹 anterior bony ampulla
3. 前庭 vestibule
4. 耳蜗 cochlea
5. 前庭窗 fenestra vestibuli
6. 蜗顶 cupula of cochlea
7. 镫骨 stapes
8. 蜗窗 fenestra cochleae
9. 后骨壶腹 posterior bony ampulla
10. 后骨半规管 posterior semicircular canal
11. 鼓膜 tympanic membrane
12. 砧骨 incus

13. 锤骨 malleus
14. 外侧半规管 lateral semicircular canal
15. 外侧骨壶腹 lateral bony ampulla
16. 总骨脚 common bony crus
17. 砧锤关节 incudomalleolar joint
18. 锤骨头 head of malleus
19. 松弛部 flaccid part
20. 锤骨前襞 anterior malleolar fold
21. 锤纹 malleolar stria
22. 黏膜 tunica mucosa
23. 鼓膜脐 umbo of tympanic membrane
24. 反射光锥 cone of reflected light

25. 紧张部 tense part
26. 纤维软骨环 fibrocartilaginous ring
27. 锤凸 malleolar prominence
28. 锤骨后襞 posterior malleolar fold
29. 砧骨体 body of incus
30. 长脚 long crus
31. 前脚 anterior crus
32. 砧镫关节 incudostapedial joint
33. 豆状突 lenticular process
34. 锤骨柄 manubrium of malleus
35. 前突 anterior process
36. 锤骨颈 neck of malleus

图 9-13　右侧骨迷路、听小骨及鼓膜
Right bony labyrinth, auditory ossicles and tympanic membrane

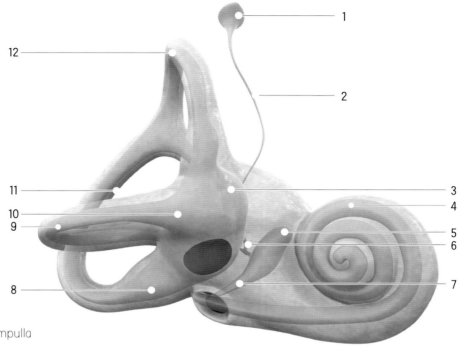

1. 内淋巴囊 endolymphatic sac
2. 内淋巴管 endolymphatic duct
3. 椭圆囊 utricle
4. 蜗管 cochlear duct
5. 球囊 saccule
6. 椭圆球囊管 utriculosaccular duct
7. 连合管 ductus reuniens
8. 后膜壶腹 posterior membranous ampulla
9. 外膜半规管 lateral semicircular duct
10. 外膜壶腹 lateral membranous ampulla
11. 后膜半规管 posterior semicircular duct
12. 前膜半规管 anterior semicircular duct
13. 前庭膜 vestibular membrane
14. 盖膜 tectorial membrane
15. 外毛细胞 outer haircell
16. 外螺旋沟 external spiral sulcus
17. 螺旋嵴 spiral crest
18. 螺旋膜 spiral membrane
19. 螺旋器隧道 Corti's tunnel
20. 内毛细胞 inner haircell
21. 内螺旋沟 internal spiral sulcus
22. 鼓阶 scala tympani
23. 蜗根 cochlear root
24. 蜗神经节 cochlear ganglion
25. 骨螺旋板 osseous spiral lamina
26. 前庭阶 scala vestibuli

右侧膜迷路 Right membranous labyrinth

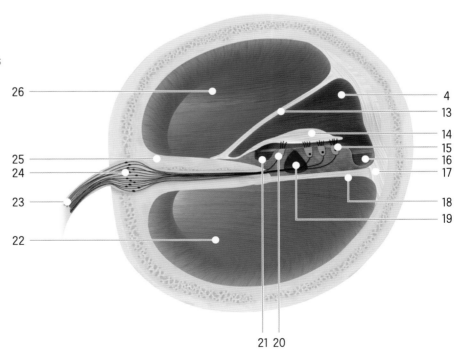

右侧螺旋器模式图 Diagram of the right spiral organ

图 9-14 右侧膜迷路及蜗管
Right membranous labyrinth and cochlear duct

第10章 周围神经系统
Peripheral Nervous System

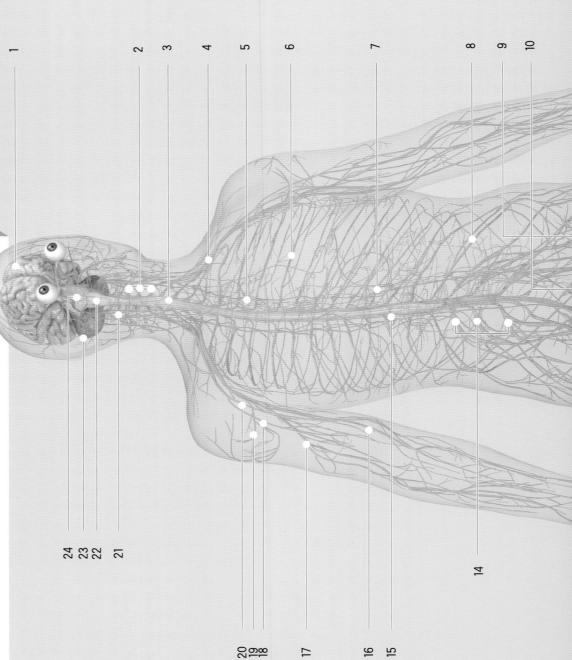

1
2
3
4
5
6
7
8
9
10

14

16
15

17

20
19
18

24
23
22
21

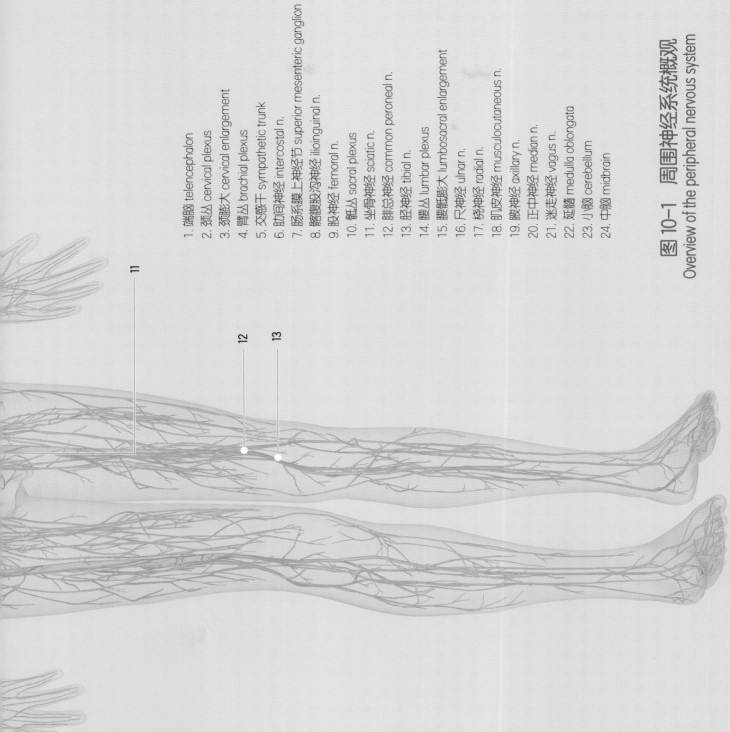

1. 端脑 telencephalon
2. 颈丛 cervical plexus
3. 颈膨大 cervical enlargement
4. 臂丛 brachial plexus
5. 交感干 sympathetic trunk
6. 肋间神经 intercostal n.
7. 肠系膜上神经节 superior mesenteric ganglion
8. 髂腹股沟神经 ilioinguinal n.
9. 股神经 femoral n.
10. 骶丛 sacral plexus
11. 坐骨神经 sciatic n.
12. 腓总神经 common peroneal n.
13. 胫神经 tibial n.
14. 腰丛 lumbar plexus
15. 腰骶膨大 lumbosacral enlargement
16. 尺神经 ulnar n.
17. 桡神经 radial n.
18. 肌皮神经 musculocutaneous n.
19. 腋神经 axillary n.
20. 正中神经 median n.
21. 迷走神经 vagus n.
22. 延髓 medulla oblongata
23. 小脑 cerebellum
24. 中脑 midbrain

图 10-1　周围神经系统概观
Overview of the peripheral nervous system

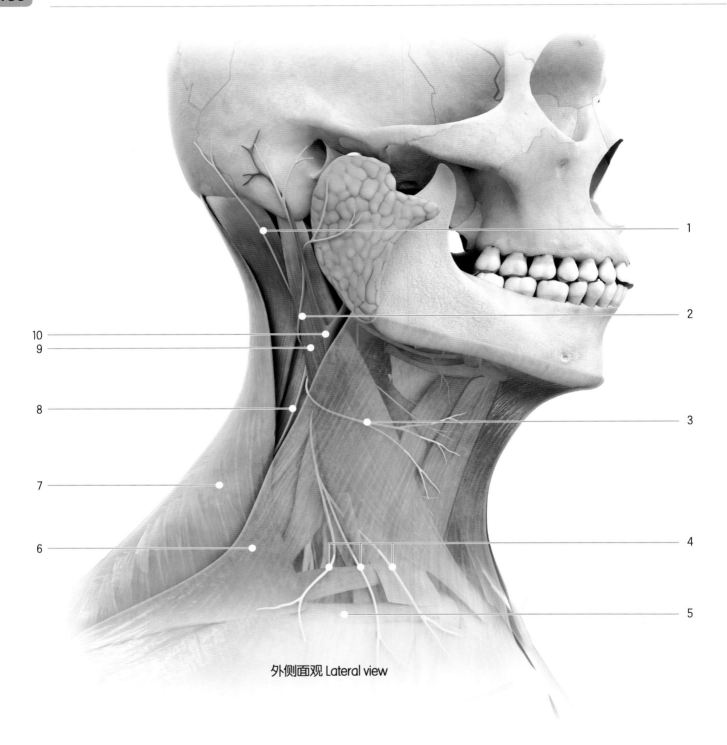

外侧面观 Lateral view

1. 枕小神经 lesser occipital n.
2. 耳大神经 great auricular n.
3. 颈横神经 transverse cervical n.
4. 锁骨上神经 supraclavicular n.
5. 锁骨 clavicle

6. 颈阔肌 platysma
7. 斜方肌 trapezius
8. 副神经 accessory n.
9. 胸锁乳突肌 sternocleidomastoid
10. 颈外静脉 external jugular v.

图 10-2　颈丛 1
Cervical plexus 1

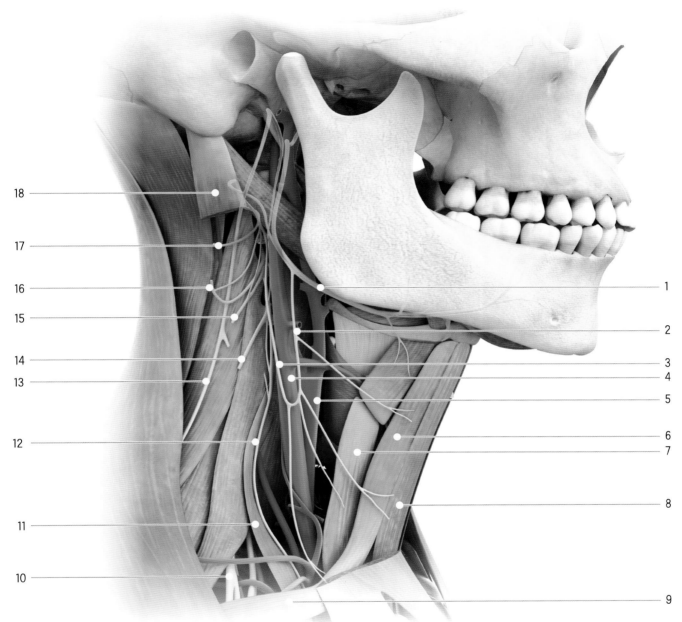

外侧面观 Lateral view

1. 舌下神经 hypoglossal n.
2. 颈袢上根 superior root of ansa cervicalis
3. 颈袢下根 inferior root of ansa cervicalis
4. 颈内静脉 internal jugular v.
5. 颈总动脉 common carotid a.
6. 肩胛舌骨肌上腹 superior belly of omohyoid
7. 胸骨甲状肌 sternothyroid
8. 胸骨舌骨肌 sternohyoid
9. 肩胛舌骨肌下腹 inferior belly of omohyoid

10. 臂丛 brachial plexus
11. 前斜角肌 scalenus anterior
12. 膈神经 phrenic n.
13. 副神经 accessory n.
14. 锁骨上神经 supraclavicular n.
15. 颈横神经 transverse cervical n.
16. 耳大神经 great auricular n.
17. 枕小神经 lesser occipital n.
18. 胸锁乳突肌（切断）sternocleidomastoid (cut)

图 10-3　颈丛 2
Cervical plexus 2

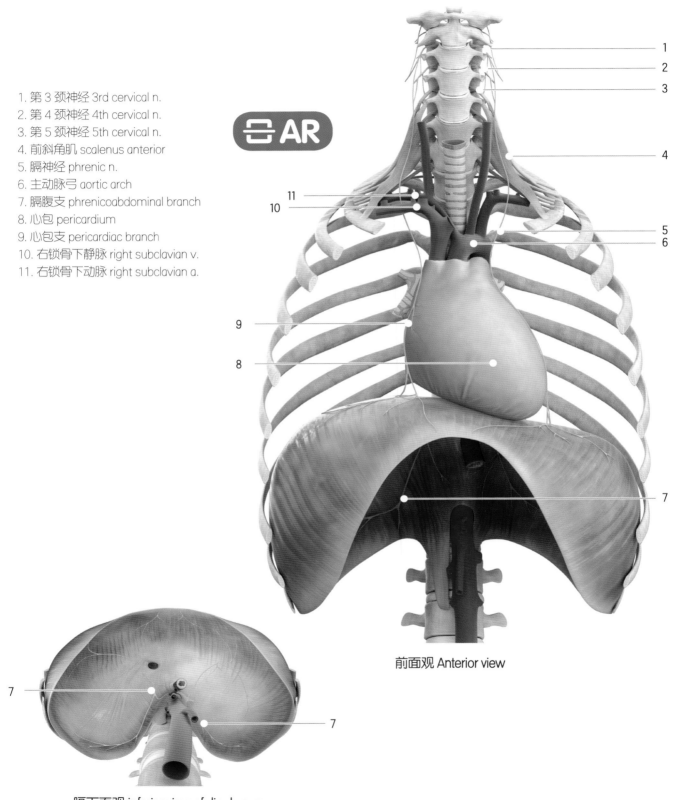

1. 第 3 颈神经 3rd cervical n.
2. 第 4 颈神经 4th cervical n.
3. 第 5 颈神经 5th cervical n.
4. 前斜角肌 scalenus anterior
5. 膈神经 phrenic n.
6. 主动脉弓 aortic arch
7. 膈腹支 phrenicoabdominal branch
8. 心包 pericardium
9. 心包支 pericardiac branch
10. 右锁骨下静脉 right subclavian v.
11. 右锁骨下动脉 right subclavian a.

前面观 Anterior view

膈下面观 inferior view of diaphragm

图 10-4　膈神经
Phrenic nerve

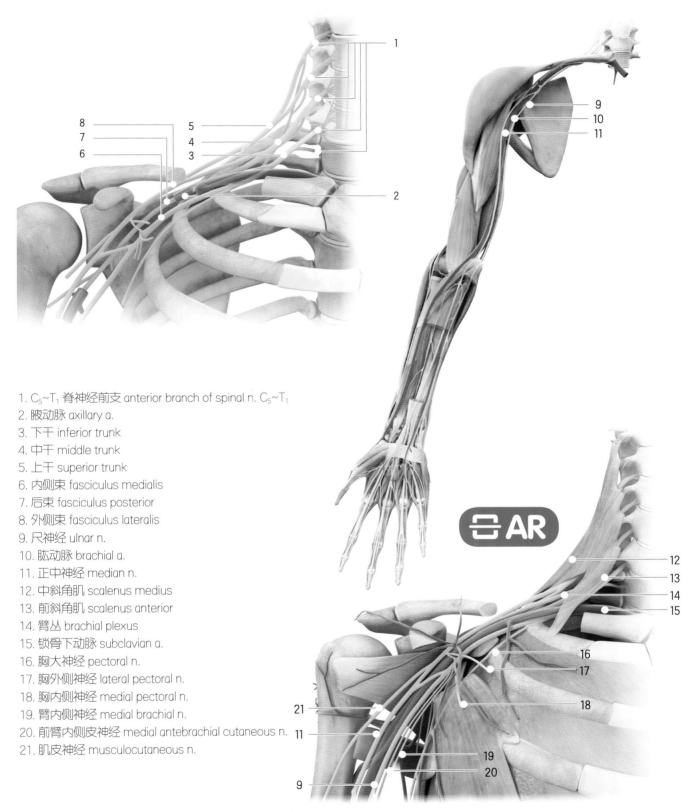

1. C$_5$~T$_1$ 脊神经前支 anterior branch of spinal n. C$_5$~T$_1$
2. 腋动脉 axillary a.
3. 下干 inferior trunk
4. 中干 middle trunk
5. 上干 superior trunk
6. 内侧束 fasciculus medialis
7. 后束 fasciculus posterior
8. 外侧束 fasciculus lateralis
9. 尺神经 ulnar n.
10. 肱动脉 brachial a.
11. 正中神经 median n.
12. 中斜角肌 scalenus medius
13. 前斜角肌 scalenus anterior
14. 臂丛 brachial plexus
15. 锁骨下动脉 subclavian a.
16. 胸大神经 pectoral n.
17. 胸外侧神经 lateral pectoral n.
18. 胸内侧神经 medial pectoral n.
19. 臂内侧神经 medial brachial n.
20. 前臂内侧皮神经 medial antebrachial cutaneous n.
21. 肌皮神经 musculocutaneous n.

前面观 Anterior view

图 10-5　臂丛及其分支
Brachial plexus and its branches

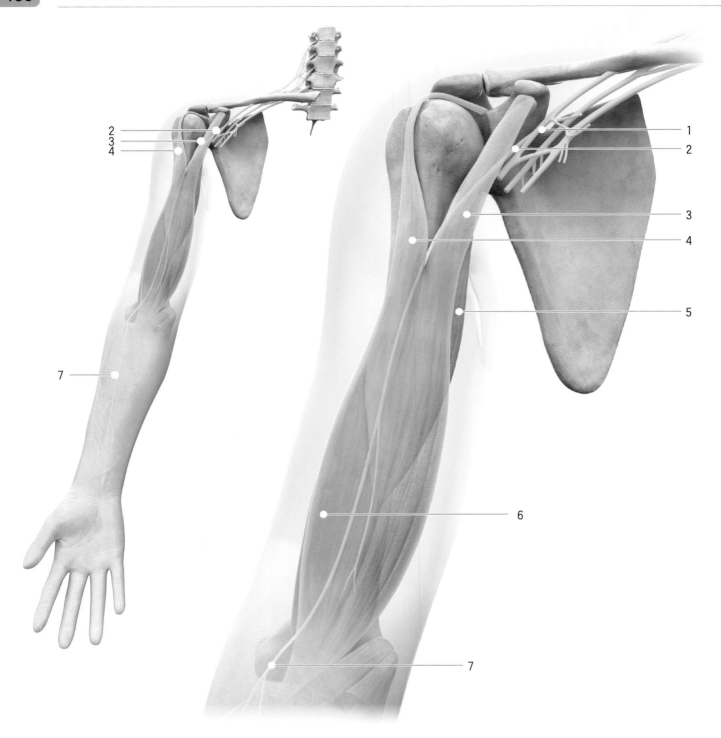

前面观 Anterior view

1. 外侧束 fasciculus lateralis
2. 肌皮神经 musculocutaneous n.
3. 肱二头肌短头 short head of biceps brachii
4. 肱二头肌长头 long head of biceps brachii

5. 喙肱肌 coracobrachialis
6. 肱肌 brachialis
7. 前臂外侧皮神经 lateral antebrachial cutaneous n.

图 10-6　肌皮神经
Musculocutaneous nerve

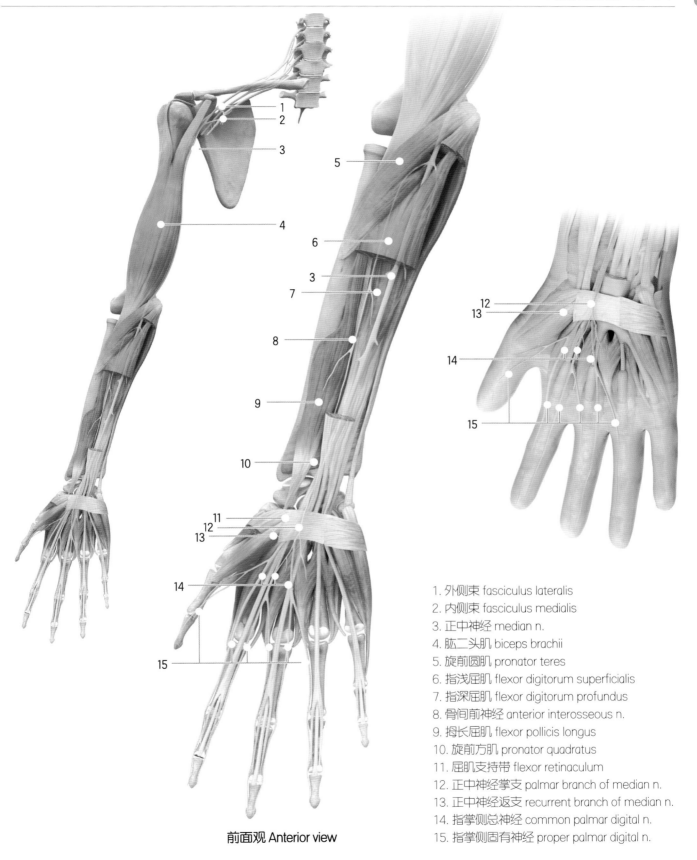

1. 外侧束 fasciculus lateralis
2. 内侧束 fasciculus medialis
3. 正中神经 median n.
4. 肱二头肌 biceps brachii
5. 旋前圆肌 pronator teres
6. 指浅屈肌 flexor digitorum superficialis
7. 指深屈肌 flexor digitorum profundus
8. 骨间前神经 anterior interosseous n.
9. 拇长屈肌 flexor pollicis longus
10. 旋前方肌 pronator quadratus
11. 屈肌支持带 flexor retinaculum
12. 正中神经掌支 palmar branch of median n.
13. 正中神经返支 recurrent branch of median n.
14. 指掌侧总神经 common palmar digital n.
15. 指掌侧固有神经 proper palmar digital n.

前面观 Anterior view

图 10-7　正中神经
Median nerve

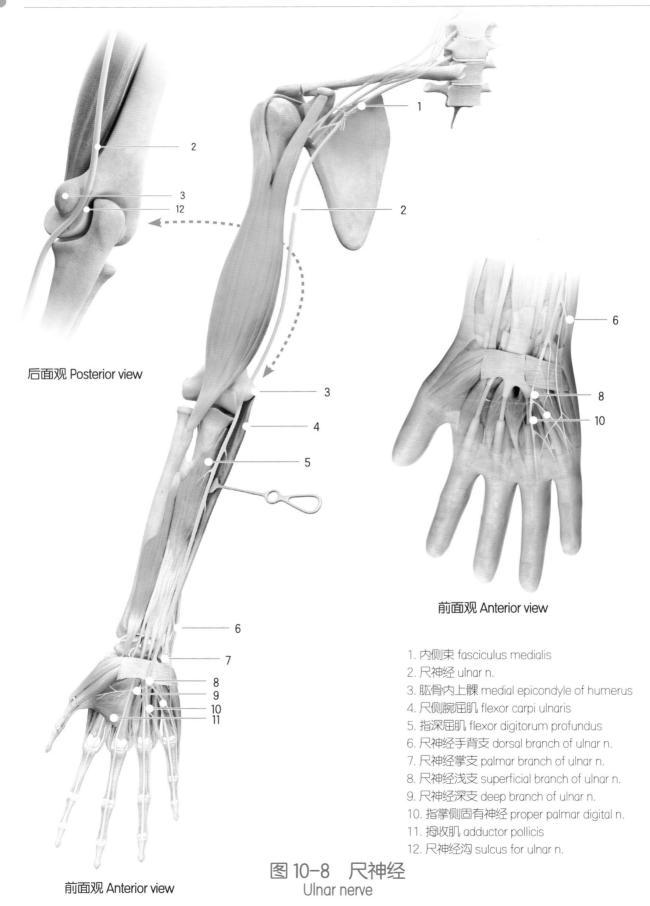

后面观 Posterior view

前面观 Anterior view

前面观 Anterior view

1. 内侧束 fasciculus medialis
2. 尺神经 ulnar n.
3. 肱骨内上髁 medial epicondyle of humerus
4. 尺侧腕屈肌 flexor carpi ulnaris
5. 指深屈肌 flexor digitorum profundus
6. 尺神经手背支 dorsal branch of ulnar n.
7. 尺神经掌支 palmar branch of ulnar n.
8. 尺神经浅支 superficial branch of ulnar n.
9. 尺神经深支 deep branch of ulnar n.
10. 指掌侧固有神经 proper palmar digital n.
11. 拇收肌 adductor pollicis
12. 尺神经沟 sulcus for ulnar n.

图 10-8 尺神经
Ulnar nerve

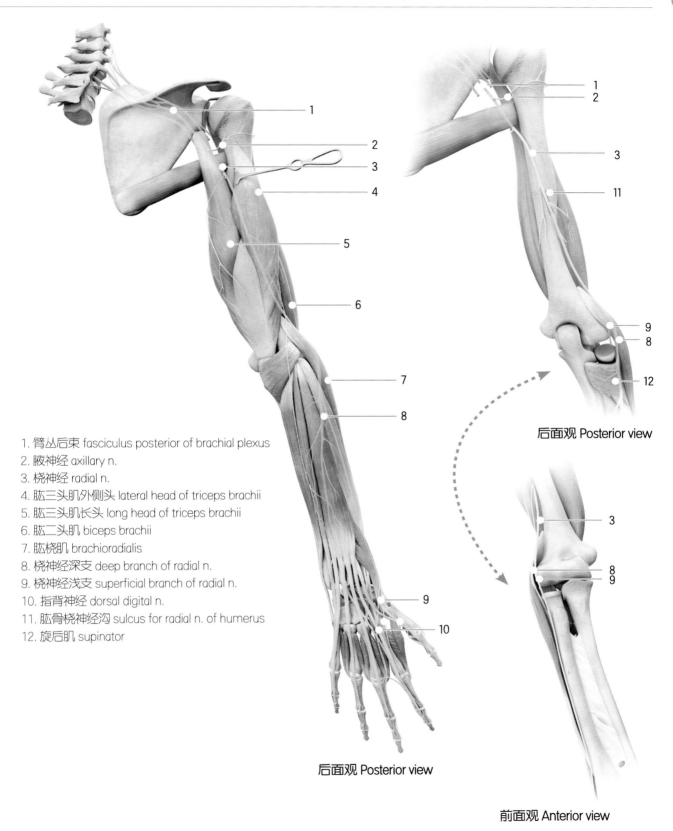

1. 臂丛后束 fasciculus posterior of brachial plexus
2. 腋神经 axillary n.
3. 桡神经 radial n.
4. 肱三头肌外侧头 lateral head of triceps brachii
5. 肱三头肌长头 long head of triceps brachii
6. 肱二头肌 biceps brachii
7. 肱桡肌 brachioradialis
8. 桡神经深支 deep branch of radial n.
9. 桡神经浅支 superficial branch of radial n.
10. 指背神经 dorsal digital n.
11. 肱骨桡神经沟 sulcus for radial n. of humerus
12. 旋后肌 supinator

后面观 Posterior view

前面观 Anterior view

后面观 Posterior view

图 10-9 桡神经及腋神经
Radial and axillary nerves

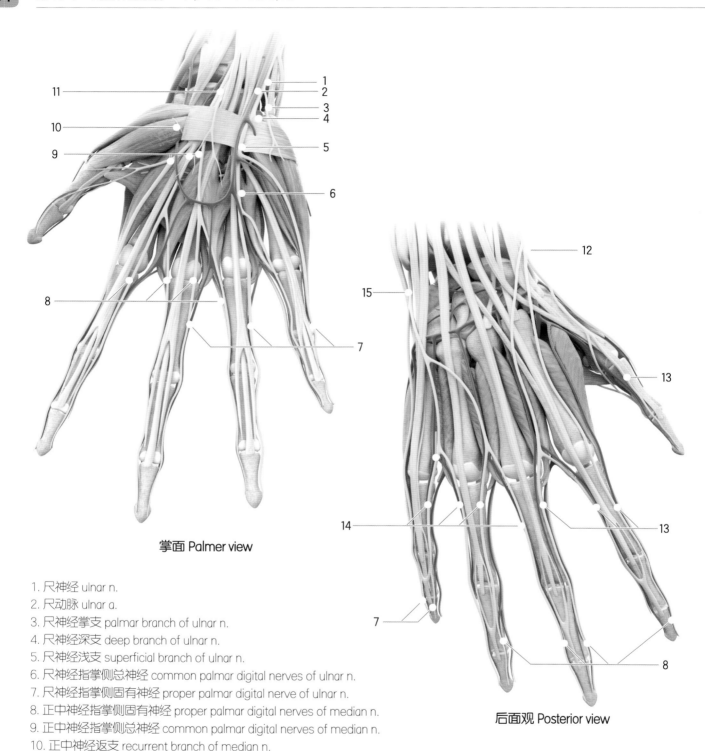

掌面 Palmer view

后面观 Posterior view

1. 尺神经 ulnar n.
2. 尺动脉 ulnar a.
3. 尺神经掌支 palmar branch of ulnar n.
4. 尺神经深支 deep branch of ulnar n.
5. 尺神经浅支 superficial branch of ulnar n.
6. 尺神经指掌侧总神经 common palmar digital nerves of ulnar n.
7. 尺神经指掌侧固有神经 proper palmar digital nerve of ulnar n.
8. 正中神经指掌侧固有神经 proper palmar digital nerves of median n.
9. 正中神经指掌侧总神经 common palmar digital nerves of median n.
10. 正中神经返支 recurrent branch of median n.
11. 正中神经 median n.
12. 桡神经浅支 superficial branch of radial n.
13. 桡神经手背支 dorsal branch of radial n.
14. 尺神经指背支 dorsal digital branch of ulnar n.
15. 尺神经手背支 dorsal branch of ulnar n.

图 10-10 手的神经
Nerves of the hand

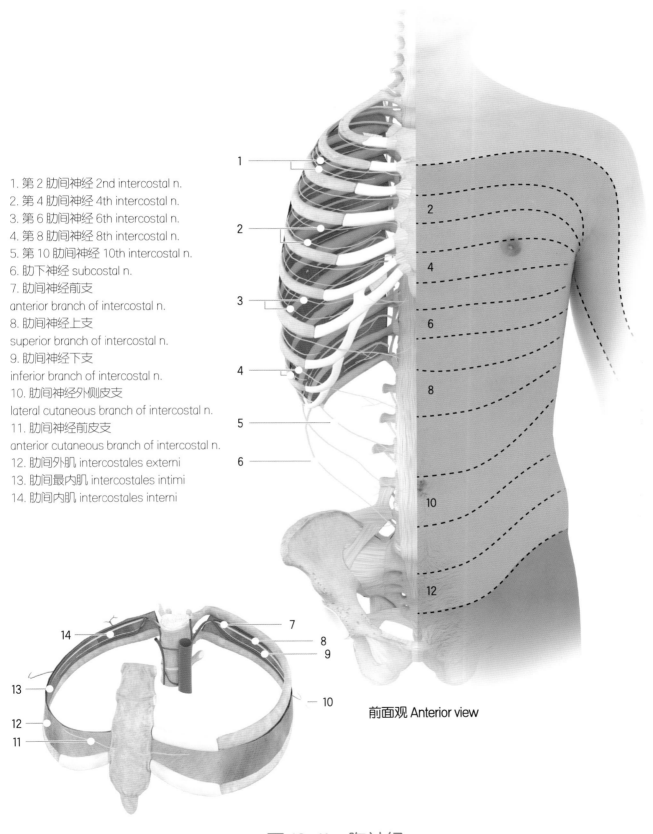

1. 第 2 肋间神经 2nd intercostal n.
2. 第 4 肋间神经 4th intercostal n.
3. 第 6 肋间神经 6th intercostal n.
4. 第 8 肋间神经 8th intercostal n.
5. 第 10 肋间神经 10th intercostal n.
6. 肋下神经 subcostal n.
7. 肋间神经前支
anterior branch of intercostal n.
8. 肋间神经上支
superior branch of intercostal n.
9. 肋间神经下支
inferior branch of intercostal n.
10. 肋间神经外侧皮支
lateral cutaneous branch of intercostal n.
11. 肋间神经前皮支
anterior cutaneous branch of intercostal n.
12. 肋间外肌 intercostales externi
13. 肋间最内肌 intercostales intimi
14. 肋间内肌 intercostales interni

前面观 Anterior view

图 10-11　胸神经
Thoracic nerves

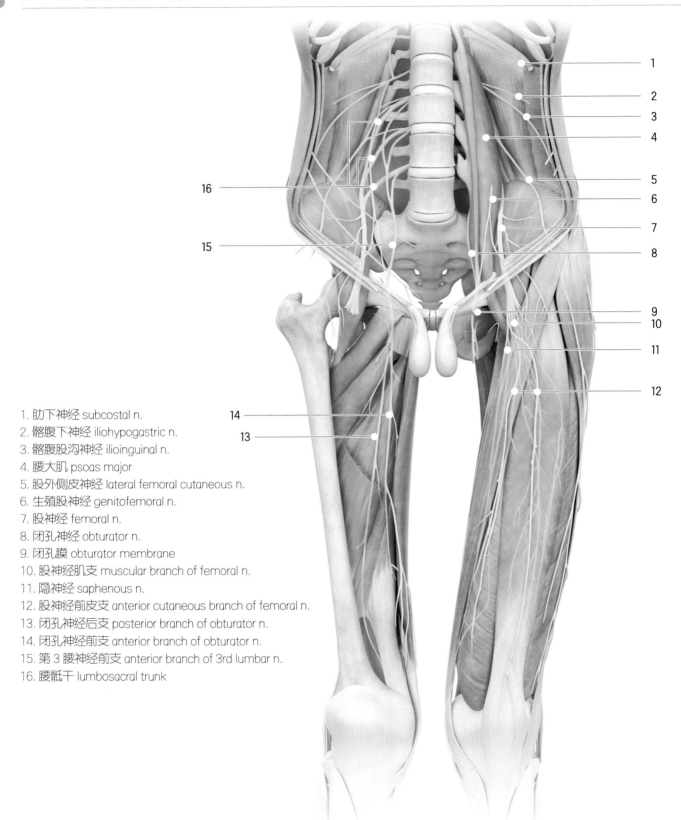

1. 肋下神经 subcostal n.
2. 髂腹下神经 iliohypogastric n.
3. 髂腹股沟神经 ilioinguinal n.
4. 腰大肌 psoas major
5. 股外侧皮神经 lateral femoral cutaneous n.
6. 生殖股神经 genitofemoral n.
7. 股神经 femoral n.
8. 闭孔神经 obturator n.
9. 闭孔膜 obturator membrane
10. 股神经肌支 muscular branch of femoral n.
11. 隐神经 saphenous n.
12. 股神经前皮支 anterior cutaneous branch of femoral n.
13. 闭孔神经后支 posterior branch of obturator n.
14. 闭孔神经前支 anterior branch of obturator n.
15. 第 3 腰神经前支 anterior branch of 3rd lumbar n.
16. 腰骶干 lumbosacral trunk

前面观 Anterior view

图 10-12　腰丛及其分支
Lumbar plexus and its branches

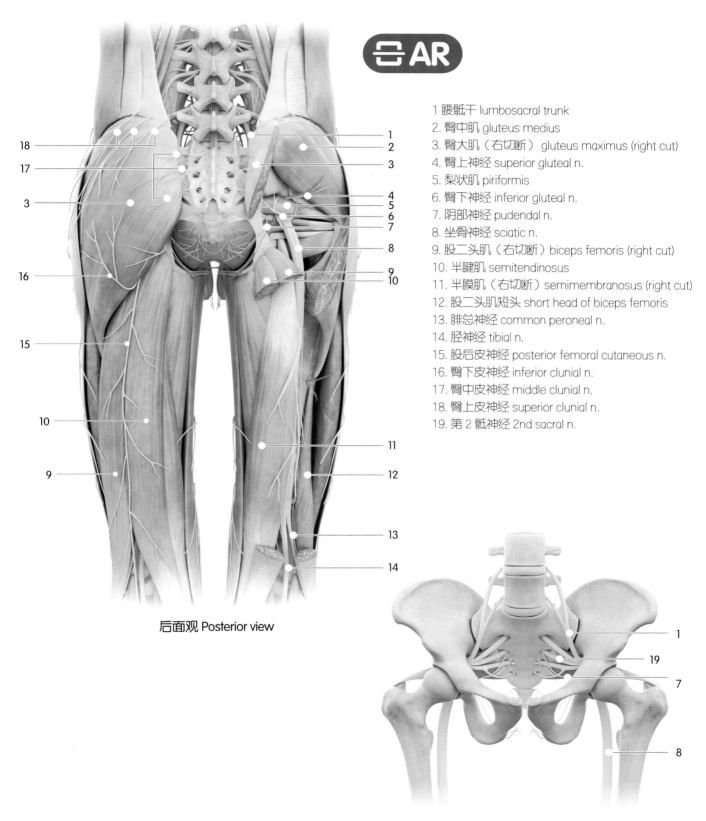

1 腰骶干 lumbosacral trunk
2. 臀中肌 gluteus medius
3. 臀大肌（右切断）gluteus maximus (right cut)
4. 臀上神经 superior gluteal n.
5. 梨状肌 piriformis
6. 臀下神经 inferior gluteal n.
7. 阴部神经 pudendal n.
8. 坐骨神经 sciatic n.
9. 股二头肌（右切断）biceps femoris (right cut)
10. 半腱肌 semitendinosus
11. 半膜肌（右切断）semimembranosus (right cut)
12. 股二头肌短头 short head of biceps femoris
13. 腓总神经 common peroneal n.
14. 胫神经 tibial n.
15. 股后皮神经 posterior femoral cutaneous n.
16. 臀下皮神经 inferior clunial n.
17. 臀中皮神经 middle clunial n.
18. 臀上皮神经 superior clunial n.
19. 第 2 骶神经 2nd sacral n.

后面观 Posterior view

前面观 Anterior view

图 10-13　骶丛及其分支
Sacral plexus and its branches

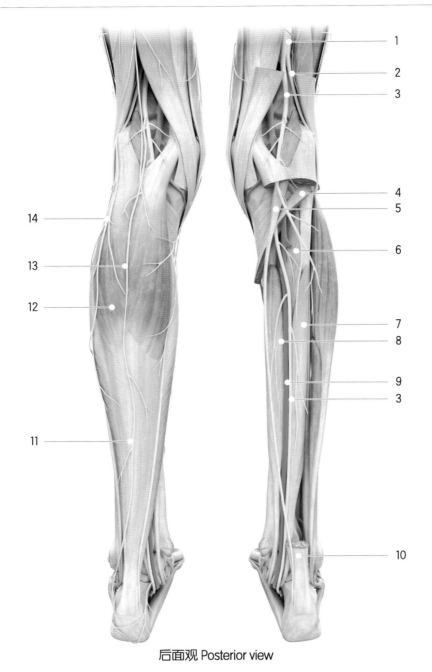

后面观 Posterior view

足底神经 Plantar nerve

1. 坐骨神经 sciatic n.
2. 腓总神经 common peroneal n.
3. 胫神经 tibial n.
4. 比目鱼肌（切断）soleus (cut)
5. 跖肌 plantaris
6. 胫骨后肌 tibialis posterior
7. 跨长屈肌 flexor hallucis longus
8. 趾长屈肌 flexor digitorum longus
9. 胫后动脉 posterior tibial a.
10. 跟腱 tendo calcaneus

11. 腓肠神经 sural n.
12. 腓肠肌 gastrocnemius
13. 腓肠内侧皮神经 medial sural cutaneous n.
14. 腓肠外侧皮神经 lateral sural cutaneous n.
15. 足底内侧神经 medial plantar n.
16. 足底外侧神经 lateral plantar n.
17. 足底外侧神经深支 deep branch of lateral plantar n.
18. 足底外侧神经浅支 superficial branch of lateral plantar n.
19. 趾足底总神经 common plantar digital n.
20. 趾足底固有神经 proper plantar digital n.

图 10-14 小腿和足底神经
Nerves of the leg and pelma

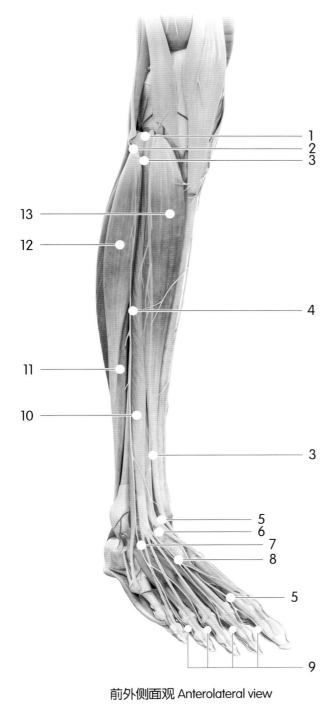

前外侧面观 Anterolateral view

1. 腓骨头 fibular head
2. 腓总神经 common peroneal n.
3. 腓深神经 deep peroneal n.
4. 腓浅神经 superficial peroneal n.
5. 腓深神经内侧支 medial branch of deep peroneal n.
6. 腓深神经外侧支 lateral branch of deep peroneal n.
7. 足背中间皮神经 intermediate dorsal cutaneous n. of foot
8. 足背内侧皮神经 medial dorsal cutaneous n. of foot
9. 趾背神经 dorsal digital nerves of foot
10. 趾长伸肌 extensor digitorum longus
11. 腓骨短肌 peroneus brevis
12. 腓骨长肌 peroneus longus
13. 胫骨前肌 tibialis anterior

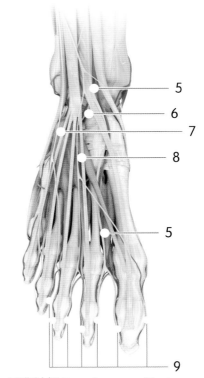

足背神经 Dorsal nerves of foot

图 10-15　小腿前外侧及足背神经
Nerves of the anterolateral region of leg and dorsum of foot

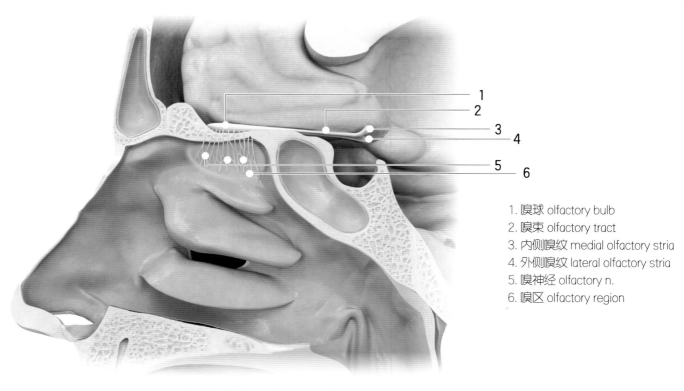

1. 嗅球 olfactory bulb
2. 嗅束 olfactory tract
3. 内侧嗅纹 medial olfactory stria
4. 外侧嗅纹 lateral olfactory stria
5. 嗅神经 olfactory n.
6. 嗅区 olfactory region

正中矢状面 Median sagittal section

图 10-16　嗅神经
Olfactory nerve

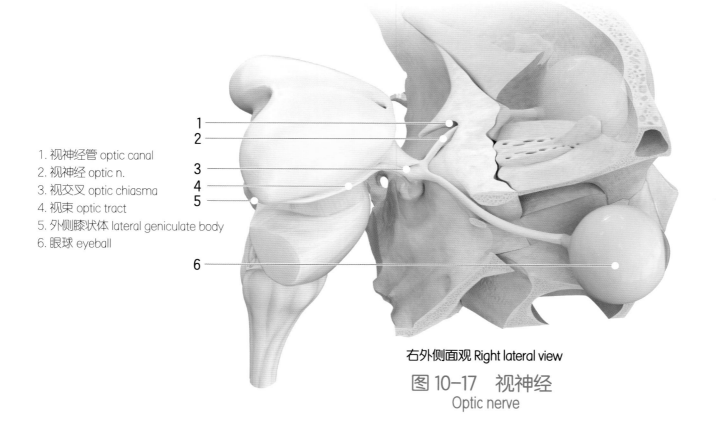

1. 视神经管 optic canal
2. 视神经 optic n.
3. 视交叉 optic chiasma
4. 视束 optic tract
5. 外侧膝状体 lateral geniculate body
6. 眼球 eyeball

右外侧面观 Right lateral view

图 10-17　视神经
Optic nerve

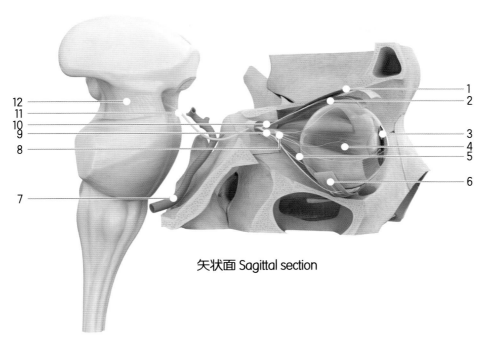

矢状面 Sagittal section

1. 上睑提肌 levator palpebrae superioris
2. 上直肌 rectus superior
3. 巩膜 sclera
4. 内直肌 rectus medialis
5. 下直肌 rectus inferior
6. 下斜肌 obliquus inferior
7. 颈内动脉 internal carotid a.
8. 睫状神经节 ciliary ganglion
9. 动眼神经下支 inferior branch of oculomotor n.
10. 动眼神经上支 superior branch of oculomotor n.
11. 动眼神经 oculomotor n.
12. 中脑 midbrain

图 10-18　动眼神经
Oculomotor nerve

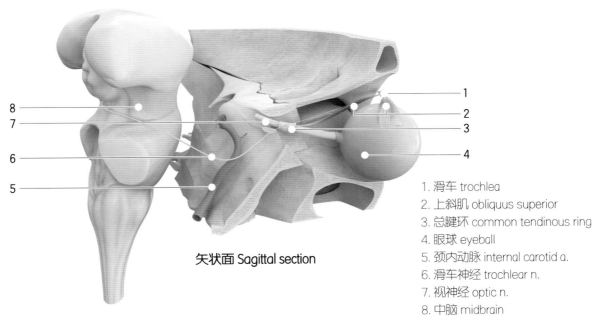

矢状面 Sagittal section

1. 滑车 trochlea
2. 上斜肌 obliquus superior
3. 总腱环 common tendinous ring
4. 眼球 eyeball
5. 颈内动脉 internal carotid a.
6. 滑车神经 trochlear n.
7. 视神经 optic n.
8. 中脑 midbrain

图 10-19　滑车神经
Trochlear nerve

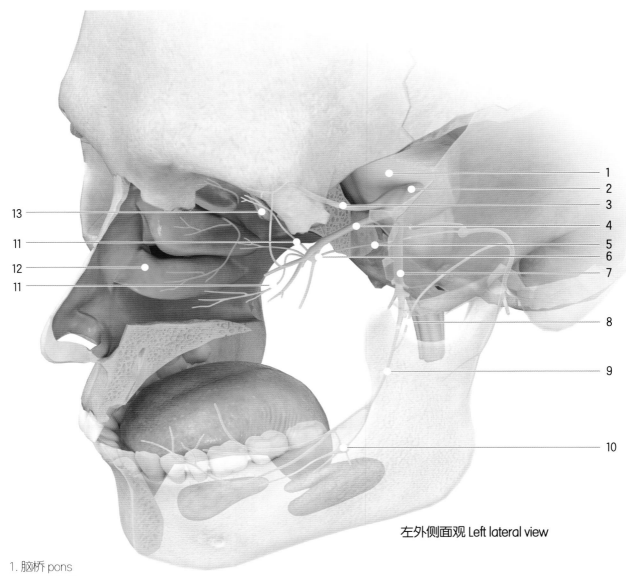

左外侧面观 Left lateral view

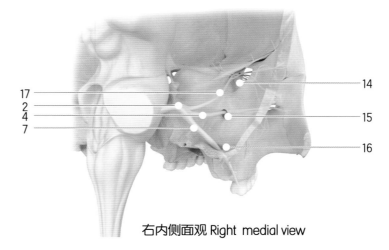

右内侧面观 Right medial view

1. 脑桥 pons
2. 三叉神经节 trigeminal ganglion
3. 眼神经 ophthalmic n.
4. 上颌神经 maxillary n.
5. 翼管神经 nerve of pterygoid canal
6. 翼腭神经节 pterygopalatine ganglion
7. 下颌神经 mandibular n.
8. 鼓索 chorda tympani
9. 舌神经 lingual n.
10. 下颌下神经节 submandibular ganglion
11. 翼腭神经 pterygopalatine n.
12. 下鼻甲 inferior nasal concha
13. 泪腺 lacrimal gland
14. 眶上裂 superior orbital fissure
15. 圆孔 foramen rotundum
16. 卵圆孔 foramen ovale
17. 眼神经 ophthalmic n.

图 10-20　三叉神经及其分支
Trigeminal nerve and its branches

1. 眶上神经 supraorbital n.
2. 眶上孔 supraorbital foramen
3. 滑车上神经 supratrochlear n.
4. 泪腺神经 lacrimal n.
5. 鼻睫神经 nasociliary n.
6. 睫状神经 ciliary nerves
7. 眶下神经 infraorbital n.
8. 眶下孔 infraorbital foramen
9. 上牙槽神经 superior alveolar nerves
10. 下颌神经 mandibular n.
11. 颧神经 zygomatic n.
12. 上颌神经 maxillary n.
13. 三叉神经节 trigeminal ganglion
14. 眼神经 ophthalmic n.
15. 睫状神经节 ciliary ganglion
16. 额神经 frontal n.

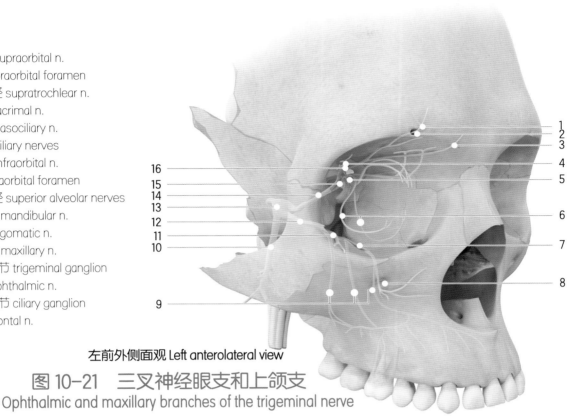

左前外侧面观 Left anterolateral view

图 10-21 三叉神经眼支和上颌支
Ophthalmic and maxillary branches of the trigeminal nerve

1. 三叉神经节 trigeminal ganglion
2. 下颌神经 mandibular n.
3. 下牙槽神经 inferior alveolar n.
4. 颏孔 mental foramen
5. 颏神经 mental n.
6. 下颌舌骨肌神经 mylohyoid n.
7. 颊神经 buccal n.
8. 舌神经 lingual n.
9. 下颌孔 mandibular foramen
10. 下牙槽神经 inferior alveolar n.

右前外侧面观 Right anterolateral view

图 10-22 三叉神经下颌支
Mandibular branch of the trigeminal nerve

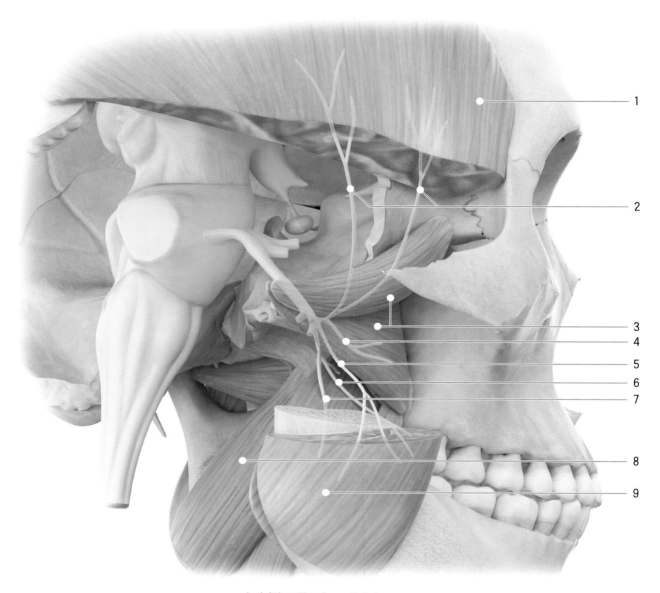

左内侧面观 Left medial view

1. 颞肌 temporalis
2. 颞支 temporal branches
3. 翼外肌 lateral pterygoid
4. 翼外肌支 lateral pterygoid branch
5. 咬肌神经 masseteric n.
6. 颊神经 buccal n.
7. 翼内肌支 medial pterygoid branch
8. 翼内肌 medial pterygoid
9. 咬肌 masseter

图 10-23　三叉神经咀嚼肌支
Masticatory branch of the trigeminal nerve

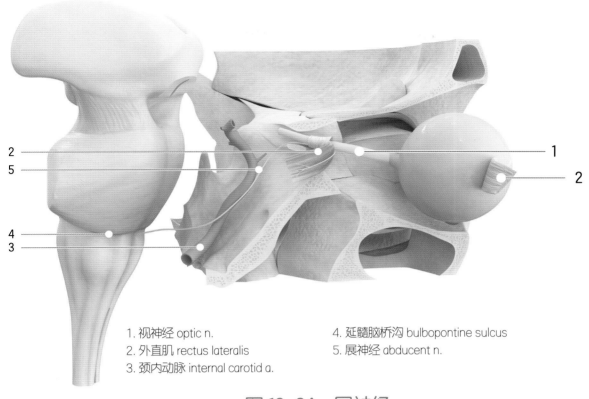

1. 视神经 optic n.
2. 外直肌 rectus lateralis
3. 颈内动脉 internal carotid a.
4. 延髓脑桥沟 bulbopontine sulcus
5. 展神经 abducent n.

图 10-24 展神经
Abducent nerve

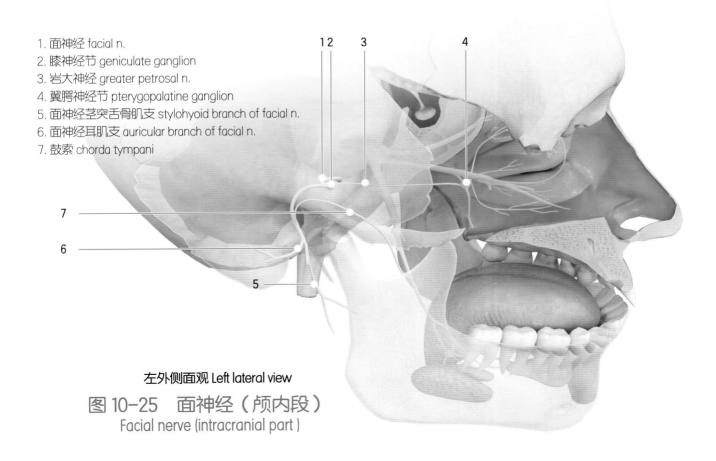

1. 面神经 facial n.
2. 膝神经节 geniculate ganglion
3. 岩大神经 greater petrosal n.
4. 翼腭神经节 pterygopalatine ganglion
5. 面神经茎突舌骨肌支 stylohyoid branch of facial n.
6. 面神经耳肌支 auricular branch of facial n.
7. 鼓索 chorda tympani

左外侧面观 Left lateral view

图 10-25 面神经（颅内段）
Facial nerve (intracranial part)

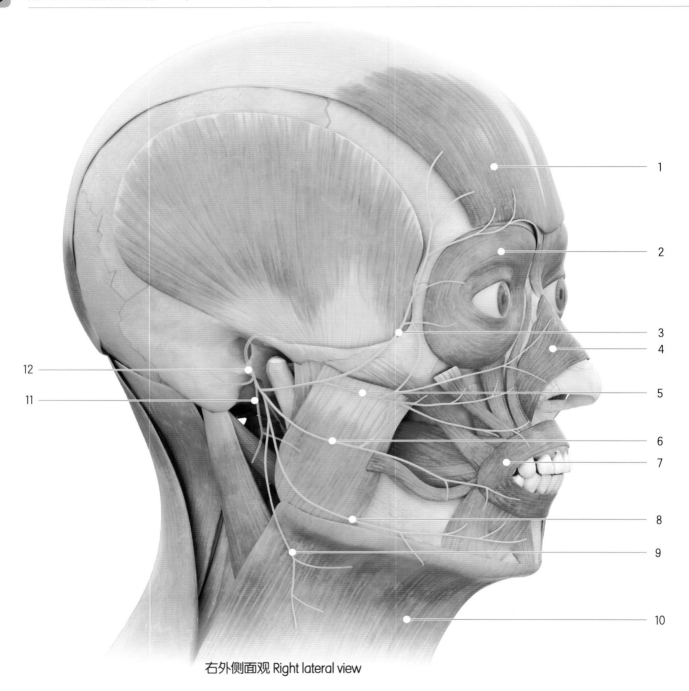

右外侧面观 Right lateral view

1. 枕额肌 occipitofrontalis
2. 眼轮匝肌 orbicularis oculi
3. 面神经颞支 temporal branch of facial n.
4. 鼻肌 nasalis
5. 面神经颧支 zygomatic branch of facial n.
6. 面神经颊支 buccal branch of facial n.
7. 口轮匝肌 orbicularis oris
8. 面神经下颌缘支 marginal mandibular branch of facial n.
9. 面神经颈支 cervical branch of facial n.
10. 颈阔肌 platysma
11. 面神经茎突舌骨肌支 stylohyoid branch
12. 面神经 facial n.

图 10-26 面神经在面部的分支
Branches of the facial nerve in the face

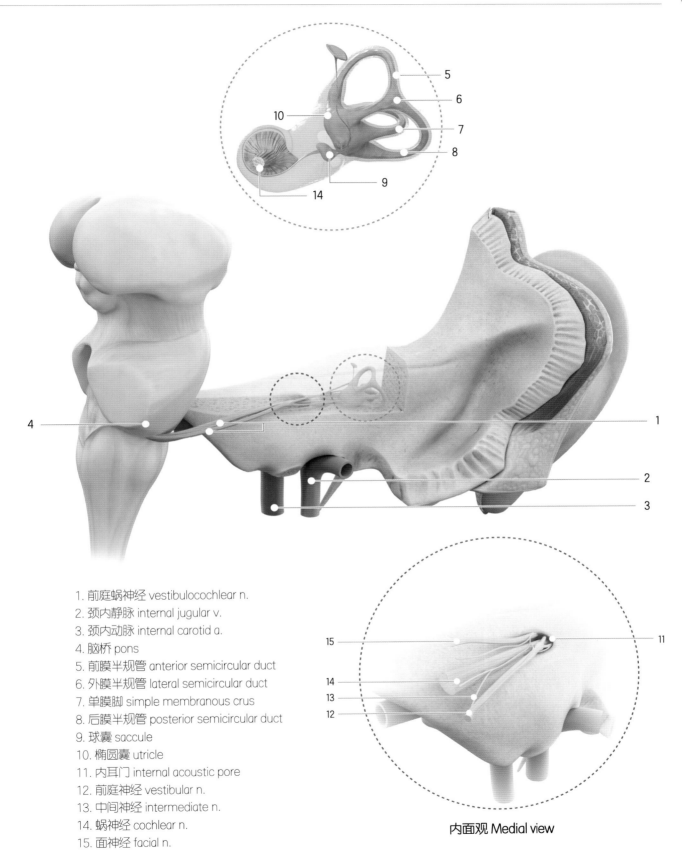

1. 前庭蜗神经 vestibulocochlear n.
2. 颈内静脉 internal jugular v.
3. 颈内动脉 internal carotid a.
4. 脑桥 pons
5. 前膜半规管 anterior semicircular duct
6. 外膜半规管 lateral semicircular duct
7. 单膜脚 simple membranous crus
8. 后膜半规管 posterior semicircular duct
9. 球囊 saccule
10. 椭圆囊 utricle
11. 内耳门 internal acoustic pore
12. 前庭神经 vestibular n.
13. 中间神经 intermediate n.
14. 蜗神经 cochlear n.
15. 面神经 facial n.

内面观 Medial view

图 10-27　前庭蜗神经
Vestibulocochlear nerve

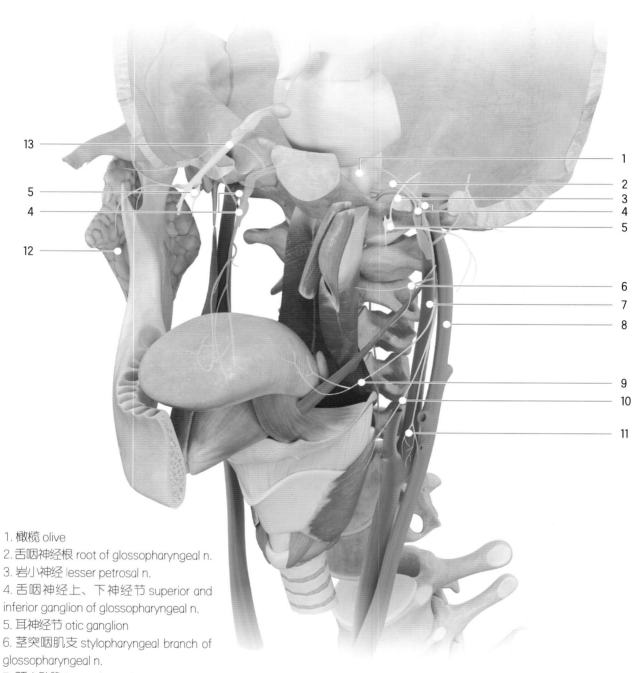

1. 橄榄 olive
2. 舌咽神经根 root of glossopharyngeal n.
3. 岩小神经 lesser petrosal n.
4. 舌咽神经上、下神经节 superior and inferior ganglion of glossopharyngeal n.
5. 耳神经节 otic ganglion
6. 茎突咽肌支 stylopharyngeal branch of glossopharyngeal n.
7. 颈内动脉 internal carotid a.
8. 颈内静脉 internal jugular v.
9. 舌支 lingual branch
10. 咽支 pharyngeal branch
11. 颈动脉支 carotid branch
12. 腮腺 parotid gland
13. 下颌神经 mandibular n.

右前外侧面观 Right anterolateral view

图 10-28　舌咽神经
Glossopharyngeal nerve

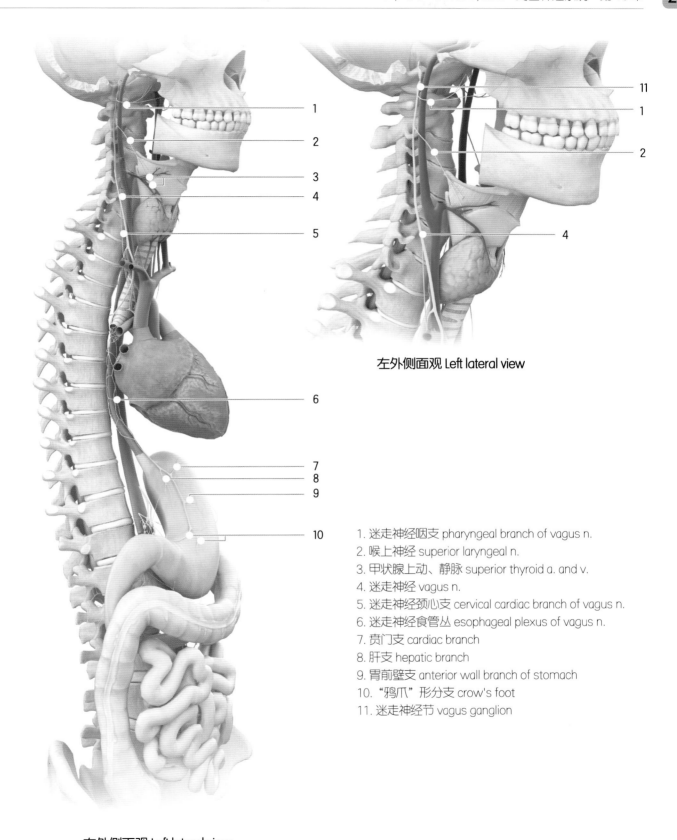

左外侧面观 Left lateral view

左外侧面观 Left lateral view

1. 迷走神经咽支 pharyngeal branch of vagus n.
2. 喉上神经 superior laryngeal n.
3. 甲状腺上动、静脉 superior thyroid a. and v.
4. 迷走神经 vagus n.
5. 迷走神经颈心支 cervical cardiac branch of vagus n.
6. 迷走神经食管丛 esophageal plexus of vagus n.
7. 贲门支 cardiac branch
8. 肝支 hepatic branch
9. 胃前壁支 anterior wall branch of stomach
10. "鸦爪"形分支 crow's foot
11. 迷走神经节 vagus ganglion

图 10-29　迷走神经 1
Vagus nerve 1

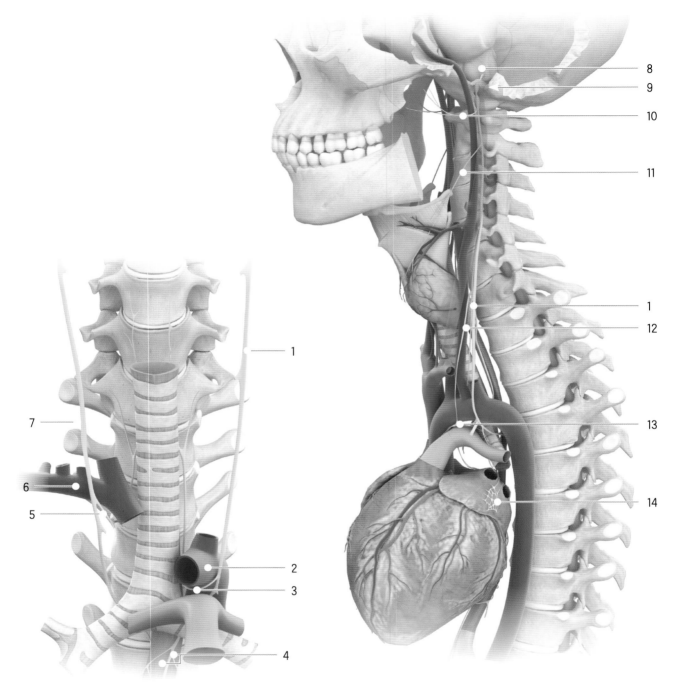

前面观 Anterior view

1. 左迷走神经 left vagus n.
2. 主动脉弓 aortic arch
3. 左喉返神经 left recurrent laryngeal n.
4. 食管及食管丛 esophagus and esophageal plexus
5. 右喉返神经 right recurrent laryngeal n.
6. 右锁骨下动脉 right subclavian a.
7. 右迷走神经 right vagus n.

右外侧面观 Right lateral view

8. 延髓 medulla oblongata
9. 颈静脉孔 jugular foramen
10. 迷走神经咽支 pharyngeal branch of vagus n.
11. 喉上神经 superior laryngeal n.
12. 颈心支 cervical cardiac branch
13. 心浅丛 superficial cardiac plexus
14. 心深丛 deep cardiac plexus

图 10-30 迷走神经 2
Vagus nerve 2

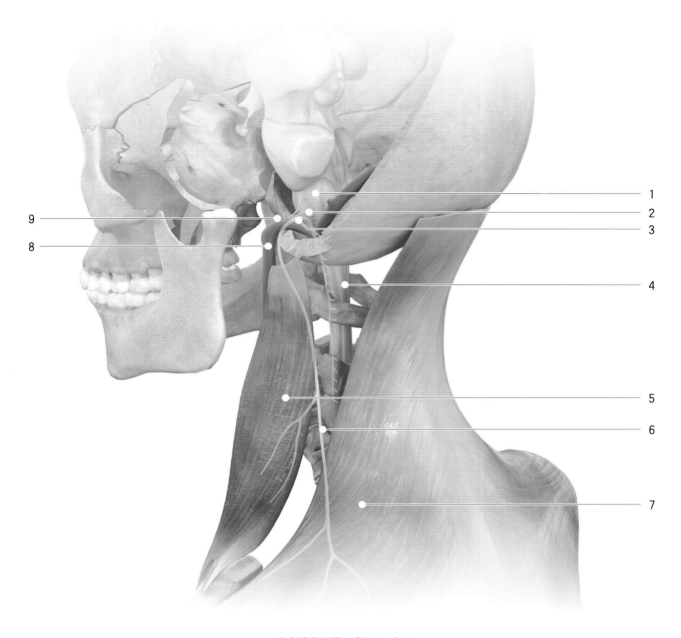

左外侧面观 Left lateral view

1. 延髓 medulla oblongata
2. 副神经颅根 cranial root of accessory n.
3. 副神经脊髓根 spinal root of accessory n.
4. 脊髓 spinal cord
5. 胸锁乳突肌 sternocleidomastoid
6. 副神经 accessory n.
7. 斜方肌 trapezius
8. 颈内静脉 internal jugular v.
9. 颈静脉孔 jugular foramen

图 10-31　副神经
Accessory nerve

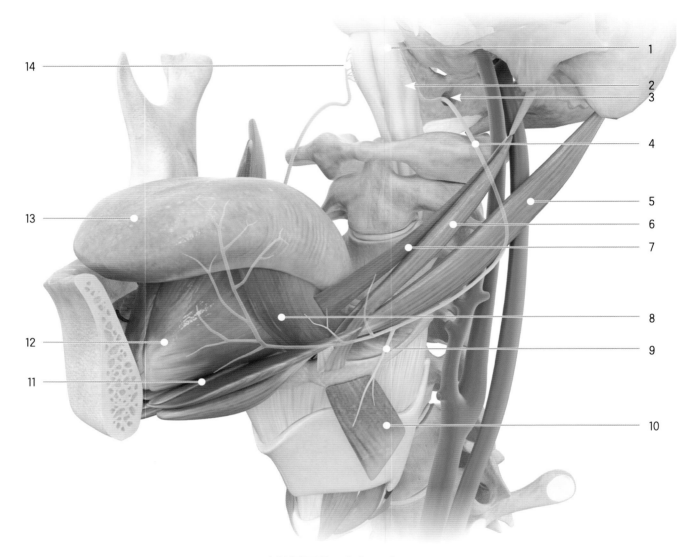

右外侧面观 Right lateral view

1. 延髓锥体 pyramid of medulla oblongata
2. 外侧沟 lateral sulcus
3. 舌下神经管下口 inferior opening of hypoglossal canal
4. 舌下神经 hypoglossal n.
5. 二腹肌后腹 posterior belly of digastric
6. 茎突舌骨肌 stylohyoid
7. 茎突舌肌 styloglossus
8. 舌骨舌肌 hyoglossus
9. 甲状舌骨肌支 thyrohyoid branch
10. 甲状舌骨肌 thyrohyoid
11. 颏舌骨肌 geniohyoid
12. 颏舌肌 genioglossus
13. 舌 tongue
14. 舌下神经根 root of hypoglossal n.

图 10-32　舌下神经
Hypoglossal nerve

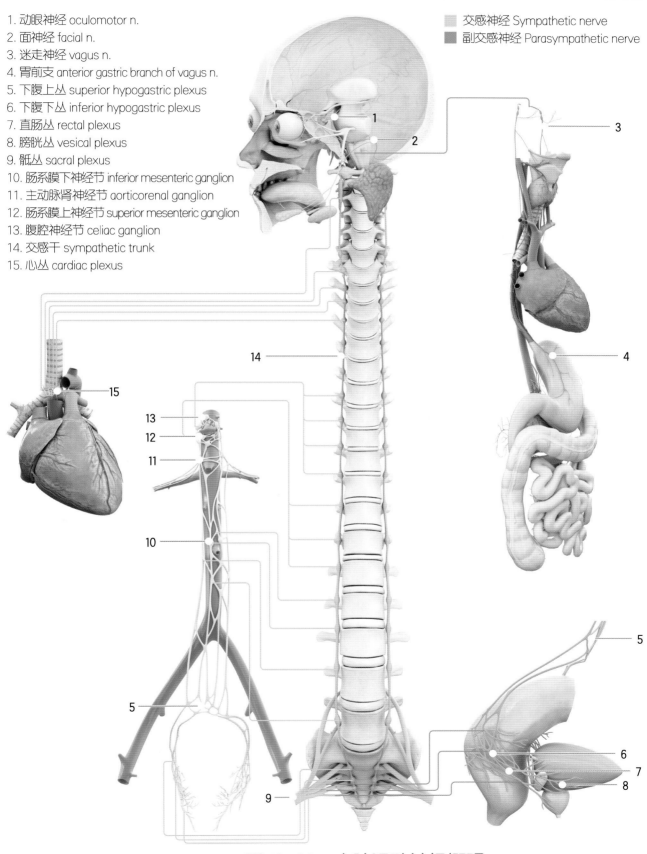

1. 动眼神经 oculomotor n.
2. 面神经 facial n.
3. 迷走神经 vagus n.
4. 胃前支 anterior gastric branch of vagus n.
5. 下腹上丛 superior hypogastric plexus
6. 下腹下丛 inferior hypogastric plexus
7. 直肠丛 rectal plexus
8. 膀胱丛 vesical plexus
9. 骶丛 sacral plexus
10. 肠系膜下神经节 inferior mesenteric ganglion
11. 主动脉肾神经节 aorticorenal ganglion
12. 肠系膜上神经节 superior mesenteric ganglion
13. 腹腔神经节 celiac ganglion
14. 交感干 sympathetic trunk
15. 心丛 cardiac plexus

交感神经 Sympathetic nerve
副交感神经 Parasympathetic nerve

图 10-33　内脏运动神经概观
Overview of the visceral motor nerve

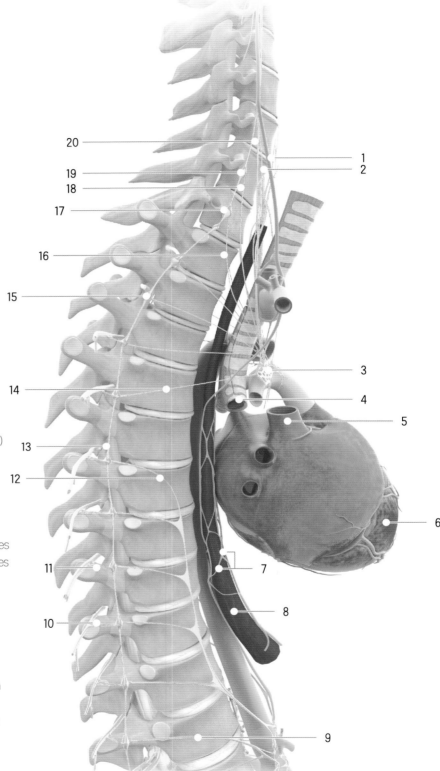

1. 右迷走神经 right vagus n.
2. 颈心支 cervical cardiac branch
3. 心深丛 deep cardiac plexus
4. 右主支气管 right principal bronchus
5. 升主动脉（切断）ascending aorta (cut)
6. 心 heart
7. 迷走神经食管丛 esophageal plexus
of vagus n.
8. 食管 esophagus
9. 内脏小神经 lesser splanchnic n.
10. 灰交通支 grey communicating branches
11. 白交通支 white communicating branches
12. 内脏大神经 greater splanchnic n.
13. 交感干 sympathetic trunk
14. 胸心神经 thoracic cardiac n.
15. 胸交感神经节 thoracic sympathetic
ganglion
16. 心下神经 inferior cardiac n.
17. 颈下神经节 inferior cervical ganglion
18. 心中神经 middle cardiac n.
19. 颈中神经节 middle cervical ganglion
20. 心上神经 superior cardiac n.

右外侧面观 Right lateral view

图 10-34　胸部内脏神经
Thoracic splanchnic nerves

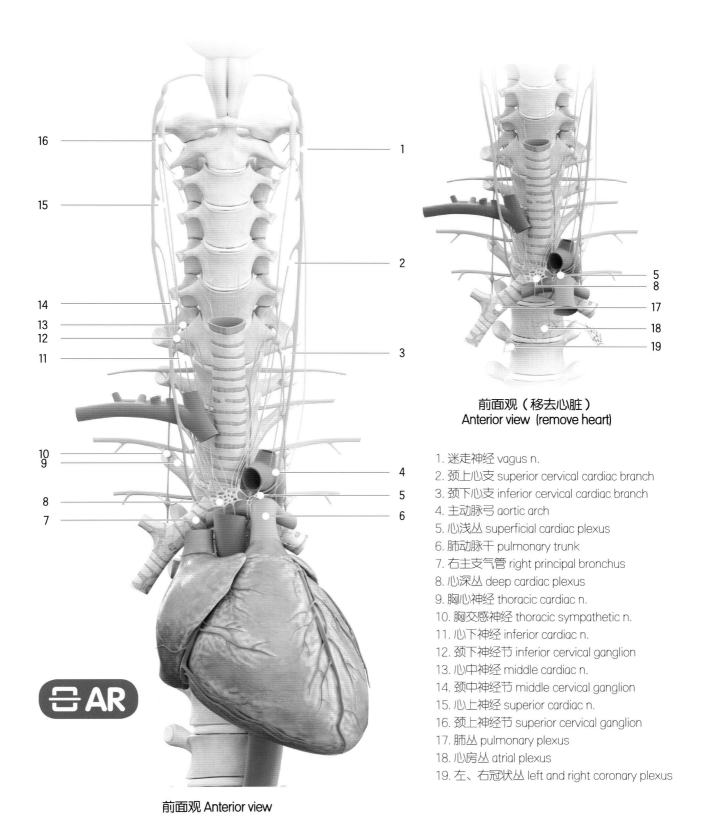

前面观（移去心脏）
Anterior view (remove heart)

1. 迷走神经 vagus n.
2. 颈上心支 superior cervical cardiac branch
3. 颈下心支 inferior cervical cardiac branch
4. 主动脉弓 aortic arch
5. 心浅丛 superficial cardiac plexus
6. 肺动脉干 pulmonary trunk
7. 右主支气管 right principal bronchus
8. 心深丛 deep cardiac plexus
9. 胸心神经 thoracic cardiac n.
10. 胸交感神经 thoracic sympathetic n.
11. 心下神经 inferior cardiac n.
12. 颈下神经节 inferior cervical ganglion
13. 心中神经 middle cardiac n.
14. 颈中神经节 middle cervical ganglion
15. 心上神经 superior cardiac n.
16. 颈上神经节 superior cervical ganglion
17. 肺丛 pulmonary plexus
18. 心房丛 atrial plexus
19. 左、右冠状丛 left and right coronary plexus

前面观 Anterior view

图 10-35　心丛及其分支
Cardiac plexus and its branches

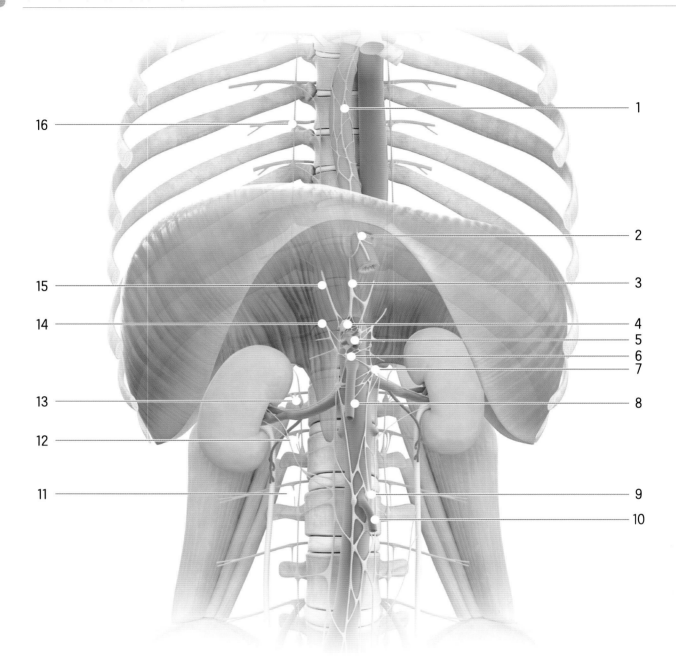

前面观 Anterior view

1. 食管前丛 anterior esophageal plexus
2. 迷走神经前干 anterior vagal trunk
3. 迷走神经后干 posterior vagal trunk
4. 腹腔神经节 celiac ganglion
5. 腹腔干 celiac trunk
6. 肠系膜上神经节 superior mesenteric ganglion
7. 主动脉肾神经节 aorticorenal ganglion
8. 肠系膜上动脉 superior mesenteric a.
9. 肠系膜下神经节 inferior mesenteric ganglion
10. 肠系膜下动脉 inferior mesenteric a.
11. 灰交通支 grey communicating branches
12. 灰、白交通支 grey and white communicating branches
13. 腰神经节 lumbar ganglion
14. 内脏小神经 lesser splanchnic n.
15. 内脏大神经 greater splanchnic n.
16. 胸神经节 thoracic ganglion

图 10-36　腹部内脏神经
Abdominal visceral nerves

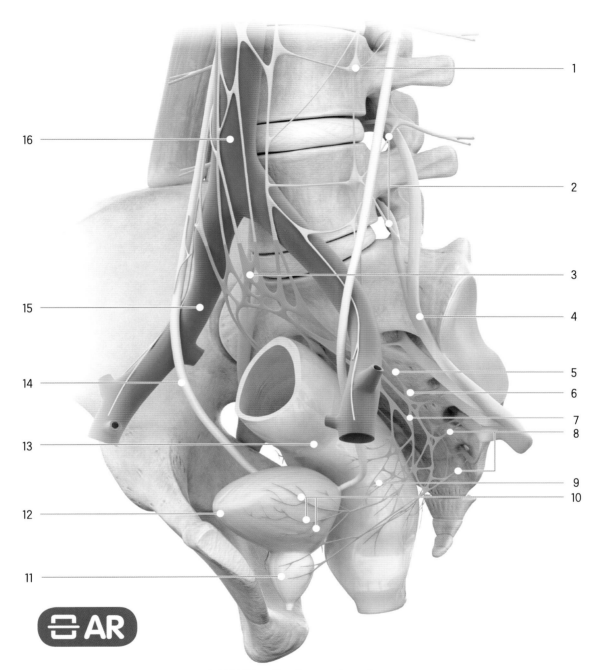

左前外侧面观 Left anterolateral view

1. 腰神经节 lumbar ganglion
2. 灰交通支 grey communicating branches
3. 上腹下丛 superior hypogastric plexus
4. 腰骶干 lumbosacral trunk
5. 骶交感干 sacral sympathetic trunk
6. 骶神经节 sacral ganglion
7. 下腹下丛 inferior hypogastric plexus
8. 盆部内脏神经 pelvic splanchnic nerves
9. 直肠丛 rectal plexus
10. 膀胱丛 vesical plexus
11. 前列腺 prostate
12. 膀胱 urinary bladder
13. 直肠 rectum
14. 输尿管 ureter
15. 右髂总动脉 right common iliac a.
16. 腹主动脉 abdominal aorta

图 10-37 盆部内脏神经
Pelvic splanchnic nerves

第11章 中枢神经系统
Central Nervous System

17
16
15
14
13

1. 楔前叶 precuneus
2. 扣带回 cingulate gyrus
3. 顶枕沟 parietooccipital sulcus
4. 胼胝体干 trunk of corpus callosum
5. 楔叶 cuneus
6. 胼胝体压部 splenium of corpus callosum
7. 距状沟 calcarine sulcus
8. 上丘 superior colliculus
9. 下丘 inferior colliculus
10. 中脑 midbrain
11. 小脑蚓 vermis
12. 延髓 medulla oblongata
13. 小脑半球 cerebellar hemisphere
14. 脑桥 pons
15. 侧脑室 lateral ventricle
16. 尾状核 caudate nucleus
17. 豆状核 lentiform nucleus

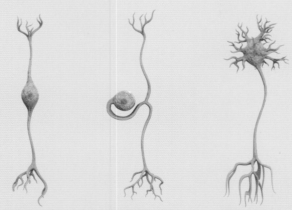

双极神经元
Bipolar neuron

假单极神经元
Pseudounipolar neuron

多极神经元
Multipolar neuron

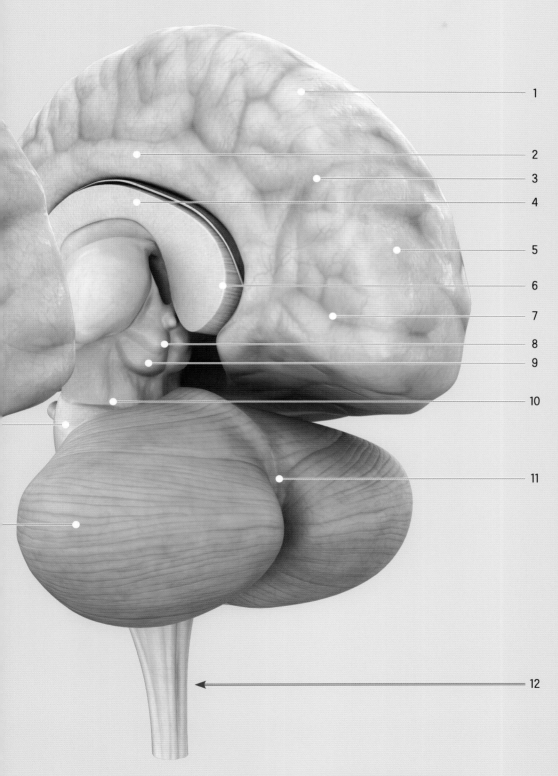

1

2

3

4

5

6

7

8

9

10

11

12

图 11-1　中枢神经系统概观
Overview of the central nervous system

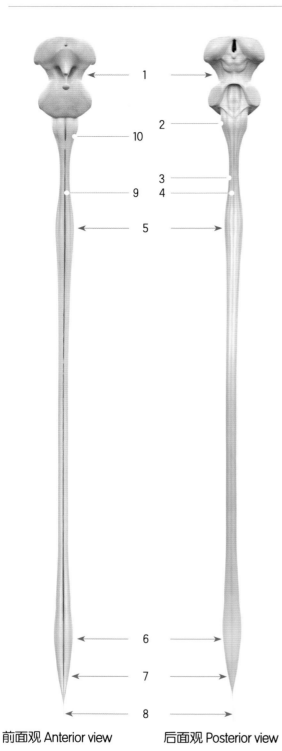

前面观 Anterior view　　后面观 Posterior view

1. 脑干 brain stem
2. 后外侧沟 posterolateral sulcus
3. 后中间沟 posterior intermediate sulcus
4. 后正中沟 posterior median sulcus
5. 颈膨大 cervical enlargement
6. 腰骶膨大 lumbosacral enlargement
7. 脊髓圆锥 conus medullaris
8. 终丝 filum terminale
9. 前正中裂 anterior median fissure
10. 前外侧沟 anterolateral sulcus

图 11-2　脊髓外形及其横切面
External features and transverse section of the spinal cord

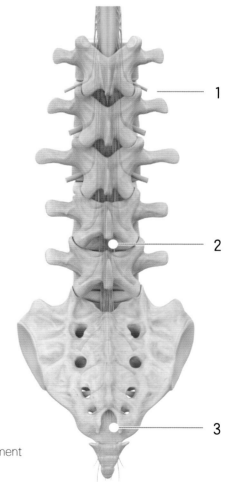

1. 后根 posterior root
2. 前根 anterior root
3. 脊神经 spinal n.
4. 脊神经节 spinal ganglion

图 11-3　脊髓和脊神经根
Spinal cord and spinal nerve root

1. 脊神经 spinal n.
2. 马尾 cauda equina
3. 终丝 filum terminale

图 11-4　马尾
Cauda equina

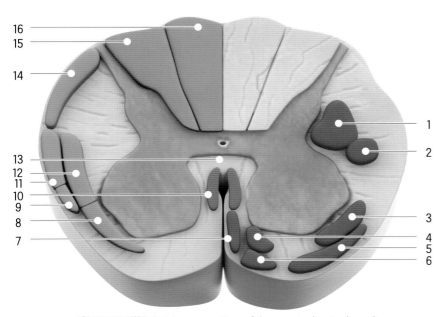

脊髓颈段横切面 Cross section of the cervical spinal cord

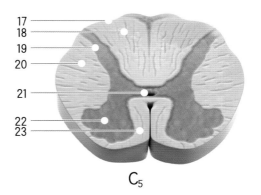

C₅

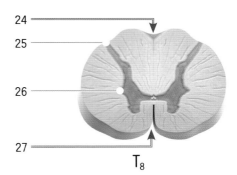

T₈

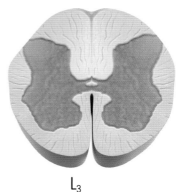

L₃

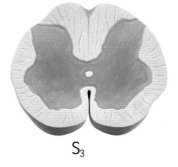

S₃

1. 皮质脊髓侧束 lateral corticospinal tract
2. 红核脊髓束 rubrospinal tract
3. 外侧网状脊髓束 lateral reticulospinal tract
4. 脑桥网状脊髓束 reticulospinal tract of pons
5. 前庭脊髓束 vestibulospinal tract
6. 顶盖脊髓束 tectospinal tract
7. 皮质脊髓前束 anterior corticospinal tract
8. 脊髓丘脑侧束 lateral spinothalamic tract
9. 脊髓橄榄束 spinoolivary tract
10. 内侧纵束 medial longitudinal fasciculus
11. 脊髓小脑前束 anterior spinocerebellar tract
12. 脊髓丘脑前束 anterior spinothalamic tract
13. 白质前连合 anterior white commissure
14. 脊髓小脑后束 posterior spinocerebellar tract
15. 楔束 fasciculus cuneatus
16. 薄束 fasciculus gracilis
17. 后中间沟 posterior intermediate sulcus
18. 后索 posterior funiculus
19. 后角 posterior horn
20. 侧索 lateral funiculus
21. 中央管 central canal
22. 前角 anterior horn
23. 前索 anterior funiculus
24. 后正中沟 posterior median sulcus
25. 后外侧沟 posterolateral sulcus
26. 侧索 lateral funiculus
27. 前正中裂 anterior median fissure

图 11-5　脊髓横切面
Transverse section of the spinal cord

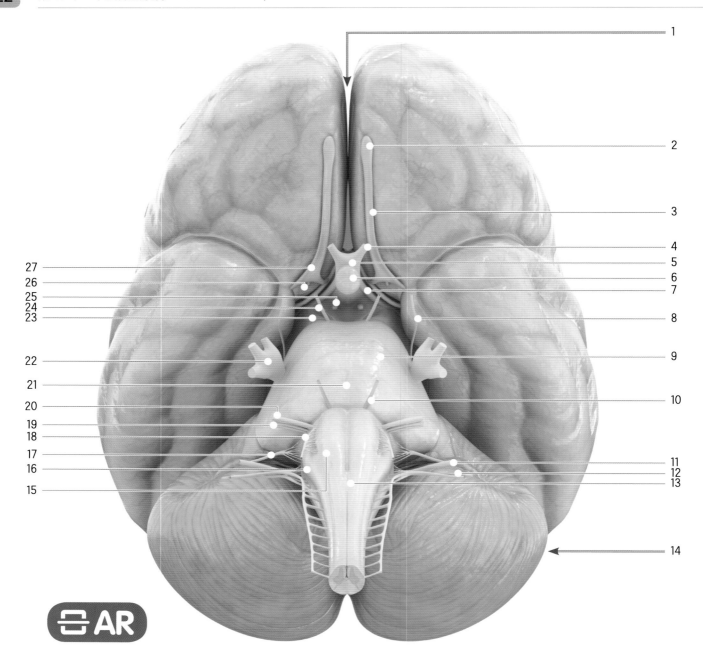

1. 大脑纵裂 cerebral longitudinal fissure
2. 嗅球 olfactory bulb
3. 嗅束 olfactory tract
4. 视神经 optic n.
5. 视交叉 optic chiasma
6. 垂体 hypophysis
7. 视束 optic tract
8. 滑车神经 trochlear n.
9. 脑桥 pons

10. 展神经 abducent n.
11. 迷走神经 vagus n.
12. 副神经 accessory n.
13. 锥体交叉 decussation of pyramid
14. 小脑 cerebellum
15. 锥体 pyramid
16. 橄榄 olive
17. 舌咽神经 glossopharyngeal n.
18. 舌下神经 hypoglossal n.

19. 前庭蜗神经 vestibulocochlear n.
20. 面神经 facial n.
21. 基底沟 basilar sulcus
22. 三叉神经 trigeminal n.
23. 大脑脚 cerebral peduncle
24. 动眼神经 oculomotor n.
25. 乳头体 mamillary body
26. 前穿质 anterior perforated substance
27. 嗅三角 olfactory trigone

图 11-6 脑的底面观
Basal surface of the brain

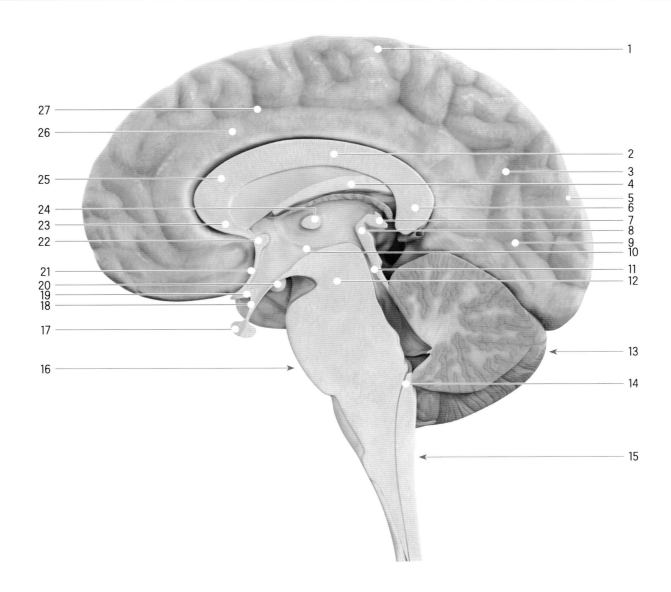

1. 中央旁小叶 paracentral lobule
2. 胼胝体干 trunk of corpus callosum
3. 顶枕沟 parietooccipital sulcus
4. 穹窿 fornix
5. 楔叶 cuneus
6. 胼胝体压部 splenium of corpus callosum
7. 松果体 pineal body
8. 后连合 posterior commissure
9. 距状沟 calcarine sulcus
10. 下丘脑沟 hypothalamic sulcus
11. 中脑水管 mesencephalic aqueduct
12. 大脑脚 cerebral peduncle
13. 小脑 cerebellum
14. 中央管 central canal

15. 延髓 medulla oblongata
16. 脑桥 pons
17. 垂体 hypophysis
18. 漏斗 infundibulum
19. 视交叉 optic chiasma
20. 乳头体 mamillary body
21. 终板 lamina terminalis
22. 前连合 anterior commissure
23. 胼胝体嘴 rostrum of corpus callosum
24. 丘脑间黏合 interthalamic adhesion
25. 胼胝体膝 genu of corpus callosum
26. 扣带回 cingulate gyrus
27. 扣带沟 cingulate sulcus

图 11-7 脑的正中矢状面
Median sagittal section of the brain

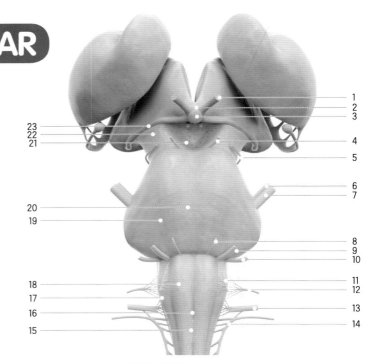

1. 视神经 optic n.
2. 视交叉 optic chiasma
3. 垂体 hypophysis
4. 动眼神经 oculomotor n.
5. 滑车神经 trochlear n.
6. 三叉神经运动根 motor root of trigeminal n.
7. 三叉神经感觉根 sensory root of trigeminal n.
8. 展神经 abducent n.
9. 面神经 facial n.
10. 前庭蜗神经 vestibulocochlear n.
11. 舌下神经 hypoglossal n.
12. 舌咽神经 glossopharyngeal n.
13. 迷走神经 vagus n.
14. 副神经 accessory n.
15. 锥体交叉 decussation of pyramid
16. 前正中沟 anteromedian groove
17. 橄榄 olive
18. 锥体 pyramid
19. 脑桥 pons
20. 基底沟 basilar sulcus
21. 脚间窝 interpeduncular fossa
22. 大脑脚 cerebral peduncle
23. 视束 optic tract
24. 尾状核 caudate nucleus
25. 背侧丘脑 dorsal thalamus
26. 豆状核 lentiform nucleus
27. 杏仁体 amygdaloid body
28. 蓝斑 locus ceruleus
29. 界沟 terminal sulcus
30. 面神经丘 facial colliculus
31. 正中沟 median sulcus
32. 髓纹 medullary stria
33. 舌下神经三角 hypoglossal triangle
34. 楔束结节 cuneate tubercle
35. 迷走神经三角 vagal triangle
36. 闩 obex
37. 薄束结节 gracile tubercle
38. 后正中沟 posterior median sulcus
39. 小脑下脚 inferior cerebellar peduncle
40. 前庭区 vestibular area
41. 小脑中脚 middle cerebellar peduncle
42. 小脑上脚 superior cerebellar peduncle
43. 上髓帆 superior medullary velum
44. 下丘 inferior colliculus
45. 上丘 superior colliculus
46. 松果体 pineal body

腹侧面观 Ventral aspect

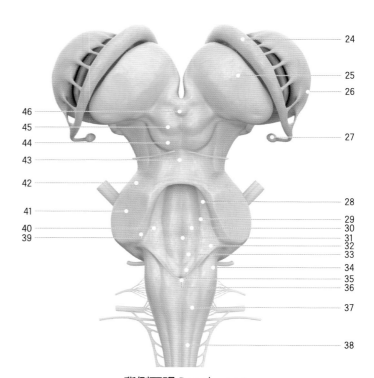

背侧面观 Dorsal aspect

图 11-8　脑干
Brain stem

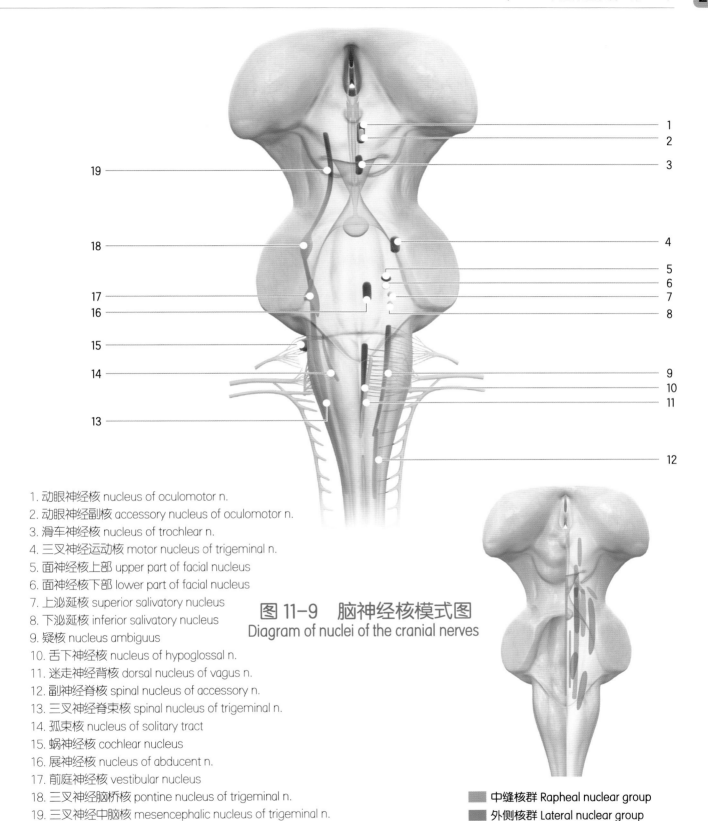

1. 动眼神经核 nucleus of oculomotor n.
2. 动眼神经副核 accessory nucleus of oculomotor n.
3. 滑车神经核 nucleus of trochlear n.
4. 三叉神经运动核 motor nucleus of trigeminal n.
5. 面神经核上部 upper part of facial nucleus
6. 面神经核下部 lower part of facial nucleus
7. 上泌涎核 superior salivatory nucleus
8. 下泌涎核 inferior salivatory nucleus
9. 疑核 nucleus ambiguus
10. 舌下神经核 nucleus of hypoglossal n.
11. 迷走神经背核 dorsal nucleus of vagus n.
12. 副神经脊核 spinal nucleus of accessory n.
13. 三叉神经脊束核 spinal nucleus of trigeminal n.
14. 孤束核 nucleus of solitary tract
15. 蜗神经核 cochlear nucleus
16. 展神经核 nucleus of abducent n.
17. 前庭神经核 vestibular nucleus
18. 三叉神经脑桥核 pontine nucleus of trigeminal n.
19. 三叉神经中脑核 mesencephalic nucleus of trigeminal n.

图 11-9　脑神经核模式图
Diagram of nuclei of the cranial nerves

中缝核群 Rapheal nuclear group
外侧核群 Lateral nuclear group
内侧核群 Medial nuclear group

图 11-10　脑干网状核团模式图
Diagram of reticular nucleus of the brain stem

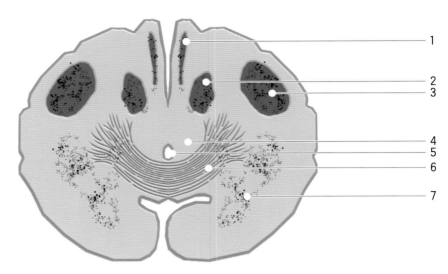

1. 薄束核 gracile nucleus
2. 楔束核 cuneate nucleus
3. 三叉神经脊束核 spinal nucleus of trigeminal n.
4. 导水管周围灰质 periaqueductal gray matter
5. 中央管 central canal
6. 锥体交叉 decussation of pyramid
7. 副神经核 accessory nucleus

图 11-11　延髓横切面（经锥体交叉）
Transverse section of the medulla oblongata (through the decussation of pyramid)

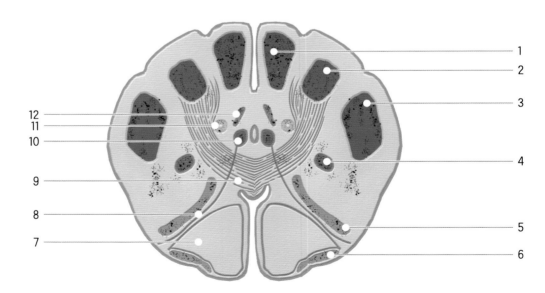

1. 薄束核 gracile nucleus
2. 楔束核 cuneate nucleus
3. 三叉神经脊束核 spinal nucleus of trigeminal n.
4. 疑核 nucleus ambiguus
5. 内侧副橄榄核 medial accessory olivary nucleus
6. 弓状核 arcuate nucleus
7. 锥体束 pyramidal tract
8. 舌下神经 hypoglossal n.
9. 内侧丘系交叉 decussation of medial lemniscus
10. 舌下神经核 nucleus of hypoglossal n.
11. 孤束核 nucleus of solitary tract
12. 迷走神经背核 dorsal nucleus of vagus n.

图 11-12　延髓横切面（经内侧丘系交叉）
Transverse section of the medulla oblongata (through the decussation of medial lemniscus)

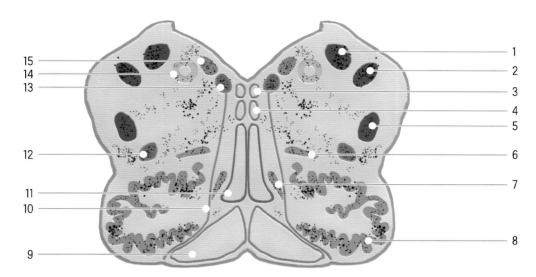

1. 前庭下核 inferior vestibular nucleus
2. 楔束副核 accessory cuneate nucleus
3. 内侧纵束 medial longitudinal fasciculus
4. 顶盖脊髓束 tectospinal tract
5. 三叉神经脊束核 spinal nucleus of trigeminal n.
6. 背侧副橄榄核 dorsal accessory olivary nucleus
7. 内侧副橄榄核 medial accessory olivary nucleus
8. 下橄榄核 inferior olivary nucleus
9. 锥体束 pyramidal tract
10. 舌下神经 hypoglossal n.
11. 内侧丘系 medial lemniscus
12. 疑核 nucleus ambiguus
13. 舌下神经核 nucleus of hypoglossal n.
14. 孤束核 nucleus of solitary tract
15. 迷走神经背核 dorsal nucleus of vagus n.

图 11-13　延髓横切面（经下橄榄核中部）
Transverse section of the medulla oblongata (through the middle part of the inferior olivary nucleus)

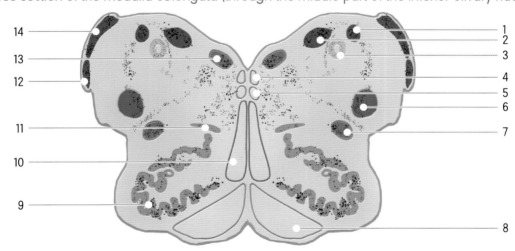

1. 前庭神经下核 inferior vestibular nucleus
2. 前庭神经内侧核 medial vestibular nucleus
3. 孤束核 nucleus of solitary tract
4. 内侧纵束 medial longitudinal fasciculus
5. 顶盖脊髓束 tectospinal tract
6. 三叉神经脊束核 spinal nucleus of trigeminal n.
7. 疑核 nucleus ambiguus
8. 锥体束 pyramidal tract
9. 下橄榄核 inferior olivary nucleus
10. 内侧丘系 medial lemniscus
11. 背侧副橄榄核 dorsal accessory olivary nucleus
12. 蜗腹侧核 ventral cochlear nucleus
13. 舌下前置核 nucleus prepositus hypoglossi
14. 蜗背侧核 dorsal cochlear nucleus

图 11-14　延髓横切面（经蜗神经核）
Transverse section of the medulla oblongata (through the cochlear nucleus)

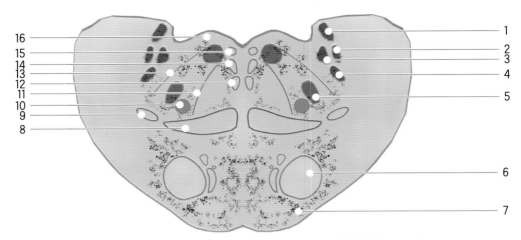

1. 前庭上核 superior vestibular nucleus
2. 前庭外侧核 lateral vestibular nucleus
3. 前庭内侧核 medial vestibular nucleus
4. 三叉神经脊束核 spinal nucleus of trigeminal n.
5. 面神经核 nucleus of facial n.
6. 锥体束 pyramidal tract
7. 脑桥核 pontine nucleus
8. 内侧丘系和斜方体 medial lemniscus and trapezoid body

9. 外侧丘系 lateral lemniscus
10. 上橄榄核 superior olivary nucleus
11. 展神经 abducent n.
12. 顶盖脊髓束 tectospinal tract
13. 面神经 facial n.
14. 内侧纵束 medial longitudinal fasciculus
15. 面神经膝 genu of facial n.
16. 面神经丘 facial colliculus

图 11-15　脑桥横切面（经面神经丘）
Transverse section of the pons (through the facial colliculus)

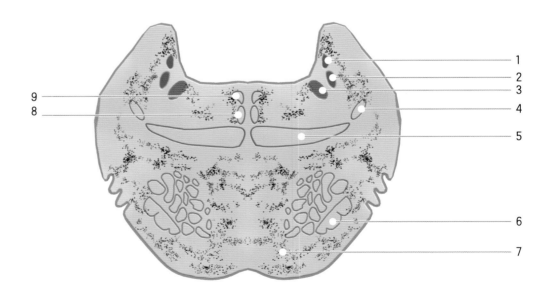

1. 三叉神经中脑核 mesencephalic nucleus of trigeminal n.
2. 三叉神经脑桥核 pontine nucleus of trigeminal n.
3. 三叉神经运动核 motor nucleus of trigeminal n.
4. 外侧丘系 lateral lemniscus
5. 内侧丘系 medial lemniscus

6. 锥体束 pyramidal tract
7. 脑桥核 pontine nucleus
8. 顶盖脊髓束 tectospinal tract
9. 内侧纵束 medial longitudinal fasciculus

图 11-16　脑桥横切面（经三叉神经运动核）
Transverse section of the pons (through the motor nucleus of trigeminal nerve)

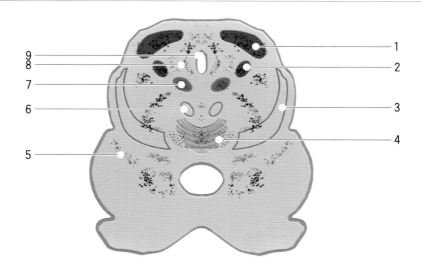

1. 下丘核 nucleus of inferior colliculus
2. 三叉神经中脑核 mesencephalic nucleus of trigeminal n.
3. 内侧丘系 medial lemniscus
4. 小脑上脚交叉 decussation of superior cerebellar peduncle
5. 黑质 substantia nigra
6. 内侧纵束 medial longitudinal fasciculus
7. 滑车神经核 nucleus of trochlear n.
8. 导水管周围灰质 periaqueductal gray matter
9. 中脑水管 mesencephalic aqueduct

图 11-17 脑桥横切面（经下丘）
Transverse section of the pons (through the inferior colliculus)

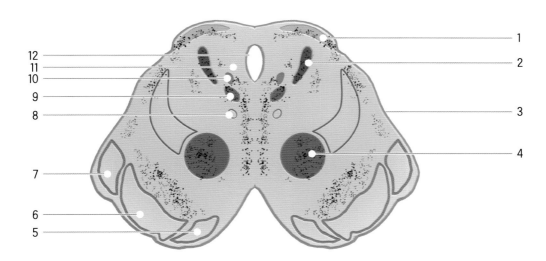

1. 上丘灰质层 gray matter layers of superior colliculus
2. 三叉神经中脑核 mesencephalic nucleus of trigeminal n.
3. 内侧丘系 medial lemniscus
4. 红核 red nucleus
5. 额桥束 frontopontine tract
6. 锥体束 pyramidal tract
7. 顶颞桥束 parietotemporopontine tract
8. 内侧纵束 medial longitudinal fasciculus
9. 动眼神经核 nucleus of oculomotor n.
10. 动眼神经副核 accessory nucleus of oculomotor n.
11. 中央灰质 central gray matter
12. 中脑水管 mesencephalic aqueduct

图 11-18 中脑横切面（经上丘）
Transverse section of the midbrain (through the superior colliculus)

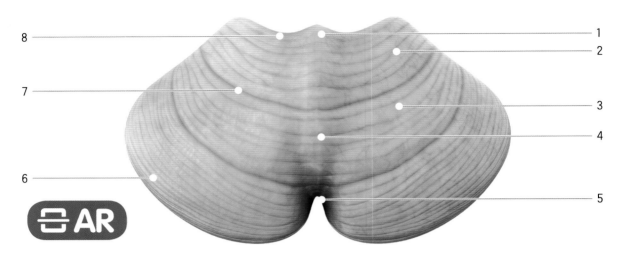

1. 中央小叶 central lobule
2. 方形小叶前部 anterior quadrangular lobule
3. 方形小叶后部 posterior quadrangular lobule
4. 小脑蚓 vermis
5. 小脑后切迹 posterior cerebellar notch
6. 小脑半球 cerebellar hemisphere
7. 原裂 primary fissure
8. 中央小叶翼 ala of central lobule

图 11-19　小脑的外形（上面）
External features of the cerebellum (superior)

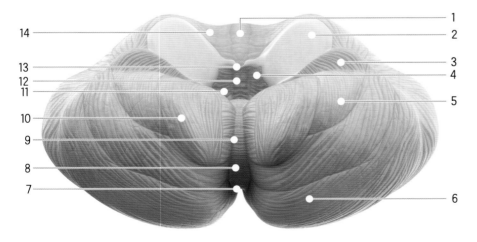

1. 中央小叶 central lobule
2. 小脑中脚 middle cerebellar peduncle
3. 绒球 flocculus
4. 小脑上脚 superior cerebellar peduncle
5. 二腹小叶 biventral lobule
6. 下半月小叶 inferior semilunar lobule
7. 蚓结节 tuber of vermis
8. 蚓锥体 pyramid of vermis
9. 蚓垂 uvula of vermis
10. 小脑扁桃体 tonsil of cerebellum
11. 小脑下脚 inferior cerebellar peduncle
12. 小结 nodule
13. 上髓帆 superior medullary velum
14. 中央小叶翼 ala of central lobule

图 11-20　小脑的外形（前面）
External features of the cerebellum (anterior)

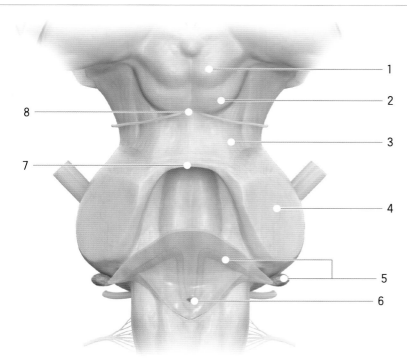

1. 上丘 superior colliculus
2. 下丘 inferior colliculus
3. 小脑上脚 superior cerebellar peduncle
4. 小脑中脚 middle cerebellar peduncle
5. 第四脑室脉络丛 choroid plexus of fourth ventricle
6. 第四脑室正中孔 median aperture of fourth ventricle
7. 上髓帆 superior medullary velum
8. 上髓帆系带 frenulum of superior medullary velum

图 11-21　第四脑室脉络组织
Tela choroidea of the fourth ventricle

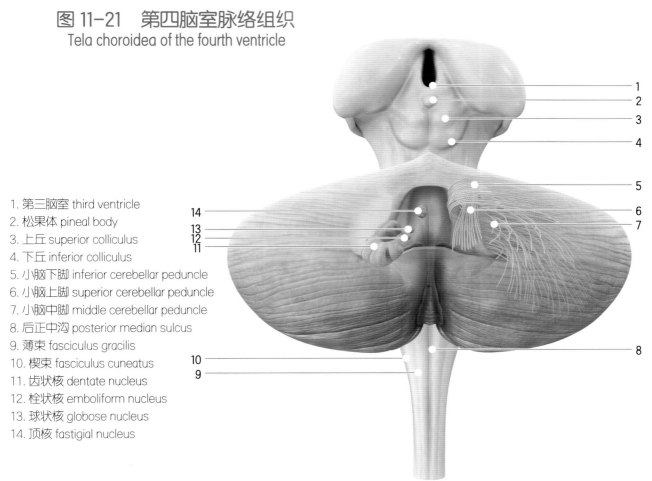

1. 第三脑室 third ventricle
2. 松果体 pineal body
3. 上丘 superior colliculus
4. 下丘 inferior colliculus
5. 小脑下脚 inferior cerebellar peduncle
6. 小脑上脚 superior cerebellar peduncle
7. 小脑中脚 middle cerebellar peduncle
8. 后正中沟 posterior median sulcus
9. 薄束 fasciculus gracilis
10. 楔束 fasciculus cuneatus
11. 齿状核 dentate nucleus
12. 栓状核 emboliform nucleus
13. 球状核 globose nucleus
14. 顶核 fastigial nucleus

图 11-22　小脑核团和小脑脚
Cerebellar nuclei and cerebellar peduncle

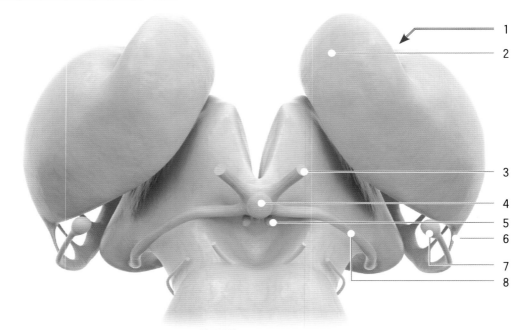

前面观 Anterior view

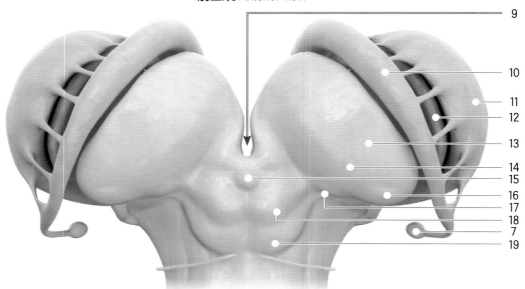

后面观 Posterior view

1. 内囊 internal capsule
2. 尾状核头 head of caudate nucleus
3. 视神经 optic n.
4. 垂体 hypophysis
5. 乳头体 mamillary body
6. 尾状核纹状体灰质桥 caudate nucleus striatum bridge of gray matter
7. 杏仁体 amygdaloid body
8. 视束 optic tract
9. 第三脑室 third ventricle
10. 尾状核体 body of caudate nucleus
11. 壳 putamen
12. 苍白球 globus pallidus
13. 背侧丘脑 dorsal thalamus
14. 丘脑枕 pulvinar
15. 松果体 pineal body
16. 外侧膝状体 lateral geniculate body
17. 内侧膝状体 medial geniculate body
18. 上丘 superior colliculus
19. 下丘 inferior colliculus

图 11-23　间脑模式图
Diagram of the diencephalon

1. 下丘脑外侧区 lateral hypothalamic region
2. 丘脑底核 subthalamic nucleus
3. 下丘脑后核 posterior hypothalamic nucleus
4. 黑质 substantia nigra
5. 红核 red nucleus
6. 弓状核 arcuate nucleus
7. 视上核 supraoptic nucleus
8. 下丘脑腹内侧核 ventromedial hypothalamic nucleus
9. 视前内侧核和视前外侧核 medial preoptic nucleus and lateral preoptic nucleus
10. 下丘脑背内侧核 dorsomedial hypothalamic nucleus
11. 前核 anterior nucleus
12. 室旁核 paraventricular nucleus
13. 穹窿 fornix

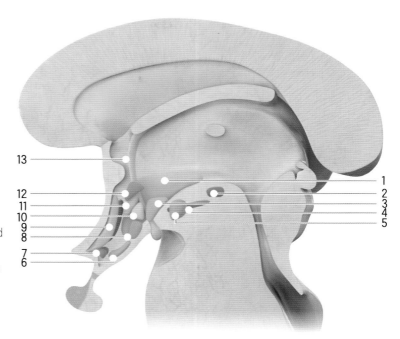

图 11-24　下丘脑核团模式图
Diagram of the hypothalamic nuclei

1. 内髓板 internal medullary lamina
2. 前核 anterior nucleus
3. 背外侧核 dorsolateral nucleus
4. 腹前核 ventral anterior nucleus
5. 腹外侧核 ventrolateral nucleus
6. 腹后外侧核 ventral posterolateral nucleus
7. 外侧膝状体 lateral geniculate body
8. 内侧膝状体 medial geniculate body
9. 丘脑枕 pulvinar
10. 后外侧核 posterolateral nucleus
11. 板内核 intralaminar nucleus
12. 背内侧核 dorsomedial nucleus
13. 腹后内侧核 ventral posteromedial nucleus
14. 内侧丘系和脊髓丘脑束 medial lemniscus and spinothalamic tract
15. 三叉丘系 trigeminal lemniscus
16. 视束 optic tract
17. 下丘臂 brachium of inferior colliculus

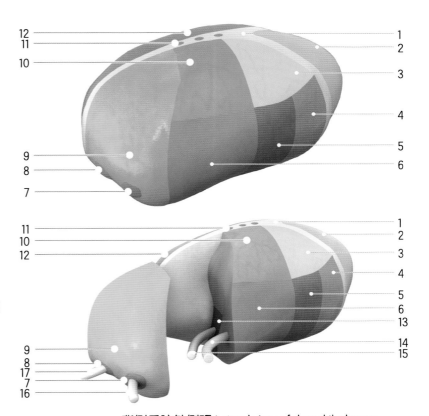

背侧丘脑外侧观 Lateral view of dorsal thalamus

图 11-25　丘脑核团模式图
Diagram of the thalamic nuclei

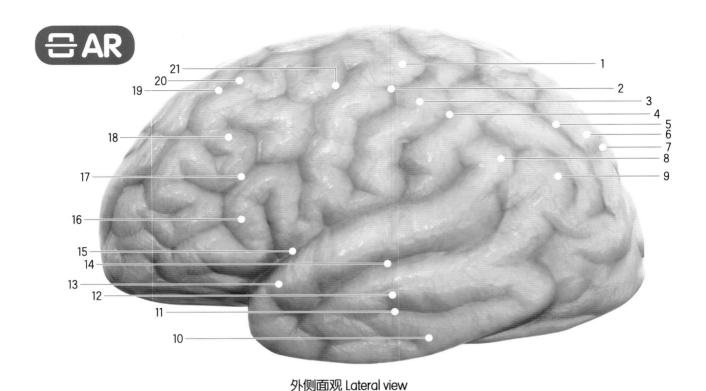

外侧面观 Lateral view

1. 中央前回 precentral gyrus
2. 中央沟 central sulcus
3. 中央后回 postcentral gyrus
4. 中央后沟 postcentral sulcus
5. 顶内沟 intraparietal sulcus
6. 顶上小叶 superior parietal lobule
7. 顶枕沟 parietooccipital sulcus
8. 缘上回 supramarginal gyrus
9. 角回 angular gyrus
10. 颞下回 inferior temporal gyrus
11. 颞下沟 inferior temporal sulcus
12. 颞中回 middle temporal gyrus
13. 颞上回 superior temporal gyrus
14. 颞上沟 superior temporal sulcus
15. 外侧沟 lateral sulcus
16. 额下回 inferior frontal gyrus
17. 额下沟 inferior frontal sulcus
18. 额中回 middle frontal gyrus
19. 额上沟 superior frontal sulcus
20. 额上回 superior frontal gyrus
21. 中央前沟 precentral sulcus

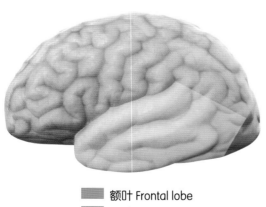

- 额叶 Frontal lobe
- 顶叶 Parietal lobe
- 枕叶 Occipital lobe
- 颞叶 Temporal lobe
- 岛叶 Insula

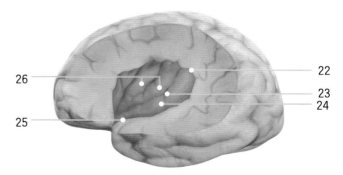

岛叶 Insula

22. 岛环状沟 circular sulcus of insula
23. 岛中央沟 central sulcus of insula
24. 岛长回 long gyrus of insula
25. 岛阈 limen of insula
26. 岛短回 short gyrus of insula

图 11-26 大脑外侧面及分叶
Lateral surface and lobes of the cerebral hemisphere

1. 中央旁小叶 paracentral lobule
2. 楔前叶 precuneus
3. 顶枕沟 parietooccipital sulcus
4. 楔叶 cuneus
5. 距状沟 calcarine sulcus
6. 舌回 lingual gyrus
7. 海马旁回 parahippocampal gyrus
8. 侧副沟 collateral sulcus
9. 枕颞内侧回 medial occipitotemporal gyrus
10. 枕颞外侧回 lateral occipitotemporal gyrus
11. 钩 uncus
12. 终板旁回 paraterminal gyrus
13. 胼胝体膝 genu of corpus callosum
14. 透明隔 septum pellucidum
15. 胼胝体干 trunk of corpus callosum
16. 扣带回 cingulate gyrus
17. 扣带沟 cingulate sulcus
18. 额上回 superior frontal gyrus

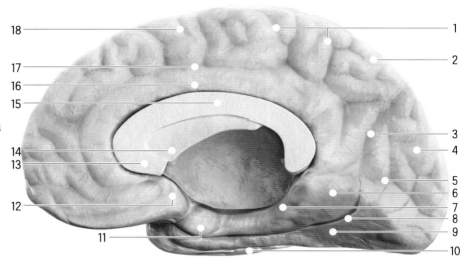

图 11-27　大脑半球内侧面
Medial surface of the cerebral hemisphere

1. 大脑纵裂 cerebral longitudinal fissure
2. 嗅球 olfactory bulb
3. 眶回 orbital gyri
4. 嗅束 olfactory tract
5. 视神经 optic n.
6. 前穿质 anterior perforated substance
7. 视束 optic tract
8. 中脑 midbrain
9. 胼胝体压部 splenium of corpus callosum
10. 枕颞沟 occipitotemporal sulcus
11. 枕颞外侧回 lateral occipitotemporal gyrus
12. 枕颞内侧回 medial occipitotemporal gyrus
13. 侧副沟 collateral sulcus
14. 海马旁回 parahippocampal gyrus
15. 乳头体 mamillary body
16. 灰结节 tuber cinereum
17. 垂体 hypophysis
18. 嗅三角 olfactory trigone
19. 直回 straight gyri

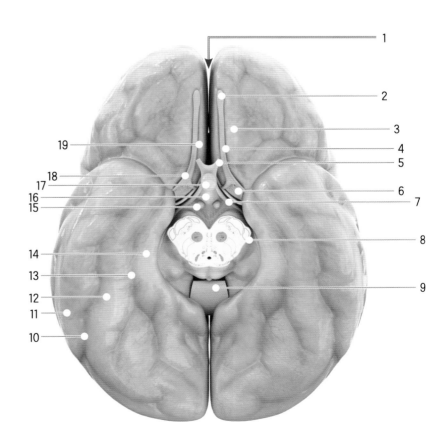

图 11-28　端脑底面
Basal surface of the telencephalon

1. 生殖器 genital organ
2. 趾 toe
3. 足 foot
4. 小腿 leg
5. 大腿 thigh
6. 躯干 trunk
7. 头 head
8. 颈 neck
9. 肩 shoulder
10. 上臂 upper arm
11. 肘 elbow
12. 前臂 forearm
13. 腕 wrist
14. 手 hand
15. 小指 little finger
16. 环指 ring finger
17. 中指 middle finger
18. 示指 index finger
19. 拇指 thumb
20. 眼 eye
21. 鼻 nose
22. 面 face
23. 上唇 upper lip
24. 上、下唇 upper and lower lips

25. 下唇 lower lip
26. 牙龈、颌 gum, jaw
27. 舌 tongue
28. 咽 pharynx
29. 腹内器官 intra-abdominal organs

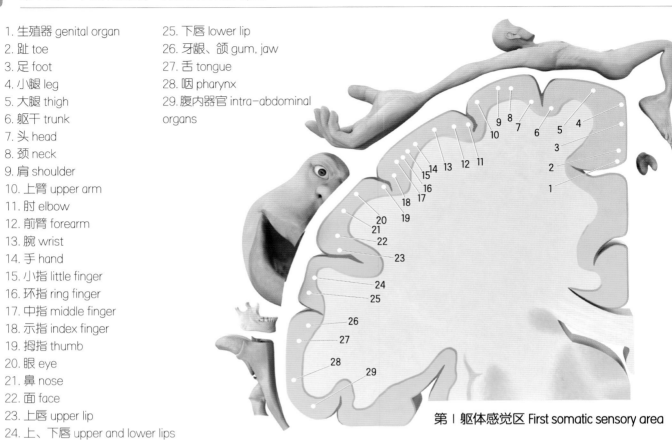

第Ⅰ躯体感觉区 First somatic sensory area

1. 趾 toe
2. 踝 malleolus
3. 膝 knee
4. 大腿 thigh
5. 躯干 trunk
6. 肩 shoulder
7. 肘 elbow
8. 腕 wrist
9. 手 hand
10. 小指 little finger
11. 环指 ring finger
12. 中指 middle finger
13. 示指 index finger
14. 拇指 thumb
15. 颈 neck
16. 额 forehead
17. 眼睑和眼球 palpebrae and eyeball
18. 面 face
19. 上、下唇 upper and lower lips
20. 颌 jaw
21. 舌 tongue

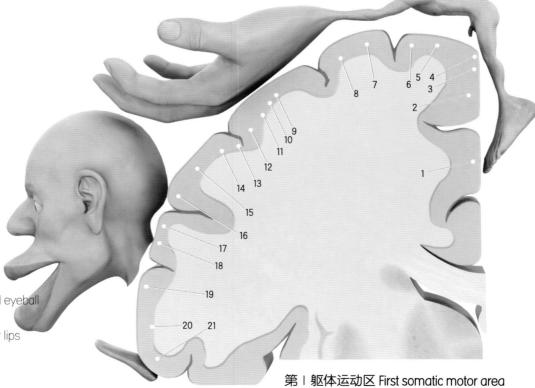

第Ⅰ躯体运动区 First somatic motor area

图 11-29　人体各部在大脑感觉区、运动区的定位
Orientation of the parts of the body in sensory and motor areas

1. 扣带回 cingulate gyrus
2. 胼胝体干
trunk of corpus callosum
3. 胼胝体压部
splenium of corpus callosum
4. 下丘 inferior colliculus
5. 上丘 superior colliculus
6. 松果体 pineal body
7. 苍白球 globus pallidus
8. 背侧丘脑 dorsal thalamus
9. 壳 putamen
10. 尾状核纹状体灰质桥
caudate nucleus striatum
bridge of gray matter
11. 屏状核 claustrum
12. 尾状核 caudate nucleus

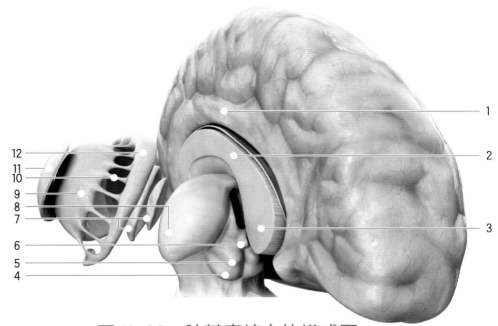

图 11-30　脑基底核立体模式图
Stereoscopic pattern of the cerebral basal nuclei

1. 前角 anterior horn
2. 尾状核头 head of caudate nucleus
3. 内囊前肢 anterior limb of internal
capsule
4. 内囊膝 genu of internal capsule
5. 壳 putamen
6. 前核 anterior nucleus
7. 腹外侧核 ventrolateral nucleus
8. 内囊后肢 posterior limb of internal
capsule
9. 内侧核 medial nucleus
10. 后角 posterior horn
11. 胼胝体压部 splenium of corpus
callosum
12. 尾状核尾 tail of caudate nucleus
13. 屏状核 claustrum
14. 外囊 external capsule
15. 最外囊 extreme capsule
16. 穹窿柱 column of fornix
17. 透明隔 septum pellucidum

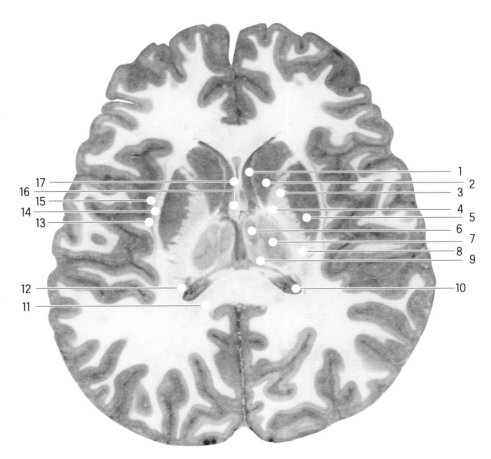

图 11-31　脑的水平切面
Horizontal section of the brain

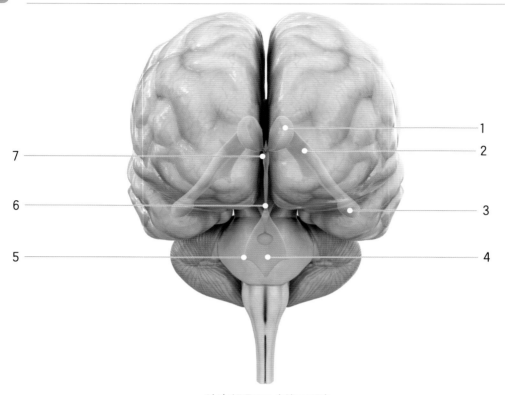

脑室投影图（前面观）
Projection map of ventricle (anterior view)

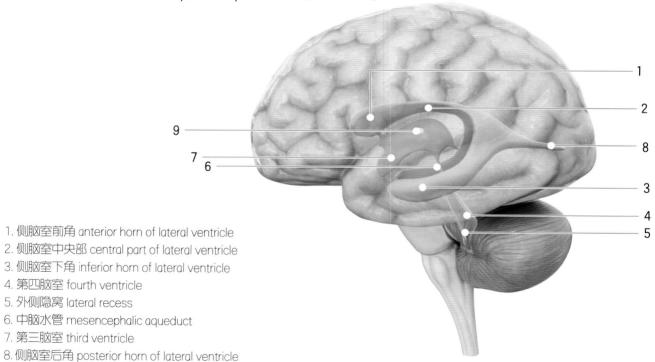

1. 侧脑室前角 anterior horn of lateral ventricle
2. 侧脑室中央部 central part of lateral ventricle
3. 侧脑室下角 inferior horn of lateral ventricle
4. 第四脑室 fourth ventricle
5. 外侧隐窝 lateral recess
6. 中脑水管 mesencephalic aqueduct
7. 第三脑室 third ventricle
8. 侧脑室后角 posterior horn of lateral ventricle
9. 丘脑间黏合 interthalamic adhesion

脑室投影图（侧面观）
Projection map of ventricle (lateral view)

图 11-32　脑室系统
Ventricular system

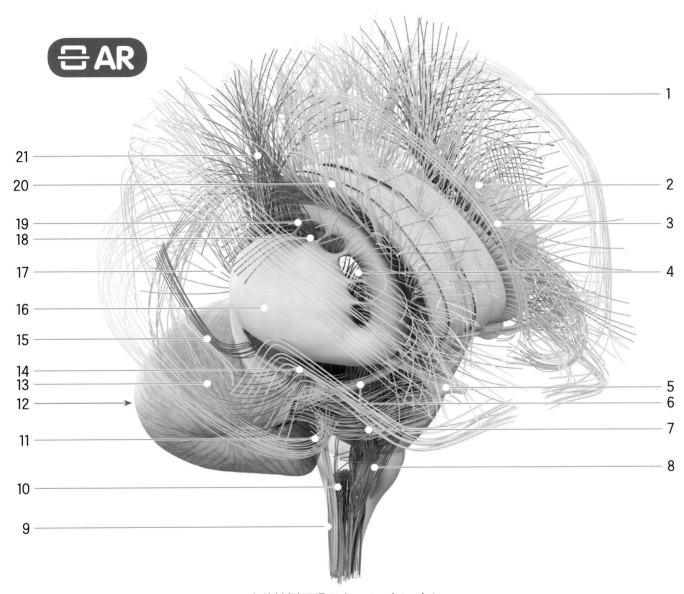

右前外侧面观 Right anterolateral view

1. 上纵束 superior longitudinal fasciculus
2. 弓状纤维 arcuate fiber
3. 扣带 cingulum
4. 额桥束 frontopontine tract
5. 视交叉 optic chiasma
6. 前联合 anterior commissure
7. 小脑中脚 middle cerebellar peduncle
8. 锥体束 pyramidal tract
9. 小脑下脚 inferior cerebellar peduncle
10. 薄束 fasciculus gracilis
11. 下纵束 inferior longitudinal fasciculus
12. 小脑 cerebellum
13. 视辐射 optic radiation
14. 钩束 uncinate fasciculus
15. 听辐射 acoustic radiation
16. 豆状核 lentiform nucleus
17. 顶枕颞桥束 parietooccipitopontine and temporopontine tract
18. 皮质核束 corticonuclear tract
19. 锥体束 pyramidal tract
20. 胼胝体 corpus callosum
21. 丘脑中央辐射 central thalamic radiation

图 11-33　大脑半球的纤维
Nerve fibers of the cerebral hemisphere

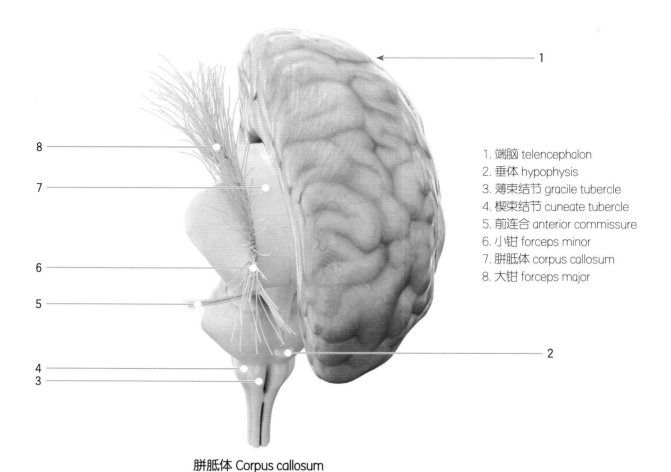

1. 端脑 telencephalon
2. 垂体 hypophysis
3. 薄束结节 gracile tubercle
4. 楔束结节 cuneate tubercle
5. 前连合 anterior commissure
6. 小钳 forceps minor
7. 胼胝体 corpus callosum
8. 大钳 forceps major

胼胝体 Corpus callosum

9. 胼胝体干 trunk of corpus callosum
10. 穹窿体 body of fornix
11. 胼胝体压部 splenium of corpus callosum
12. 穹窿连合 commissure of fornix
13. 穹窿脚 crus of fornix
14. 束状回 fasciolar gyrus
15. 海马 hippocampus
16. 海马脚 pes hippocampi
17. 乳头体 mamillary body
18. 穹窿柱 column of fornix
19. 胼胝体嘴 rostrum of corpus callosum
20. 胼胝体膝 genu of corpus callosum

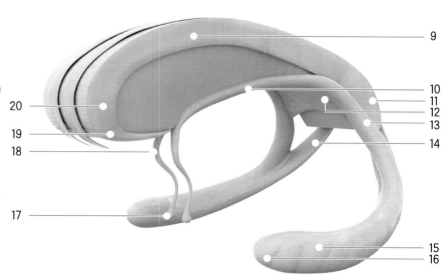

海马连合 Commissure of hippocampus

图 11-34 连合纤维
Commissural fibers

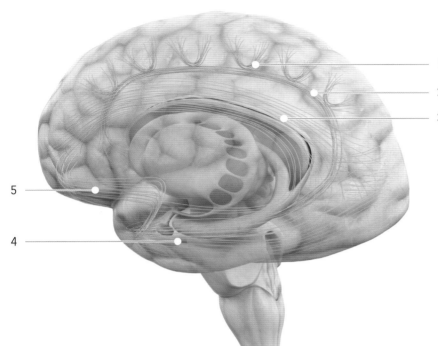

1. 弓状纤维 arcuate fibers
2. 扣带 cingulum
3. 上纵束 superior longitudinal fasciculus
4. 下纵束 inferior longitudinal fasciculus
5. 钩束 uncinate fasciculus

图 11-35 联络纤维
Association fibers

1. 胼胝体 corpus callosum
2. 额桥束 frontopontine tract
3. 尾状核 caudate nucleus
4. 垂体 hypophysis
5. 锥体束 pyramidal tract
6. 内侧丘系 medial lemniscus
7. 视辐射 optic radiation
8. 听辐射 acoustic radiation
9. 豆状核 lentiform nucleus
10. 顶枕颞桥束 parietooccipitopontine and temporopontine tract
11. 皮质核束 corticonuclear tract
12. 丘脑中央辐射 central thalamic radiation

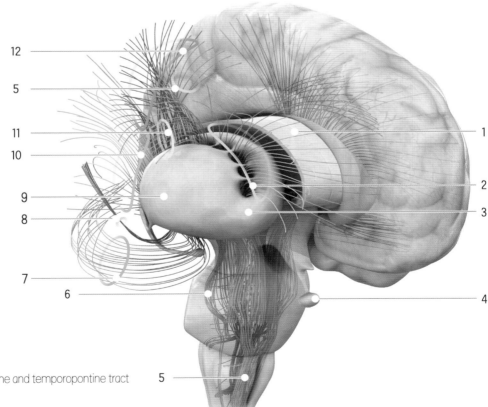

图 11-36 投射纤维
Projection fibres

第12章 神经系统传导通路

Nervous System Pathways

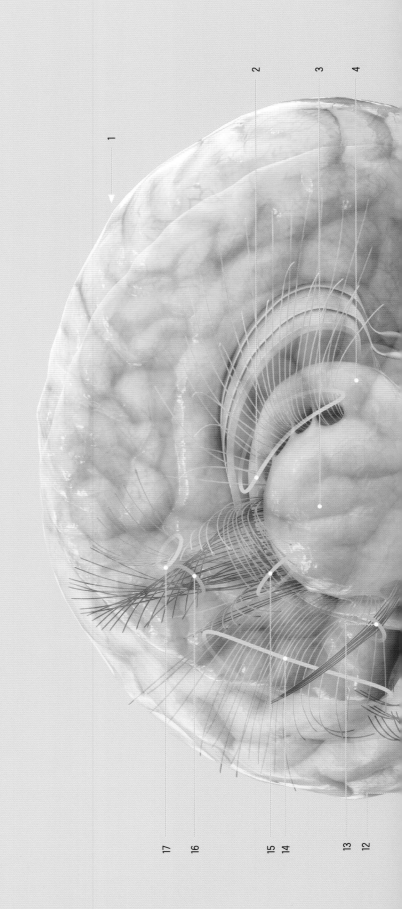

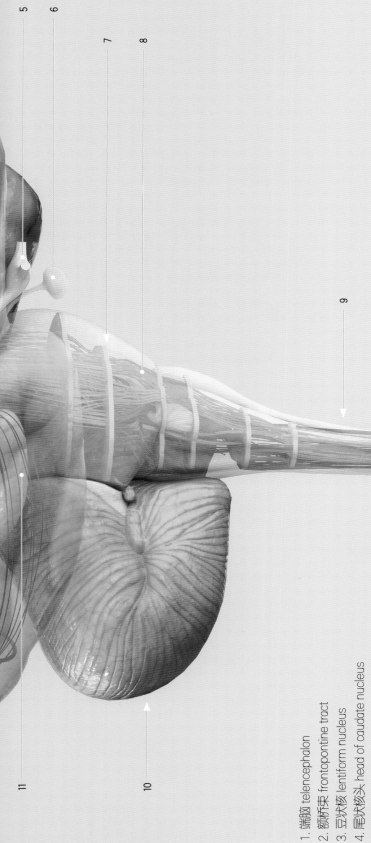

5
6
7
8
9
10
11

1. 端脑 telencephalon
2. 额桥束 frontopontine tract
3. 豆状核 lentiform nucleus
4. 尾状核头 head of caudate nucleus
5. 视交叉 optic chiasma
6. 垂体 hypophysis
7. 脑桥 pons
8. 锥体束 pyramidal tract
9. 延髓 medulla oblongata
10. 小脑 cerebellum
11. 海马 hippocampus
12. 视辐射 optic radiation
13. 听辐射 acoustic radiation
14. 顶枕颞桥束 parietooccipitopontine and temporopontine tract
15. 皮质核束 corticonuclear tract
16. 丘脑中央辐射 central thalamic radiation
17. 皮质脊髓束 corticospinal tract

图 12-1 神经系统传导通路概观
Overview of the nervous system pathways

1. 中央后回 postcentral gyrus
2. 内囊 internal capsule
3. 豆状核 lentiform nucleus
4. 腹后外侧核 ventral posterolateral nucleus
5. 内侧丘系 medial lemniscus
6. 内侧丘系交叉 decussation of medial lemniscus
7. 脊神经后根节 posterior root ganglion of spinal n.
8. 延髓 medulla oblongata
9. 楔束核 cuneate nucleus
10. 薄束核 gracile nucleus
11. 脑桥 pons
12. 中脑 midbrain
13. 背侧丘脑 dorsal thalamus
14. 中央旁小叶后部 posterior part of paracentral lobule
15. 薄束 fasciculus gracilis
16. 楔束 fasciculus cuneatus
17. 脊髓 spinal cord

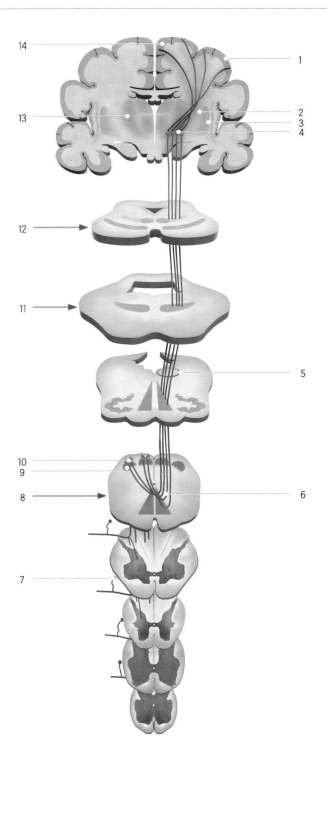

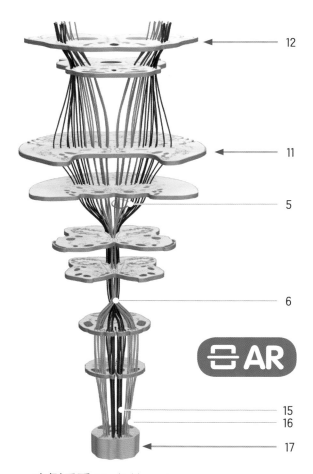

内侧丘系 Medial lemniscus

图 12-2   躯干和四肢意识性本体感觉和精细触觉传导通路
Pathway of the consious propriceptive sensibility and fine touch of the trunk and limbs

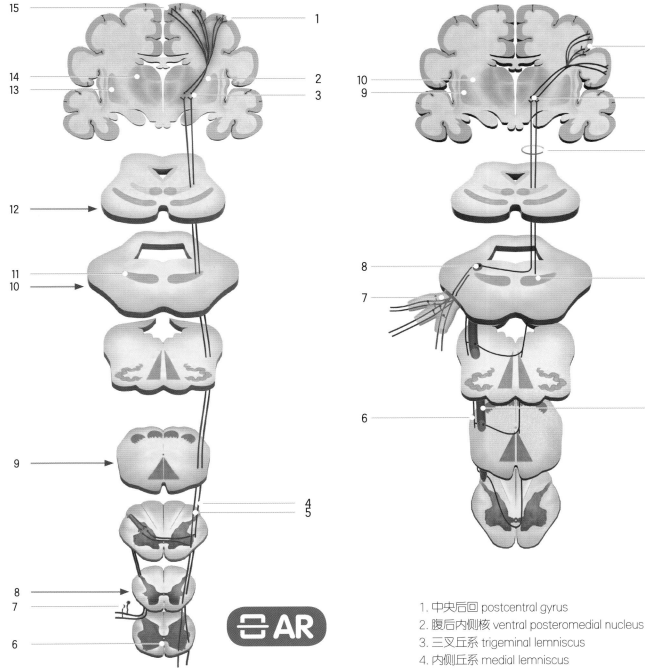

1. 中央后回 postcentral gyrus
2. 腹后内侧核 ventral posteromedial nucleus
3. 三叉丘系 trigeminal lemniscus
4. 内侧丘系 medial lemniscus
5. 三叉神经脊束核 spinal nucleus of trigeminal n.
6. 三叉神经脊束 spinal tract of trigeminal n.
7. 三叉神经节 trigeminal ganglion
8. 三叉神经脑桥核 pontine nucleus of trigeminal n.
9. 豆状核 lentiform nucleus
10. 内囊 internal capsule

1. 中央后回 postcentral gyrus
2. 内囊 internal capsule
3. 腹后外侧核 ventral posterolateral nucleus
4. 脊髓丘脑侧束 lateral spinothalamic tract
5. 脊髓丘脑前束 anterior spinothalamic tract
6. 白质前连合 anterior white commissure
7. 脊神经后根节 posterior root ganglion of spinal n.
8. 脊髓 spinal cord
9. 延髓 medulla oblongata
10. 脑桥 pons
11. 内侧丘系 medial lemniscus
12. 中脑 midbrain
13. 豆状核 lentiform nucleus
14. 背侧丘脑 dorsal thalamus
15. 中央旁小叶后部 posterior part of paracentral lobule

图 12-3　躯干和四肢浅感觉传导通路
Pathway of exteroceptive sensibility of the trunk and limbs

图 12-4　头面部浅感觉传导通路
Pathway of exteroceptive sensibility of the head and face

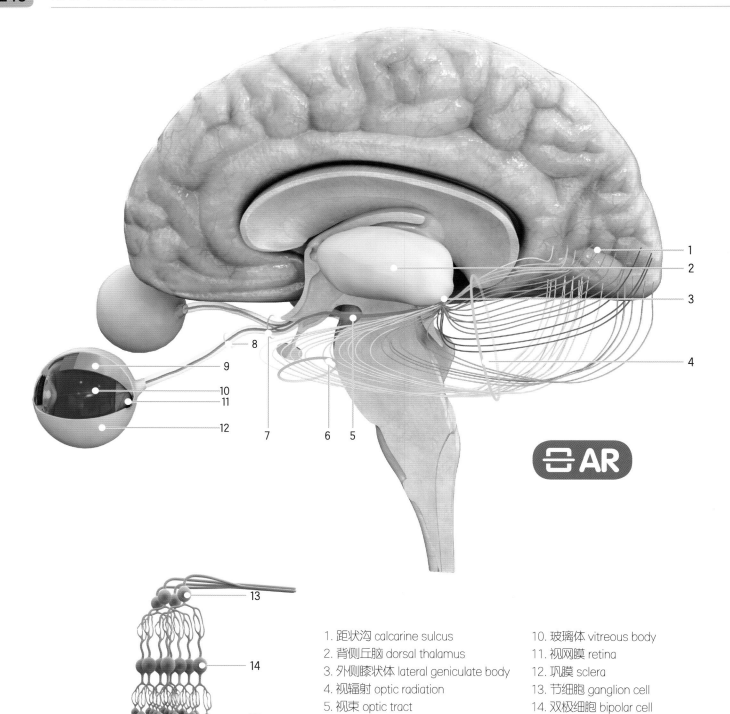

视网膜的结构模式图
Schematic diagram of the structure of the retina

1. 距状沟 calcarine sulcus
2. 背侧丘脑 dorsal thalamus
3. 外侧膝状体 lateral geniculate body
4. 视辐射 optic radiation
5. 视束 optic tract
6. 麦耶氏襻 Meyer's loop
7. 视交叉 optic chiasma
8. 视神经 optic n.
9. 脉络膜 choroid

10. 玻璃体 vitreous body
11. 视网膜 retina
12. 巩膜 sclera
13. 节细胞 ganglion cell
14. 双极细胞 bipolar cell
15. 视锥细胞 cone cell
16. 视杆细胞 rod cell
17. 色素上皮 pigment epithelium

图 12-5   视觉传导通路
Visual pathway

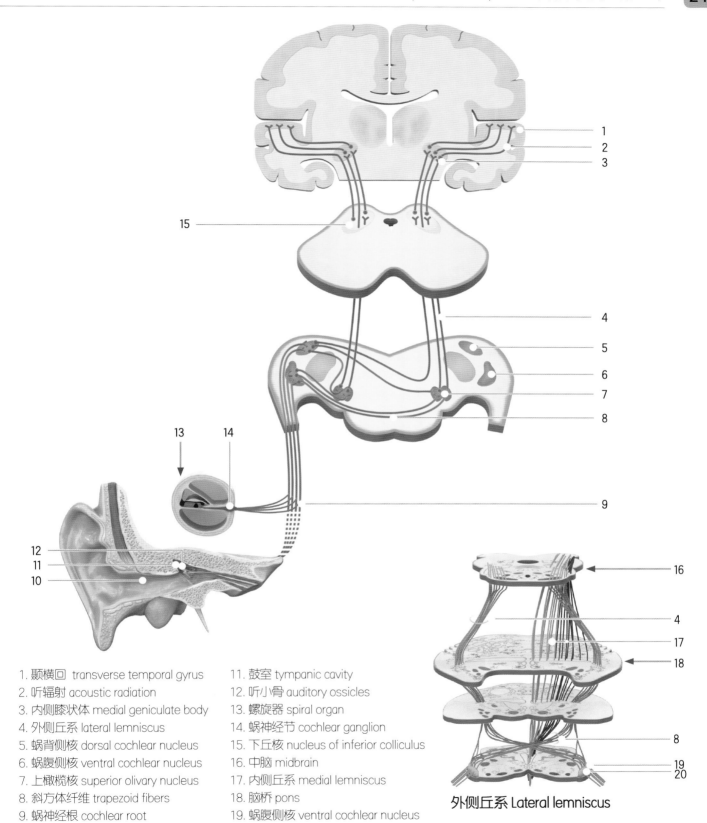

1. 颞横回 transverse temporal gyrus
2. 听辐射 acoustic radiation
3. 内侧膝状体 medial geniculate body
4. 外侧丘系 lateral lemniscus
5. 蜗背侧核 dorsal cochlear nucleus
6. 蜗腹侧核 ventral cochlear nucleus
7. 上橄榄核 superior olivary nucleus
8. 斜方体纤维 trapezoid fibers
9. 蜗神经根 cochlear root
10. 外耳道 external acoustic meatus

11. 鼓室 tympanic cavity
12. 听小骨 auditory ossicles
13. 螺旋器 spiral organ
14. 蜗神经节 cochlear ganglion
15. 下丘核 nucleus of inferior colliculus
16. 中脑 midbrain
17. 内侧丘系 medial lemniscus
18. 脑桥 pons
19. 蜗腹侧核 ventral cochlear nucleus
20. 蜗背侧核 dorsal cochlear nucleus

外侧丘系 Lateral lemniscus

图 12-6　听觉传导通路
Auditory pathway

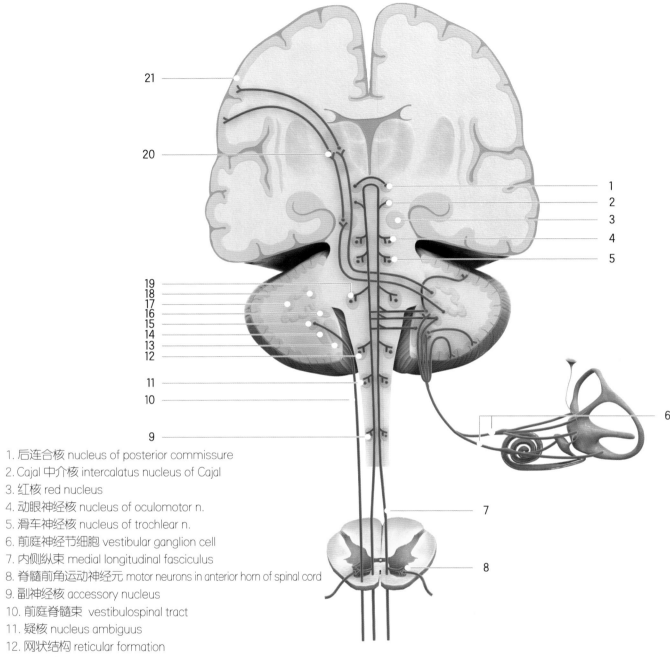

1. 后连合核 nucleus of posterior commissure
2. Cajal 中介核 intercalatus nucleus of Cajal
3. 红核 red nucleus
4. 动眼神经核 nucleus of oculomotor n.
5. 滑车神经核 nucleus of trochlear n.
6. 前庭神经节细胞 vestibular ganglion cell
7. 内侧纵束 medial longitudinal fasciculus
8. 脊髓前角运动神经元 motor neurons in anterior horn of spinal cord
9. 副神经核 accessory nucleus
10. 前庭脊髓束 vestibulospinal tract
11. 疑核 nucleus ambiguus
12. 网状结构 reticular formation
13. 前庭神经内侧核 medial vestibular nucleus
14. 前庭神经下核 inferior vestibular nucleus
15. 前庭神经外侧核 lateral vestibular nucleus
16. 前庭神经上核 superior vestibular nucleus
17. 齿状核 dentate nucleus
18. 球状核 globose nucleus
19. 展神经核 nucleus of abducent n.
20. 背侧丘脑腹后核 ventral posterior nucleus of the dorsal thalamus
21. 大脑皮质 cerebral cortex

图 12-7 平衡觉传导通路
Equilibrium pathway

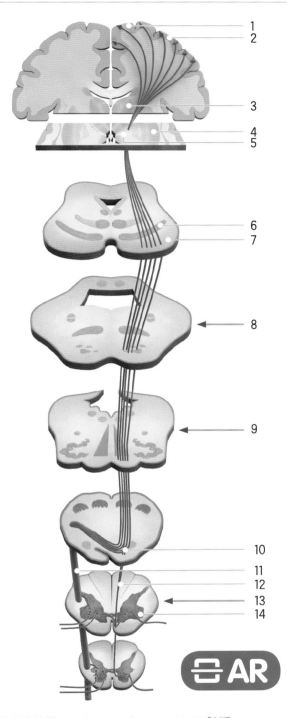
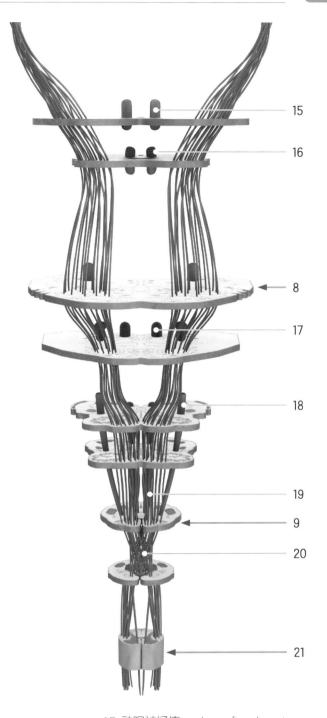

1. 中央旁小叶前部 anterior part of paracentral lobule
2. 中央前回 precentral gyrus
3. 背侧丘脑 dorsal thalamus
4. 豆状核 lentiform nucleus
5. 内囊 internal capsule
6. 黑质 substantia nigra
7. 大脑脚底 crus cerebri

8. 脑桥 pons
9. 延髓 medulla oblongata
10. 锥体交叉 decussation of pyramid
11. 皮质脊髓侧束 lateral corticospinal tract
12. 皮质脊髓前束 anterior corticospinal tract
13. 脊髓 spinal cord
14. 前角 anterior horn

15. 动眼神经核 nucleus of oculomotor n.
16. 滑车神经核 nucleus of trochlear n.
17. 展神经核 nucleus of abducent n.
18. 疑核 nucleus ambiguus
19. 锥体束 pyramidal tract
20. 锥体交叉 decussation of pyramid
21. 脊髓 spinal cord

图 12-8　锥体系（皮质脊髓束）
Pyramidal system (corticospinal tract)

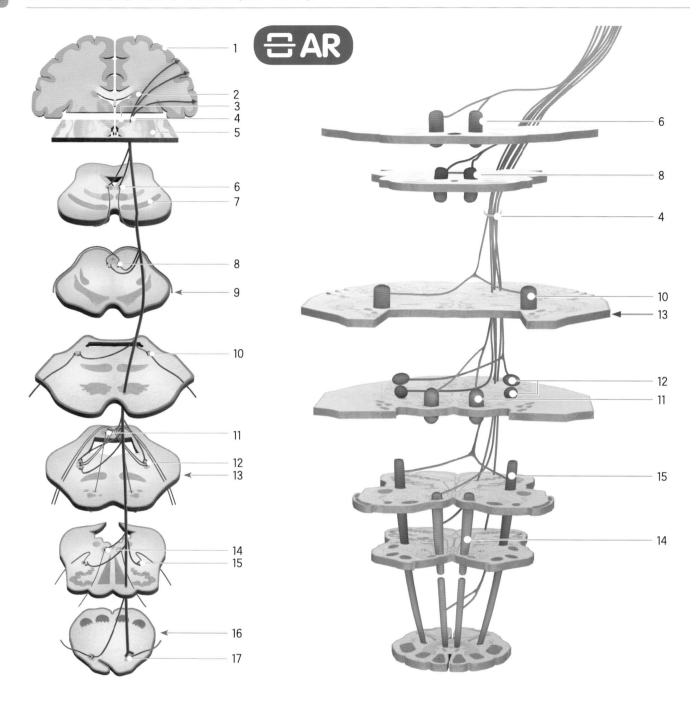

1. 中央前回 precentral gyrus
2. 内囊 internal capsule
3. 背侧丘脑 dorsal thalamus
4. 皮质核束 corticonuclear tract
5. 豆状核 lentiform nucleus
6. 动眼神经核 nucleus of oculomotor n.

7. 黑质 substantia nigra
8. 滑车神经核 nucleus of trochlear n.
9. 中脑 midbrain
10. 三叉神经运动核 motor nucleus of trigeminal n.
11. 展神经核 nucleus of abducent n.
12. 面神经核 nucleus of facial n.

13. 脑桥 pons
14. 舌下神经核 nucleus of hypoglossal n.
15. 疑核 nucleus ambiguus
16. 延髓 medulla oblongata
17. 副神经核 accessory nucleus

图 12-9　皮质核束
Corticonuclear tract

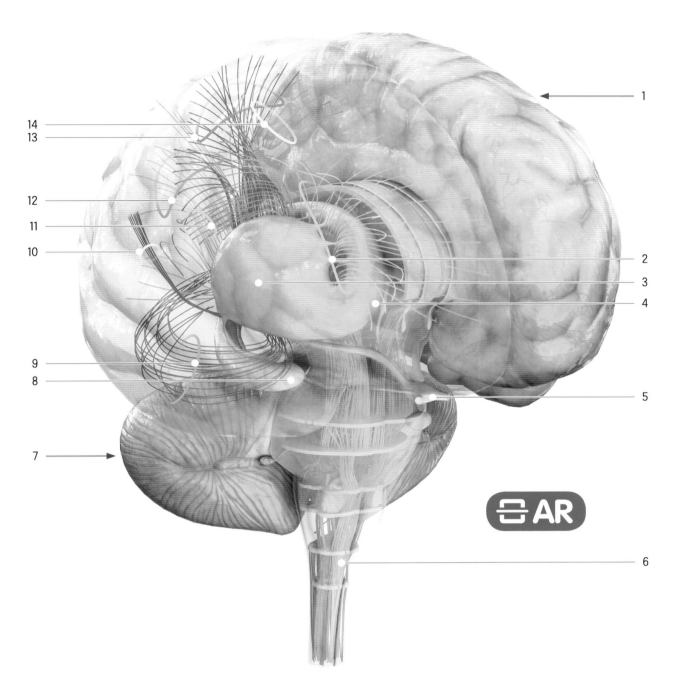

1. 端脑 telencephalon
2. 额桥束 frontopontine tract
3. 豆状核 lentiform nucleus
4. 尾状核头 head of caudate nucleus
5. 视交叉 optic chiasma
6. 锥体束 pyramidal tract
7. 小脑 cerebellum
8. 海马 hippocampus
9. 视辐射 optic radiation
10. 听辐射 acoustic radiation
11. 皮质核束 corticonuclear tract
12. 顶枕颞桥束 parietooccipitopontine and temporopontine tract
13. 丘脑中央辐射 central thalamic radiation
14. 皮质脊髓束 corticospinal tract

图 12-10　通过内囊的投射纤维
Projection fibers through the internal capsule

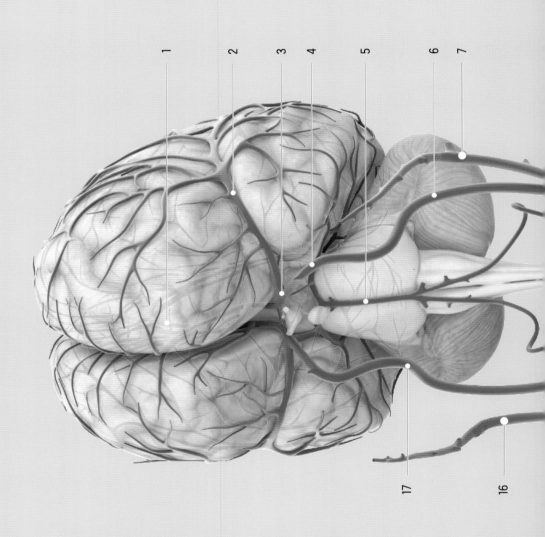

1
2
3
4
5
6
7

17
16

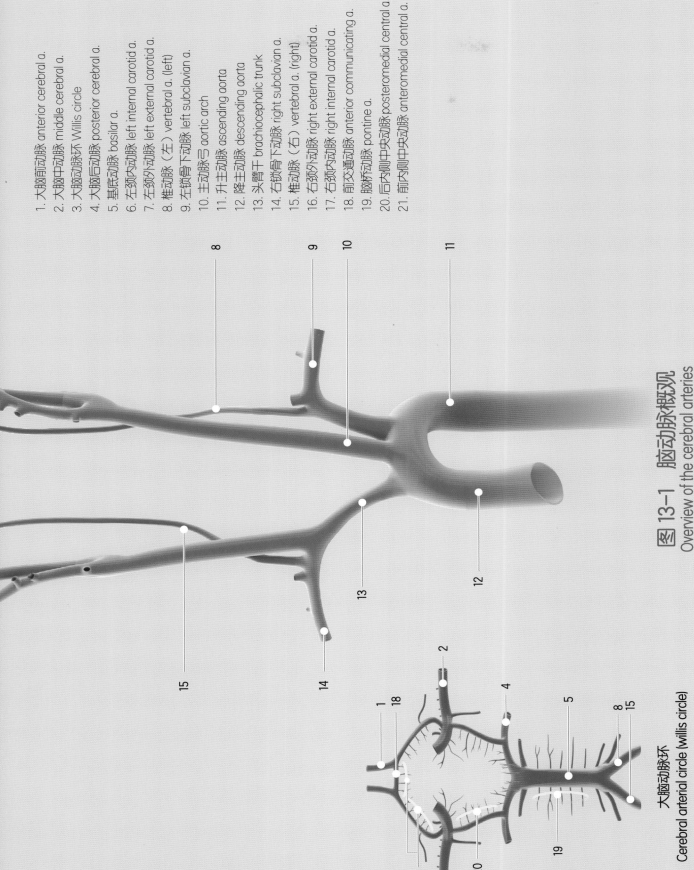

1. 大脑前动脉 anterior cerebral a.
2. 大脑中动脉 middle cerebral a.
3. 大脑动脉环 Willis circle
4. 大脑后动脉 posterior cerebral a.
5. 基底动脉 basilar a.
6. 左颈内动脉 left internal carotid a.
7. 左颈外动脉 left external carotid a.
8. 椎动脉（左）vertebral a. (left)
9. 左锁骨下动脉 left subclavian a.
10. 主动脉弓 aortic arch
11. 升主动脉 ascending aorta
12. 降主动脉 descending aorta
13. 头臂干 brachiocephalic trunk
14. 右锁骨下动脉 right subclavian a.
15. 椎动脉（右）vertebral a. (right)
16. 右颈外动脉 right external carotid a.
17. 右颈内动脉 right internal carotid a.
18. 前交通动脉 anterior communicating a.
19. 脑桥动脉 pontine a.
20. 后内侧中央动脉 posteromedial central a.
21. 前内侧中央动脉 anteromedial central a.

图 13-1 脑动脉概观
Overview of the cerebral arteries

大脑动脉环
Cerebral arterial circle (willis circle)

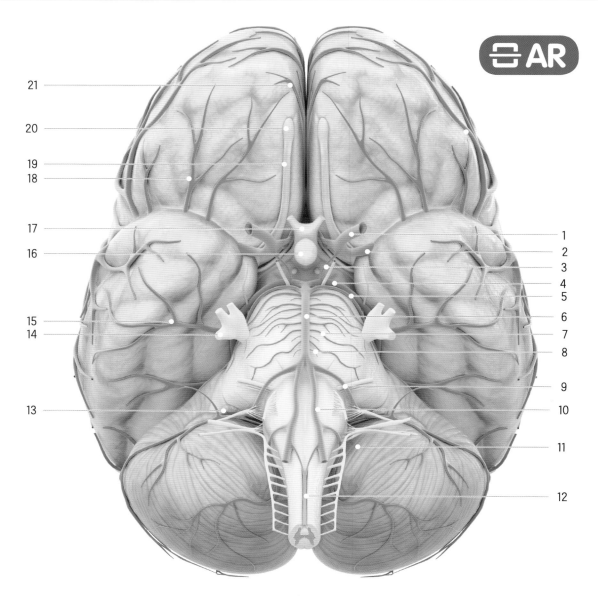

下面观 Inferior view

1. 颈内动脉 internal carotid a.
2. 大脑中动脉 middle cerebral a.
3. 后交通动脉 posterior communicating a.
4. 大脑后动脉 posterior cerebral a.
5. 小脑上动脉 superior cerebellar a.
6. 基底动脉 basilar a.
7. 脑桥动脉 pontine a.
8. 迷路动脉 labyrinthine a.
9. 小脑下前动脉 anterior inferior cerebellar a.
10. 椎动脉 vertebral a.
11. 小脑后下动脉 posterior inferior cerebellar a.
12. 脊髓前动脉 anterior spinal a.
13. 脉络丛 choroid plexus
14. 三叉神经节 trigeminal ganglion
15. 颞前支 anterior temporal branch
16. 垂体 hypophysis
17. 视交叉 optic chiasma
18. 眶额外侧动脉 lateral orbitofrontal a.
19. 嗅束 olfactory tract
20. 嗅球 olfactory bulb
21. 眶额内侧动脉 medial orbitofrontal a.

图 13-2 脑底的动脉
Arteries at the base of the brain

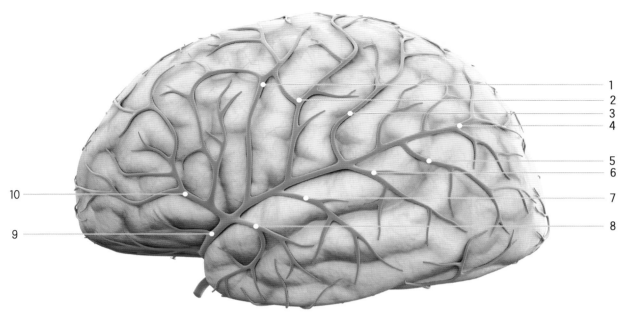

外侧面观 Lateral view

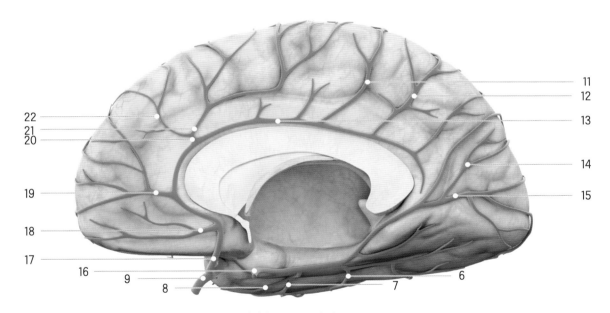

内侧面观 Medial view

1. 中央前沟动脉 precentral sulcus a.
2. 中央沟动脉 central sulcus a.
3. 中央后沟动脉 postcentral sulcus a.
4. 顶后动脉 posterior parietal a.
5. 角回动脉 angular gyrus a.
6. 颞叶后动脉 posterior temporal a.
7. 颞叶中动脉 middle temporal a.
8. 颞叶前动脉 anterior temporal a.

9. 大脑中动脉 middle cerebral a.
10. 额叶底外侧动脉 lateral frontobasal a.
11. 旁中央动脉 paracentral a.
12. 楔前动脉 precuneal a.
13. 胼胝体周围动脉 pericallosal a.
14. 顶枕支 parietooccipital branch
15. 距状沟支 calcarine branch
16. 大脑后动脉 posterior cerebral a.

17. 大脑前动脉 anterior cerebral a.
18. 额叶底内侧动脉 medial frontobasal a.
19. 额叶前内侧支 anteromedial frontal branch
20. 胼胝体缘动脉 callosomarginal a.
21. 额叶后内侧支 posteromedial frontal branch
22. 额叶中内侧支 mediomedial frontal branch

图 13-3 大脑半球的动脉
Arteries of the cerebral hemisphere

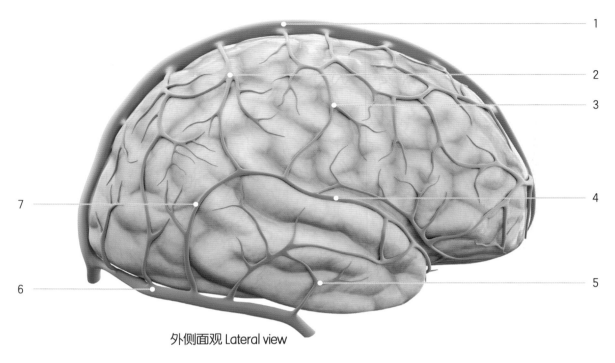

外侧面观 Lateral view

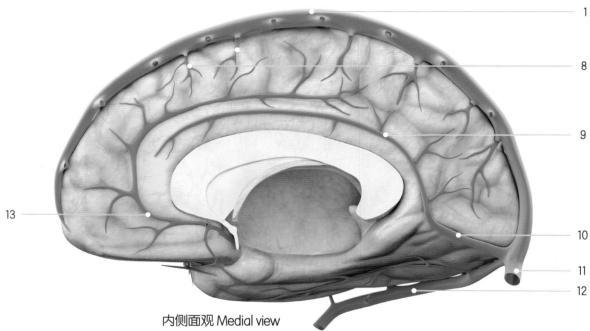

内侧面观 Medial view

1. 上矢状窦 superior sagittal sinus
2. 大脑上静脉 superior cerebral v.
3. 上吻合静脉 superior anastomotic v.
4. 大脑中浅静脉 superficial middle cerebral v.
5. 大脑下静脉 inferior cerebral v.
6. 横窦 transverse sinus
7. 下吻合静脉 inferior anastomotic v.

8. 大脑浅静脉 superficial cerebral v.
9. 下矢状窦 inferior sagittal sinus
10. 直窦 straight sinus
11. 窦汇 confluence of sinuses
12. 乙状窦 sigmoid sinus
13. 大脑前静脉 anterior cerebral v.

图 13-4 大脑半球的静脉
Veins of the cerebral hemisphere

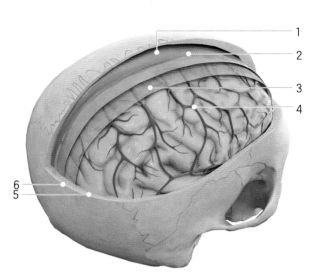

右后外侧面观 Right posterolateral view

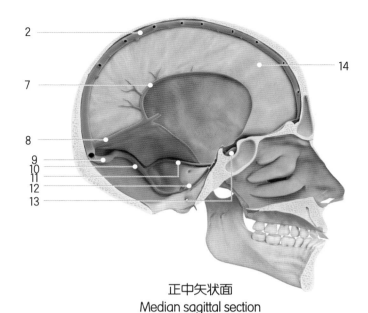

正中矢状面
Median sagittal section

1. 硬脑膜 cerebral dura mater
2. 上矢状窦 superior sagittal sinus
3. 蛛网膜 arachnoid mater
4. 大脑浅静脉 superficial cerebral v.
5. 板障 diploe
6. 外板 outer plate
7. 下矢状窦 inferior sagittal sinus
8. 直窦 straight sinus
9. 横窦 transverse sinus
10. 乙状窦 sigmoid sinus
11. 岩上窦 superior petrosal sinus
12. 岩下窦 inferior petrosal sinus
13. 海绵窦 cavernous sinus
14. 大脑镰 cerebral falx
15. 视神经 optic n.
16. 颈内动脉 internal carotid a.
17. 海绵间窦 intercavernous sinus
18. 基底静脉丛 basilar venous plexus
19. 脑膜动脉 meningeal a.
20. 小脑幕 tentorium of cerebellum
21. 三叉神经节 trigeminal ganglion

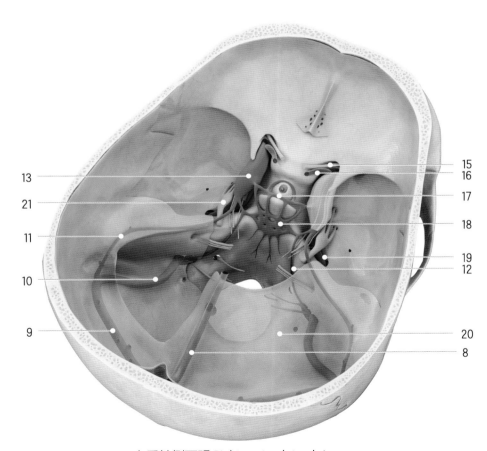

右后外侧面观 Right posterolateral view

图 13-5　脑被膜及硬脑膜窦
Meninges of the brain and sinuses of dura mater

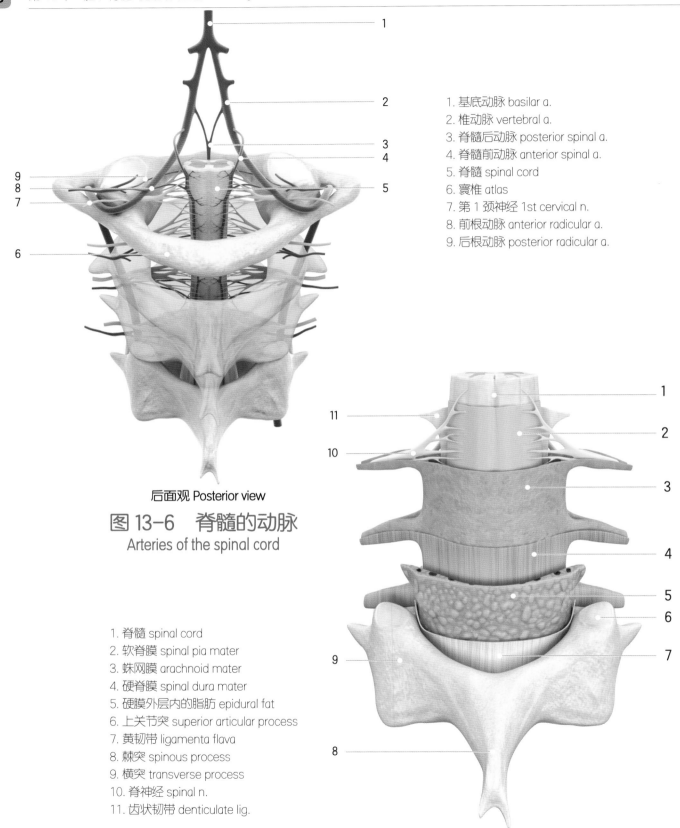

后面观 Posterior view

图 13-6 脊髓的动脉
Arteries of the spinal cord

1. 基底动脉 basilar a.
2. 椎动脉 vertebral a.
3. 脊髓后动脉 posterior spinal a.
4. 脊髓前动脉 anterior spinal a.
5. 脊髓 spinal cord
6. 寰椎 atlas
7. 第 1 颈神经 1st cervical n.
8. 前根动脉 anterior radicular a.
9. 后根动脉 posterior radicular a.

1. 脊髓 spinal cord
2. 软脊膜 spinal pia mater
3. 蛛网膜 arachnoid mater
4. 硬脊膜 spinal dura mater
5. 硬膜外层内的脂肪 epidural fat
6. 上关节突 superior articular process
7. 黄韧带 ligamenta flava
8. 棘突 spinous process
9. 横突 transverse process
10. 脊神经 spinal n.
11. 齿状韧带 denticulate lig.

后面观 Posterior view

图 13-7 脊髓被膜
Meninges of the spinal cord

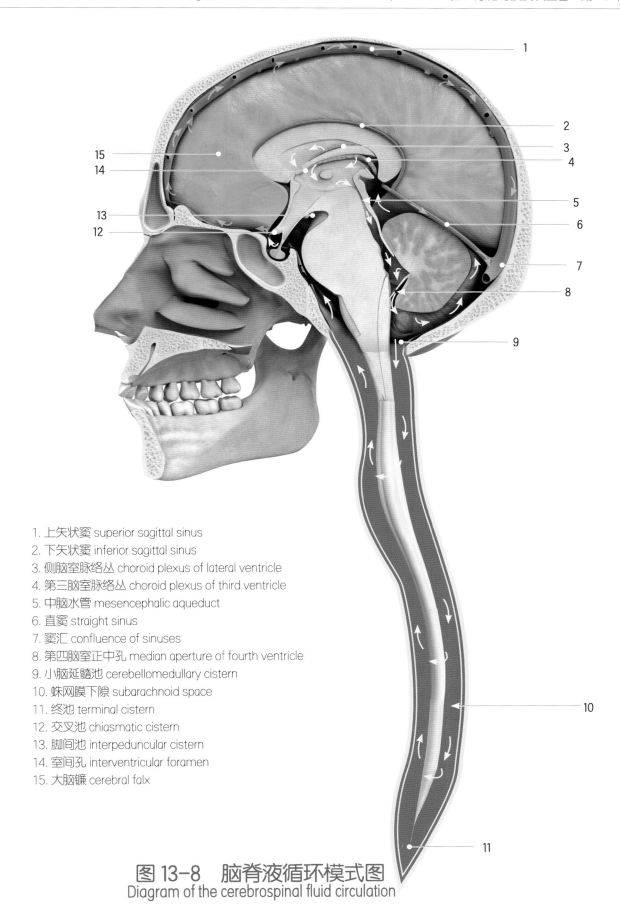

1. 上矢状窦 superior sagittal sinus
2. 下矢状窦 inferior sagittal sinus
3. 侧脑室脉络丛 choroid plexus of lateral ventricle
4. 第三脑室脉络丛 choroid plexus of third ventricle
5. 中脑水管 mesencephalic aqueduct
6. 直窦 straight sinus
7. 窦汇 confluence of sinuses
8. 第四脑室正中孔 median aperture of fourth ventricle
9. 小脑延髓池 cerebellomedullary cistern
10. 蛛网膜下隙 subarachnoid space
11. 终池 terminal cistern
12. 交叉池 chiasmatic cistern
13. 脚间池 interpeduncular cistern
14. 室间孔 interventricular foramen
15. 大脑镰 cerebral falx

图 13-8　脑脊液循环模式图
Diagram of the cerebrospinal fluid circulation

第14章 内分泌系统
Endocrine System

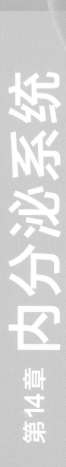

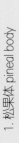

1. 松果体 pineal body
2. 垂体 hypophysis
3. 脑干 brain stem
4. 延髓 medulla oblongata
5. 甲状腺 thyroid gland
6. 胸腺 thymus
7. 心包 pericardium
8. 胰 pancreas
9. 腹主动脉 abdominal aorta
10. 睾丸 testis
11. 右髂总动脉 right common iliac a.
12. 下腔静脉 inferior vena cava
13. 肾 kidney
14. 肾上腺 suprarenal gland
15. 卵巢 ovary

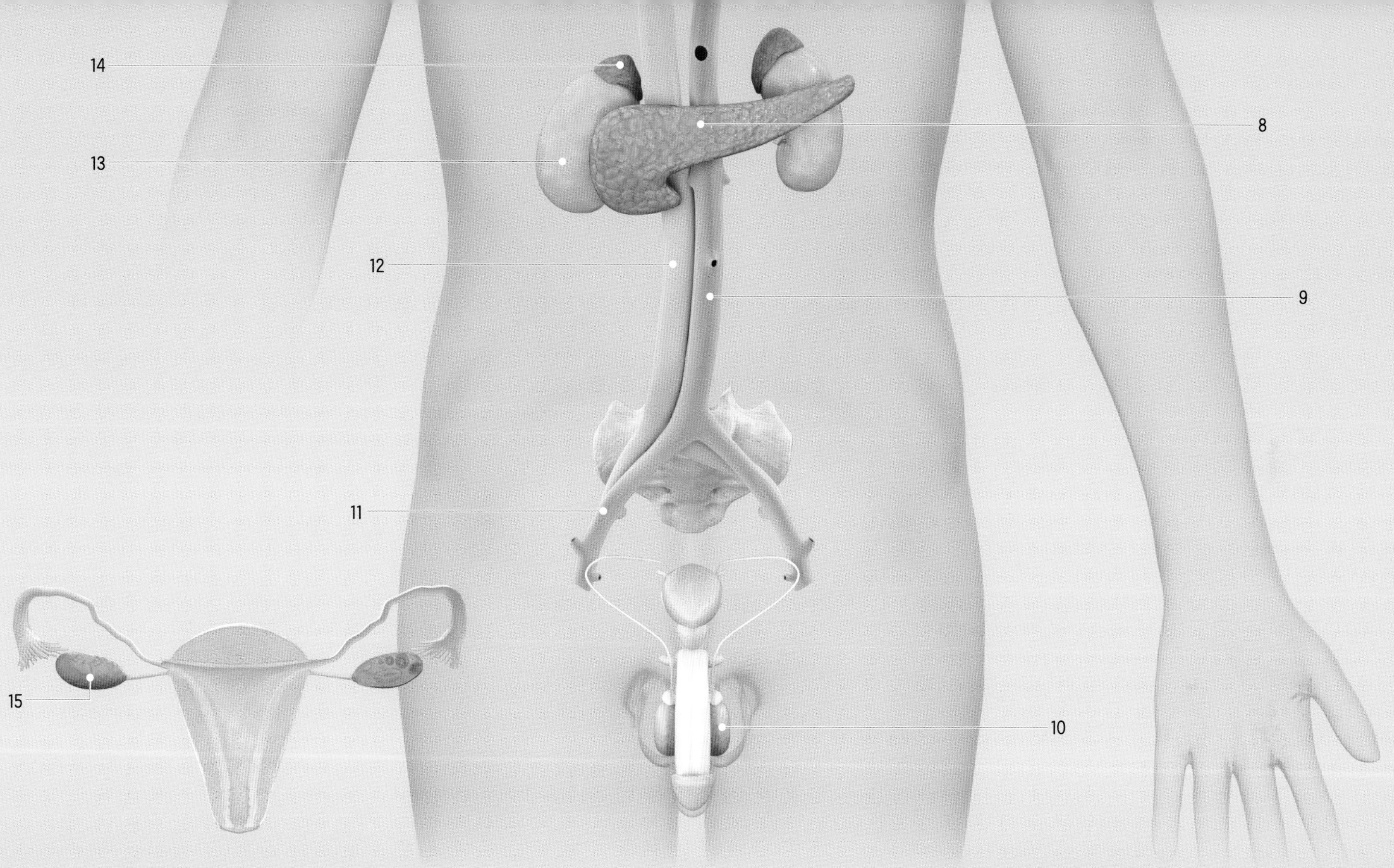

图 14-1 内分泌腺概观
Overview of the endocrine gland

中英文名词对照索引

T